Dietary DRI Reference Intakes

Dietary DRI Reference Intakes

The Essential Guide to Nutrient Requirements

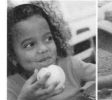 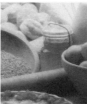 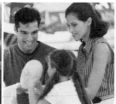 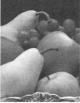 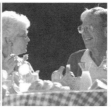

Jennifer J. Otten, Jennifer Pitzi Hellwig, Linda D. Meyers,

Editors

INSTITUTE OF MEDICINE
OF THE NATIONAL ACADEMIES

THE NATIONAL ACADEMIES PRESS
Washington, D.C.
www.nap.edu

THE NATIONAL ACADEMIES PRESS 500 Fifth Street, N.W. Washington, DC 20001

NOTICE: The project that is the subject of this report was approved by the Governing Board of the National Research Council, whose members are drawn from the councils of the National Academy of Sciences, the National Academy of Engineering, and the Institute of Medicine.

This project was supported by Contract No. 4500096095 between the National Academy of Sciences and Health Canada and by the National Research Council. Any opinions, findings, conclusions, or recommendations expressed in this publication are those of the author(s) and do not necessarily reflect the view of the organizations or agencies that provided support for this project.

Library of Congress Cataloging-in-Publication Data

Dietary reference intakes : the essential guide to nutrient requirements / Jennifer J. Otten, Jennifer Pitzi Hellwig, Linda D. Meyers, editors.
    p. cm.
  Includes bibliographical references and index.
   ISBN 0-309-10091-7 (hardback) — ISBN 0-309-65646-X (pdfs) 1. Nutrition. 2. Nutrition—Evaluation. 3. Reference values (Medicine) I. Otten, Jennifer J. II. Hellwig, Jennifer Pitzi. III. Meyers, Linda D.
  QP141.D5296 2006
  612.3—dc22
                             2006015626

Additional copies of this report are available from the National Academies Press, 500 Fifth Street, N.W., Lockbox 285, Washington, DC 20055; (800) 624-6242 or (202) 334-3313 (in the Washington metropolitan area); Internet, http://www.nap.edu.

For more information about the Institute of Medicine, visit the IOM home page at: **www.iom.edu.**

The serpent has been a symbol of long life, healing, and knowledge among almost all cultures and religions since the beginning of recorded history. The serpent adopted as a logotype by the Institute of Medicine is a relief carving from ancient Greece, now held by the Staatliche Museen in Berlin.

"Knowing is not enough; we must apply.
Willing is not enough; we must do."
—Goethe

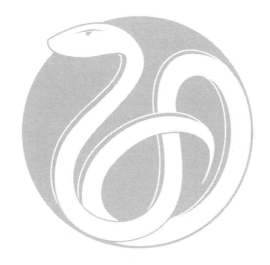

INSTITUTE OF MEDICINE
OF THE NATIONAL ACADEMIES

Advising the Nation. Improving Health.

THE NATIONAL ACADEMIES
Advisers to the Nation on Science, Engineering, and Medicine

The **National Academy of Sciences** is a private, nonprofit, self-perpetuating society of distinguished scholars engaged in scientific and engineering research, dedicated to the furtherance of science and technology and to their use for the general welfare. Upon the authority of the charter granted to it by the Congress in 1863, the Academy has a mandate that requires it to advise the federal government on scientific and technical matters. Dr. Ralph J. Cicerone is president of the National Academy of Sciences.

The **National Academy of Engineering** was established in 1964, under the charter of the National Academy of Sciences, as a parallel organization of outstanding engineers. It is autonomous in its administration and in the selection of its members, sharing with the National Academy of Sciences the responsibility for advising the federal government. The National Academy of Engineering also sponsors engineering programs aimed at meeting national needs, encourages education and research, and recognizes the superior achievements of engineers. Dr. Wm. A. Wulf is president of the National Academy of Engineering.

The **Institute of Medicine** was established in 1970 by the National Academy of Sciences to secure the services of eminent members of appropriate professions in the examination of policy matters pertaining to the health of the public. The Institute acts under the responsibility given to the National Academy of Sciences by its congressional charter to be an adviser to the federal government and, upon its own initiative, to identify issues of medical care, research, and education. Dr. Harvey V. Fineberg is president of the Institute of Medicine.

The **National Research Council** was organized by the National Academy of Sciences in 1916 to associate the broad community of science and technology with the Academy's purposes of furthering knowledge and advising the federal government. Functioning in accordance with general policies determined by the Academy, the Council has become the principal operating agency of both the National Academy of Sciences and the National Academy of Engineering in providing services to the government, the public, and the scientific and engineering communities. The Council is administered jointly by both Academies and the Institute of Medicine. Dr. Ralph J. Cicerone and Dr. Wm. A. Wulf are chair and vice chair, respectively, of the National Research Council.

www.national-academies.org

PREFACE

This book is a selective summary of the series of publications on *Dietary Reference Intakes* (DRIs). Its goal is to serve as a practical, hands-on reference to help guide health professionals in the United States and Canada in their day-to-day task of assessing and planning for the nutrient needs of individuals and groups of people. The book also provides educators with a tool for guiding students in the understanding of the DRI concept and use of the reference values. It is derived from work authored by the Food and Nutrition Board (FNB) of the Institute of Medicine (IOM).

This book is not meant to replace the original DRI series of nutrient reference values published between 1997 and 2005 nor is it intended to be a thorough representation of the series. Based on material from the original DRI series, this book stays true to the findings and recommendations from the original reports. Without introducing new data or conclusions, this document recasts essential ideas from the original reports in an accessible and more compact form.

The DRI values and paradigm replace the former Recommended Dietary Allowances (RDAs) for the United States and Recommended Nutrient Intakes (RNIs) for Canada. In the past, RDAs and RNIs were the primary values available to U.S. and Canadian health professionals for planning and assessing the diets of individuals and groups. The DRIs represent a more complete set of values. They were developed in recognition of the growing and diverse uses of quantitative reference values and the availability of more sophisticated approaches for dietary planning and assessment purposes.

Although all reference values in this book are based on data, available data were often sparse or drawn from studies with significant limitations in addressing various questions confronted by the original DRI panel and subcommittees. Thus, although governed by scientific rationale, informed judgments were often required in setting reference values. Where data were available, criteria of nutritional adequacy were carefully identified; these criteria are listed in tables in each nutrient chapter.

Readers are urged to recognize that the DRI process is iterative in character. We expect that the DRI conceptual framework will continue to evolve and be improved as new information becomes available and is applied to an expanding list of nutrients and other food components. Thus, because the DRI activity is ongoing, comments were solicited widely and received on the originally published reports of this series. With more experience, the proposed models for establishing reference intakes of nutrients and other food components that play significant roles in promoting and sustaining health and optimal functioning will be refined. Also, as new information or new methods of analysis are adopted, these reference values undoubtedly will be reassessed. This book will be updated in the future as the original series is revised.

This book has been reviewed in draft form by individuals chosen for their diverse perspectives and technical expertise, in accordance with procedures approved by the National Research Council's Report Review Committee. The purpose of this independent review is to provide candid, confidential, and critical comments that will assist the institution in making its published book as sound as possible and to ensure that the book meets institutional standards. We wish to thank the following individuals for their review of this report: Lawrence Appel, Johns Hopkins Medical Institutions; Stephanie A. Atkinson, McMaster University; Susan I. Barr, University of British Columbia; Ann M. Coulston, Ely Lilly and Co.; John W. Erdman, University of Illinois at Urbana-Champaign; Norman I. Krinsky, Tufts University; Joanne R. Lupton, Texas A&M University; Suzanne Murphy, University of Hawaii; Roy M. Pitkin, University of California, Los Angeles; Robert M. Russell, Tufts University.

Although these reviewers provided many constructive comments and suggestions, they were not asked to endorse nor did they see the final draft of the book before its release and publication. The review of this report was overseen by Clyde J. Behney, who was responsible for making certain that an independent examination of this report was carried out in accordance with institutional procedures and that all review comments were carefully considered.

The Institute of Medicine gratefully acknowledges Health Canada's support and participation in this initiative. This close collaboration represents a pioneering step in the harmonization of nutrient reference intakes in North America. In particular, the Food and Nutrition Board wishes to extend special thanks to our Health Canada partners who helped refine drafts and provided invaluable comments that vastly improved the project: Mary Bush, Danielle Brulé, Margaret Cheney, Krista Esslinger, Linda Greene-Finestone, and Sylvie St-Pierre. We also express our gratitude and thanks to Health Canada for permitting incorporation of materials on the Dietary Reference Intakes extracted from *The Canadian Community Health Survey 2.2, Nutrition Focus: A Guide to Accessing and Interpreting the Data,* published by Health Canada in 2006.

The consultants for this project—Johanna T. Dwyer, Rachel K. Johnson, Rena Mendelson, Esther F. Myers, Sharon M. Nickols-Richardson, Linda G. Snetselaar, Huguette Turgeon-O'Brien, and Susan Whiting—ably performed their work under severe time pressures (see Appendix B for biographical sketches). All gave their time and effort willingly and without financial reward; the public and the science and practice of nutrition are among the major beneficiaries of their dedication. This project would not have been undertaken and completed without the dedicated work of the project staff, in particular, Jennifer Otten who co-wrote and managed the project and its many iterations, Jennifer Pitzi Hellwig who co-wrote and copyedited parts of the book, Mary Kalamaras who guided initial plans and copyedited a very complex and complicated manuscript, and Linda D. Meyers who oversaw the project and never hesitated to assist when help was needed. The intellectual and managerial contributions made by these individuals to the project were critical. Sincere thanks also go to other IOM and National Academies staff, including Ricky Washington, Gerri Kennedo, Ann Merchant, Virginia Bryant, Barbara Kline Pope, Estelle Miller, Will Mason, Lara Andersen, Sally Stanfield, Charles Baum, Sally Groom, Dorothy Lewis, Stephen Mautner, Marc Gold, Linda Kilroy, Anton Bandy, Gary Walker, Vivian Tillman, Bronwyn Schrecker Jamrok, Tyjen Tsai, and Sandra Amamoo-Kakra.

I also want to extend my personal gratitude to the many volunteers who served the Institute of Medicine and the nation as members of the Food and Nutrition Board, members of the committees who prepared the DRI series and reviewers of the draft reports in that series. Their dedication and expertise in reviewing, interpreting, and translating scientific evidence into nutrient reference values is a substantial contribution to the public's health.

Harvey V. Fineberg, M.D., Ph.D.
President, Institute of Medicine

CONTENTS

---

*Full references, which also appear in the parent report series, the *Dietary Reference Intakes,* are not printed in this book but are provided online at http://www.nap.edu/catalog/11537.html.

INTRODUCTION

For more than half a century, the Recommended Dietary Allowances (RDAs) of the United States and the Dietary Standards/Recommended Nutrient Intakes (RNIs) of Canada have served as the chief components for nutrition policy in their respective countries, playing dominant roles in the task of meeting the known nutritional needs of healthy people in North America.

Revised and updated many times throughout their history, the RDAs and RNIs generally reflected changes resulting from the broader evolution taking place in the field of nutrition science. However, by the 1990s, a number of important developments had occurred that dramatically altered the nutrition research landscape and ultimately challenged the RDA and RNI status quo. Among them were the significant gains made in scientific knowledge regarding the link between diet, health, and chronic disease, and the emergence of advanced technologies that could measure small changes in individual adaptations to various nutrient intakes. Additionally, the use of fortified or enriched foods and the increased consumption of nutrients in pure form, either singly or in combination with others outside of the context of food, prompted the closer examination of the potential effects of excess nutrient intake.

In 1994, in response to these and other important considerations, the Food and Nutrition Board of the National Academies' Institute of Medicine, with support from the U.S. and Canadian governments and others, embarked on an initiative to develop a new, broader set of dietary reference values, known as the Dietary Reference Intakes (DRIs). The DRIs expand upon and replace the RDAs and RNIs with four categories of values intended to help individuals optimize their health, prevent disease, and avoid consuming too much of a nutrient. These dietary reference values were subsequently published in a series of reports released between 1997 and 2005, titled the *Dietary Reference Intakes*.

Recognizing the groundbreaking nature of the series and its impact on the nutrition community, the Food and Nutrition Board and Health Canada came together again in 2005 in an effort to extend the reach of the original reports to a wider audience. *Dietary Reference Intakes: The Essential Guide to Nutrient Requirements* is the result of their collaboration. Based on the key concepts and recommendations set forth in the original DRI series, this book serves as a practical, hands-on reference to help guide health professionals in the United States and Canada in their day-to-day task of assessing and planning for the nutrient needs of individuals and groups of people. This book also provides educators with a tool for guiding students in the understanding of the DRI concept and use of the reference values.

The book is divided into four parts: Part I provides a foundation for understanding how and why the DRIs were developed, definitions of the DRI categories, and specific guidance on their appropriate uses. Part II presents discussions on reference values for dietary carbohydrate, fiber, total fat, fatty acids, cholesterol, protein, amino acids, and water. Major new approaches and findings included in this section are formulas for estimating energy requirements; recommended physical activity levels; the definition of dietary fiber; and Acceptable Macronutrient Distribution Ranges (AMDRs), which have been introduced as a percentage of energy intake for fat, carbohydrate, protein, and linoleic and α-linolenic acids. Also included is information on the relationship between macronutrients and chronic disease.

Part III profiles 35 individual nutrients. In addition to providing reference values, each profile reviews the function of a given nutrient in the human body; summarizes the known effects of deficiencies and excessive intakes; describes how a nutrient may be related to chronic disease or developmental abnormalities; and provides the indicator of adequacy for determining the nutrient requirements.

A comprehensive set of appendixes, including a glossary and summary tables of DRI values appear in Part IV. Full references, which also appear in the parent report series, the *Dietary Reference Intakes,* are provided online at http://www.nap.edu/catalog/11537.html.

PART I
DEVELOPMENT AND APPLICATION

The Dietary Reference Intakes (DRIs) represent a radical new approach toward nutrition assessment and dietary planning, and therefore necessitate a thorough understanding of their origin, purpose, and intended applications. Part I of this book first addresses these areas, then follows with practical guidance on the correct application of the DRI values to the task of assessing and planning the diets of individuals and groups.

"Introduction to the Dietary Reference Intakes" provides a history of the creation of the DRIs, along with an introduction to the four categories they comprise: the Estimated Average Requirement (EAR), the Recommended Dietary Allowance (RDA), the Adequate Intake (AI), the Tolerable Upper Intake Level (UL), as well as the new Acceptable Macronutrient Distribution Ranges (AMDRs). The values are defined and their appropriate uses are discussed in detail, as are the parameters that were used to develop them, such as life stage groups and applicable populations. Also discussed are how the values differ from each other, as well as from the previous Recommended Dietary Allowances (RDAs) and Canada's Recommended Nutrient Intakes (RNIs).

"Applying the Dietary Reference Intakes" provides guidance on how to use and interpret the DRI values when assessing and planning the nutrient intakes of both individuals and groups. It summarizes pertinent information taken from two DRI reports published by the Food and Nutrition Board of the National Academies' Institute of Medicine. They are *Dietary Reference Intakes: Applications in Dietary Assessment* (2000) and *Dietary Reference Intakes: Applications in Dietary Planning* (2003). The chapter is divided into two main sections, "Working with Individuals" and "Working with Groups," which are each subdivided into assessment and planning sections. The sections on assessment also include explanations of the methods and equations that are used to determine whether individuals and groups are consuming adequate levels of nutrients. In addition, the chapter summary includes a quick-reference table on the appropriate uses of DRI values for specific aspects of nutrition assessment and planning.

INTRODUCTION TO THE DIETARY REFERENCE INTAKES

In 1941, the National Research Council issued its first set of Recommended Dietary Allowances (RDAs) for vitamins, minerals, protein, and energy. Developed initially by the forerunner of the Food and Nutrition Board of the Institute of Medicine, the recommendations were intended to serve as a guide for good nutrition and as a "yardstick" by which to measure progress toward that goal. Since then, RDAs have served as the basis for almost all federal and state food and nutrition programs and policies. By 1989, they had been revised nine times and expanded from a coverage of 8 original nutrients to 27 nutrients.

In 1938, the Canadian Council on Nutrition prepared the first dietary standard designed specifically for use in Canada. The *Dietary Standard for Canada* was revised in 1950, 1963, 1975, and 1983 and published by Health Canada and its predecessors. The 1983 revision was renamed *Recommended Nutrient Intakes (RNIs) for Canadians*. In the late 1980s, it was decided to incorporate considerations of the prevention of chronic diseases as well as nutritional deficiencies into the revision of the RNIs. In 1990, *Nutrition Recommendations: The Report of the Scientific Review Committee* was published. The report contained updated RNIs and recommendations on the selection of a dietary pattern that would supply all essential nutrients, while reducing risk of chronic diseases.

Both RDA and RNI values have been widely used for planning diets, assessing the adequacy of diets in individuals and populations, providing nutrition education and guidance, and as a standard for nutrition labeling and fortification. However, the former RDAs and RNIs were not always well suited for these applications and the need for new values was recognized. Also of note, the RNIs and RDAs differed from each other in their definition, revision and publication dates, and how their data have been interpreted by both U.S. and Canadian scientific committees.

Beginning in 1994, the Food and Nutrition Board, with support from the U.S. and Canadian governments and others, set out to develop and implement a new paradigm to establish recommended nutrient intakes that replaced and expanded upon the RDAs and RNIs. Reflecting updated scientific and statistical understandings, this decade-long review resulted in the development of the family of reference values collectively known as the Dietary Reference Intakes (DRIs). In contrast to the creation of the RDAs and RNIs, which involved establishing single values for each nutrient, adjusted for age, sex, and physiological condition, the DRIs feature four reference values, only one of which, the RDA, is familiar to the broad nutrition community (although the method by which it is derived has changed). The DRIs are a common set of reference values for Canada and the United States and are based on scientifically grounded relationships between nutrient intakes and indicators of adequacy, as well as the prevention of chronic diseases, in apparently healthy populations.

The development of the DRIs publication series (see Box 1 for a list of publications in the series) was undertaken by the standing Committee on the Scientific Evaluation of Dietary Reference Intakes, two standing subcommittees (the Subcommittee on Upper Reference Levels of Nutrients and the Subcommittee on Uses and Interpretation of Dietary Reference Intakes), and a series of expert panels. Each of the panels was responsible for reviewing the requirements for a specific group of nutrients.

Totaling nearly 5,000 pages, these reports summarize what is known about how nutrients function in the human body; the selection of indicators of adequacy on which to determine nutrient requirements; the factors that may affect how nutrients are utilized and therefore affect requirements; and how nutrients may be related to the prevention of chronic disease across all age groups. They also provide specific guidance on how to use the appropriate values to assess and plan the diets of groups and individuals.

A NEW APPROACH TO NUTRIENT REFERENCE VALUES

Collectively referred to as the Dietary Reference Intakes, the DRIs include four nutrient-based reference values that are used to assess and plan the diets of healthy people. The reference values include the Estimated Average Requirement (EAR), the Recommended Dietary Allowance (RDA), the Adequate Intake (AI), and the Tolerable Upper Intake Level (UL). (Brief definitions of the DRI categories are provided in Box 2.) Developed for vitamins, minerals, macronutrients, and energy, these reference values replace and expand upon the previous nutrient reference values for the United States and Canada. New to the nutrition world, the DRIs represent a significant paradigm shift in the way dietary reference values are established and used by practitioners, educators, and researchers. Unlike the RDAs and RNIs (prior to 1990), which focused primarily on reducing the incidence of diseases of deficiency, the DRI values are also

---

BOX 1 The DRI Publications

Nutrient-specific reports:
- *DRIs for Calcium, Phosphorus, Magnesium, Vitamin D, and Fluoride* (1997)
- *DRIs for Thiamin, Riboflavin, Niacin, Vitamin B$_6$, Folate, Vitamin B$_{12}$, Pantothenic Acid, Biotin, and Choline* (1998)
- *DRIs for Vitamin C, Vitamin E, Selenium, and Carotenoids* (2000)
- *DRIs for Vitamin A, Vitamin K, Arsenic, Boron, Chromium, Copper, Iodine, Iron, Manganese, Molybdenum, Nickel, Silicon, Vanadium, and Zinc* (2001)
- *DRIs for Energy, Carbohydrate, Fiber, Fat, Fatty Acids, Cholesterol, Protein, and Amino Acids* (2002/2005)
- *DRIs for Water, Potassium, Sodium, Chloride, and Sulfate* (2005)

Reports that explain appropriate uses:
- *DRIs: Applications in Dietary Assessment* (2000)
- *DRIs: Applications in Dietary Planning* (2003)

Related or derivative reports:
- *DRIs: Proposed Definition and Plan for Review of Dietary Antioxidants and Related Compounds* (1998)
- *DRIs: A Risk Assessment Model for Establishing Upper Intake Levels for Nutrients* (1998)
- *DRIs: Proposed Definition of Dietary Fiber* (2001)
- *DRIs: Guiding Principles for Nutrition Labeling and Fortification* (2003), prepared as a separate activity

http://www.nap.edu/catalog/dri

---

intended to help individuals optimize their health, prevent disease, and avoid consuming too much of a nutrient. Specifically, the DRIs differ from the former RDAs and RNIs in several key ways:

- When available, data on a nutrient's safety and role in health are considered in the formulation of a recommendation, taking into account the potential reduction in the risk of chronic degenerative disease or developmental abnormality, rather than just the absence of signs of deficiency.

BOX 2 DRI Definitions

Estimated Average Requirement (EAR): The average daily nutrient intake level that is estimated to meet the requirements of half of the healthy individuals in a particular life stage and gender group.[a]

Recommended Dietary Allowance (RDA): The average daily dietary nutrient intake level that is sufficient to meet the nutrient requirements of nearly all (97–98 percent) healthy individuals in a particular life stage and gender group.

Adequate Intake (AI): The recommended average daily intake level based on observed or experimentally determined approximations or estimates of nutrient intake by a group (or groups) of apparently healthy people that are assumed to be adequate; used when an RDA cannot be determined.

Tolerable Upper Intake Level (UL): The highest average daily nutrient intake level that is likely to pose no risk of adverse health effects to almost all individuals in the general population. As intake increases above the UL, the potential risk of adverse effects may increase.

---

[a] In the case of energy, an Estimated Energy Requirement (EER) is provided. The EER is the average dietary energy intake that is predicted to maintain energy balance in a healthy adult of a defined age, gender, weight, height, and level of physical activity consistent with good health. In children and pregnant and lactating women, the EER is taken to include the needs associated with the deposition of tissues or the secretion of milk at rates consistent with good health.

- The concepts of probability and risk explicitly underpin the determination of the DRIs and inform their application in assessment and planning.
- Greater emphasis is placed on the distribution of nutrient requirements within a population, rather than on a single value (like the former RDAs and RNIs).
- Where data exist, upper levels of intake have been established regarding the risk of adverse health effects.
- Compounds found naturally in foods that may not meet the traditional concept of a nutrient, but have a potential risk or possible benefit to health, are reviewed and, if sufficient data exist, reference intakes are established.

As discussed earlier, the previous RDAs and RNIs were originally only intended to plan nutritional adequacy for groups. But because previous RDAs and RNIs were the only values available to health professionals, they were also used to assess and plan the diets of individuals and to make judgments about excess intakes for both individuals and groups. However, they were not ideally suited for these purposes. To prevent further misapplication, the expansion to the DRI framework included methodologies for appropriate uses of the nutrient values with individuals and groups.

The four primary uses of the DRIs are to assess the intakes of individuals, assess the intakes of population groups, plan diets for individuals, and plan diets for groups. Some of the dietary planning activities that are most relevant to DRI use include dietary guidance, institutional food planning, military food and nutrition planning, planning for food-assistance programs, food labeling, food fortification, developing new or modified food products, and food-safety assurance.

THE DRI CATEGORIES

Most nutrients have a set of DRIs. Often, a nutrient has an Estimated Average Requirement (EAR) from which the Recommended Dietary Allowance (RDA) is mathematically derived. When an EAR for a nutrient cannot be determined (thus precluding the setting of an RDA), then an Adequate Intake (AI) is often developed. Many nutrients also have a Tolerable Upper Intake Level (UL).

The values for the EAR and AI are defined by using specific criteria for nutrient adequacy and answer the question "adequate for what?". For example, values for vitamin C were set based on the amount of vitamin C that would nearly saturate leukocytes without leading to excessive urinary loss, rather than the level necessary to prevent scurvy. The UL is defined by using a specific indicator of excess, if one is available. Where data were available, the chosen criteria have been identified in each nutrient chapter.

In some cases, various intake levels can produce a range of benefits. For example, one criterion, or indicator, of adequacy may be the most appropriate one to use when determining an individual's risk of becoming deficient in the nutrient, while another criterion of adequacy may be more applicable to reducing one's risk of chronic diseases or conditions, such as certain neurodegenerative diseases, cardiovascular disease, cancer, diabetes mellitus, or age-related macular degeneration.

It is also important to note that each reference value refers to average daily nutrient intake. Some deviation around this average value is expected over a number of days. In fact, it is the average mean intake over this time frame that serves as the nutritionally important reference value. In most cases, the amounts derived from day-to-day intake may vary substantially without ill effect.

Estimated Average Requirement

The Estimated Average Requirement (EAR) is the average daily nutrient intake level that is estimated to meet the nutrient needs of half of the healthy individuals in a life stage or gender group. Although the term "average" is used, the EAR actually represents an estimated median requirement. As such, the EAR exceeds the needs of half of the group and falls short of the needs of the other half.

The EAR is the primary reference point for assessing the adequacy of estimated nutrient intakes of groups and is a tool for planning intakes for groups. It is also the basis for calculating the RDA. Although it can also be used to examine the probability that usual intake is inadequate for individuals (in conjunction with information on the variability of requirements), it is not meant to be used as a goal for daily intake by individuals. In the case of energy, an estimated energy requirement called the Estimated Energy Requirement (EER) is provided.

Recommended Dietary Allowance

The Recommended Dietary Allowance (RDA) is an estimate of the daily average dietary intake that meets the nutrient needs of nearly all (97–98 percent) healthy members of a particular life stage and gender group. The RDA thus exceeds the requirements of nearly all members of the group. It can be used as a guide for daily intake by individuals, and because it falls above the requirements of most people, intakes below the RDA cannot be assessed as being inadequate. Usual intake at the RDA should have a low probability of inadequacy.

If an EAR cannot be set due to data limitations, no RDA will be calculated. For nutrients that have a statistically normal requirement distribution, the RDA is set by adding two standard deviations (SD) to the EAR. Thus,

$$RDA = EAR + 2SD$$

For nutrients with skewed requirement distributions (most notably, iron in menstruating women) the RDA is set between the 97th and 98th percentile of the requirement distribution. (See Part I, "Applying the Dietary Reference Intakes" for more information on calculating RDAs when nutrient requirements are skewed.)

Adequate Intake

If sufficient or adequate scientific evidence is not available to establish an EAR and thus an RDA, an AI is usually derived for the nutrient instead. An AI is

Acceptable Macronutrient Distribution Ranges (AMDR)

A growing body of evidence indicates that an imbalance in macro-nutrients (e.g., low or high percent of energy), particularly with certain fatty acids and relative amounts of fat and carbohydrates, can increase risk of several chronic diseases. Based on this evidence, Acceptable Macronutrient Distribution Ranges (AMDRs) have been estimated for individuals. An AMDR is the range of intakes of an energy source that is associated with a reduced risk of chronic disease, yet can provide adequate amounts of essential nutrients.

The AMDR is expressed as a percentage of total energy intake. A key feature of each AMDR is that it has a lower and upper boundary. For example, the AMDR for carbohydrates ranges from 45 to 65 percent of total energy intake. Intakes that fall below or above this range increase the potential for an elevated risk of chronic diseases. Intakes outside of the range also raise the risk of inadequate consumption of essential nutrients. The AMDRs are discussed in more detail in Part II, "Macronutrients, Healthful Diets, and Physical Activity."

based on fewer data and incorporates more judgment than is used in establishing an EAR and subsequently the RDA. The setting of an AI usually indicates that more research is needed to determine, with some degree of confidence, the mean and distribution of requirements for that specific nutrient.

The AI is a recommended average daily nutrient intake level based on observed or experimentally determined approximations or estimates of nutrient intake by a group (or groups) of apparently healthy people who are assumed to be maintaining an adequate nutritional state. Examples of adequate nutritional states include normal growth, maintenance of normal levels of nutrients in plasma, and other aspects of nutritional well-being or general health.

The AI is expected to meet or exceed the needs of most individuals in a specific life stage and gender group. When an RDA is not available for a nutrient (because an EAR could not be developed), the AI can be used as the guide for an individual's intake. However, the AI has very limited uses in assessments of any type.

Tolerable Upper Intake Level

The Tolerable Upper Intake Level (UL) is the highest average daily nutrient intake level likely to pose no risk of adverse health effects for nearly all people

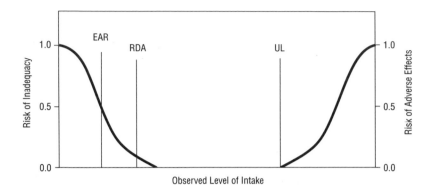

FIGURE 1 Relationship between Dietary Reference Intakes. This figure shows that the Estimated Average Requirement (EAR) is the intake at which the risk of inadequacy is 0.5 (50 percent) to an individual. The Recommended Dietary Allowance (RDA) is the intake at which the risk of inadequacy is very small—only 0.02 to 0.03 (2 to 3 percent). The Adequate Intake (AI) does not bear a consistent relationship to the EAR or the RDA because it is set without the estimate of the requirement. At intakes between the RDA and the Tolerable Upper Intake Level (UL), the risks of inadequacy and of excess are both close to zero. At intakes above the UL, the risk of adverse effects may increase.

in a particular group. As intake increases above the UL, the potential risk for adverse effects increases. The need for setting a UL grew out of two major trends: increased fortification of foods with nutrients and the use of dietary supplements by more people and in larger doses.

The UL is not a recommended level of intake, but rather the highest intake level that can be tolerated without the possibility of causing ill effects. The value applies to chronic daily use and is usually based on the total intake of a nutrient from food, water, and supplements if adverse effects have been associated with total intake. However, if adverse effects have been associated with intake from supplements or food fortificants alone, the UL is based on the nutrient intake from one or both of these sources only, rather than on total intake.

For some nutrients, not enough data were available to set a UL. However, this does not mean that consuming excess amounts poses no risks. Instead, it indicates a need for caution in consuming large amounts. See Figure 1 for a visual relationship between the DRIs.

PARAMETERS USED IN DEVELOPING DRIS

The DRIs presented in this publication apply to the healthy general population. In addition, DRI values are assigned to life stage groups that correspond to various periods of the human lifespan. Reference heights and weights for life stage and gender groups were used for extrapolations performed on the basis of body weight or size. They also indicate the extent to which intake adjustments might be made for individuals or population groups that significantly deviate from typical heights and weights.

Applicable Populations

An important principle underlying the DRIs is that they are standards for apparently healthy people and are not meant to be applied to those with acute or chronic disease or for the repletion of nutrient levels in previously deficient individuals. Meeting the recommended intakes for the nutrients would not necessarily provide enough for individuals who are already malnourished, nor would they be adequate for certain disease states marked by increase nutrient requirements. Although the RDA or AI may serve as the basis for specialized guidance, qualified medical and nutrition personnel should make the needed adjustments for individuals with specific needs.

Life Stage Groups

Where data were available, DRIs were divided into 12 life stage groups and also by gender. The life stage groups were chosen by considering variations in the requirements of all of the nutrients under review. If data were too limited to distinguish different nutrient requirements by life stage or gender groups, the analysis was then presented for a larger grouping.

INFANCY

Infancy covers the first 12 months of life and is divided into two 6-month intervals. The first 6-month interval was not subdivided because intake is relatively constant during this time. That is, as infants grow, they ingest more food; however, on a body-weight basis their intake remains the same. During the second 6 months of life, growth rate slows. As a result, total daily nutrient needs on a body-weight basis may be less than those during the first 6 months of life.

The average intake by full-term infants born to healthy, well-nourished mothers and exclusively fed human milk has been adopted as the primary basis for deriving the AI for most nutrients during the first 6 months of life. The only exception to this criterion is vitamin D, which occurs in low concentrations in human milk.

In general, special consideration was not given to possible variations in physiological need during the first month after birth or to the intake variations that result from differences in milk volume and nutrient concentration during early lactation. Specific recommended intakes to meet the needs of formula-fed infants have not been set.

- First 6 months (Ages 0 through 6 months): The AI for a nutrient for infants in this age group was calculated using two measures, the average concentration of the nutrient from 2 through 6 months of lactation and an estimated average volume of human milk intake of 0.78 L/day. The AI represents the product of these two measures. Infants are expected to consume increasing volumes of human milk as they grow.
- Second 6 months (Ages 7 through 12 months): During this time, infants experience slowed growth and gradual weaning to a mixed diet of human milk and solid foods. There is no evidence for markedly different nutrient needs, except for some nutrients such as iron and zinc, which have relatively high requirements. An EAR and RDA for iron and zinc have been derived for this age group. The AIs (again, with the exception of vitamin D) are based on the sum of the average amount of the nutrient provided by 0.6 L/day of human milk and the average amount of the nutrient provided by the usual intakes of complementary weaning foods consumed by infants at this age.

TODDLERS: AGES 1 THROUGH 3 YEARS

Toddlers experience greater velocity of growth in height compared to 4- and 5-year-olds, and this distinction provides the biological basis for establishing separate recommended intakes for this age group. Data on which to base DRIs for toddlers are sparse, and in many cases, DRIs were derived by extrapolating data taken from the studies of infants or adults (see Appendix C).

EARLY CHILDHOOD: AGES 4 THROUGH 8 YEARS

Children aged 4 through 8 or 9 years (the latter depending on puberty onset in each gender) undergo major changes in velocity of growth and endocrine status. For many nutrients, a reasonable amount of data was available on nutrient intake and various criteria for adequacy to serve as the basis for the EARs/RDAs and AIs for this group. For nutrients that lack data on the requirements of children, EARs and RDAs for children are based on extrapolations from adult values.

PUBERTY/ADOLESCENCE: AGES 9 THROUGH 13 YEARS, AND 14 THROUGH 18 YEARS

The adolescent years were divided into two categories because growth occurs in some children as late as age 20 years. For some nutrients, different EARs/

RDAs and AIs were derived for girls and boys. Several indicators support the biological appropriateness of creating two adolescent age groups and gender groups:

- Age 10 years as the mean age of onset of breast development for white females in the United States; this is a physical marker for the beginning of increased estrogen secretion (in African American girls, onset is about a year earlier, for unknown reasons).
- The female growth spurt begins before the onset of breast development, thereby supporting the grouping of 9 through 13 years.
- The mean age of onset of testicular development in males is 10.5 through 11 years.
- The male growth spurt begins 2 years after the start of testicular development, thereby supporting the grouping of 14 through 18 years.

Young Adulthood and Middle Age: Ages 19 through 30 Years, and 31 through 50 Years

Adulthood was divided into two age groups to account for the possible value of achieving optimal genetic potential for peak bone mass with the consumption of higher nutrient intakes during early adulthood rather than later in life. Moreover, mean energy expenditure decreases from ages 19 through 50 years, and nutrient needs related to energy metabolism may also decrease.

Adulthood and Older Adults: Ages 51 through 70 Years, and over 70 Years

The age period of 51 through 70 years spans active work years for most adults. After age 70, people of the same age increasingly display different levels of physiological functioning and physical activity. Age-related declines in nutrient absorption and kidney function also may occur.

Pregnancy and Lactation

Nutrient recommendations are set for these life stages because of the many unique changes in physiology and nutrition needs that occur during pregnancy and lactation.

In setting EARs/RDAs and AIs, consideration was given to the following factors:

- The needs of the fetus during pregnancy and the production of milk during lactation

- Adaptations to increased nutrient demand, such as increased absorption and greater conservation of many nutrients
- Net loss of nutrients due to physiological mechanisms, regardless of intake, such as seen with calcium in lactation

Due to the last two factors, for some nutrients there may not be a basis for setting EAR/RDA or AI values for pregnant or lactating women that differ from the values set for other women of comparable age.

Reference Heights and Weights

Reference heights and weights for life stage and gender groups are useful when more specificity about body size and nutrient requirements is needed than that provided by life stage categories. For example, while an EAR may be developed for 4- to 8-year-olds, it could be assumed that a 4-year-old girl small for her age might require less than the EAR for her age group. Conversely, an 8-year-old boy who is big for his age might require more than the EAR for his age group. However, based on the model for establishing RDAs, the RDA (and AI) should meet the needs of both.

There are other reasons for using reference heights and weights in determining requirements. Data regarding nutrient requirements that are reported on a body-weight basis (such as with protein) necessitate the use of reference heights and weights to transform the data for comparison purposes. Or, frequently, the only available data are those regarding adult requirements. In these situations, extrapolating the data on the basis of body weight or size is a possible option to arrive at values for other age groups. Thus, when data are not available, the EARs or ULs for children or pregnant women may be established by extrapolating from adult values on the basis of body weight or, depending on the nutrient, on the basis of relative energy expenditure.

The reference heights and weights used in the more recent DRI reports are shown in Table 1. Earlier reports used slightly different reference heights and weights. (For more information on previous reference heights and weights see Appendix B of the report titled *Dietary Reference Intakes for Energy, Carbohydrate, Fiber, Fat, Fatty Acids, Cholesterol, Protein, and Amino Acids,* 2002/2005.) The new charts include reference heights and weights that are more representative of U.S. and Canadian populations.

TABLE 1 Reference Heights and Weights for Children and Adults

Gender	Age	Median Body Mass Index[a] (kg/m²)	Median Reference Height,[a] cm (in)	Reference Weight,[b] kg (lb)
Males/females	2–6 mo	—	62 (24)	6 (13)
	7–12 mo	—	71 (28)	9 (20)
	1–3 y	—	86 (34)	12 (27)
	4–8 y	15.3	115 (45)	20 (44)
Males	9–13 y	17.2	144 (57)	36 (79)
	14–18 y	20.5	174 (68)	61 (134)
	19–30 y[c]	22.5	177 (70)	70 (154)
Females	9–13 y	17.4	144 (57)	37 (81)
	14–18 y	20.4	163 (64)	54 (119)
	19–30 y[c]	21.5	163 (64)	57 (126)

[a] Taken from data on male and female median body mass index and height-for-age data from the Centers for Disease Control and Prevention (CDC)/National Center for Health Statistics (NCHS) Growth Charts.

[b] Calculated from CDC/NCHS Growth Charts; median body mass index and median height for ages 4 through 19 years.

[c] Since there is no evidence that weight should change as adults age, if activity is maintained, the reference weights for adults aged 19 through 30 years are applied to all adult age groups.

SUMMARY

The Dietary Reference Intakes (DRIs) replace and expand upon the previous revisions of the RDAs and RNIs and represent a new approach to setting nutrient values by greatly extending the scope and application of previous nutrient standards.

DRIs are a family of quantitative estimates of nutrient intakes intended for use in assessing and planning diets for healthy people. The DRI concept goes beyond the goal of former RDAs and RNIs of ensuring healthy diets, quantifying the relationship between a nutrient and the risk of disease, including chronic disease that results from either inadequate or excess intake.

The next chapter, "Applying the Dietary Reference Intakes," provides helpful guidelines and methods on how to accurately apply the DRI values when assessing and planning the diets of both individuals and groups.

APPLYING THE DIETARY REFERENCE INTAKES

The goal of dietary assessment is to determine if the nutrient intakes of an individual or group are meeting the needs of that individual or group. The goal of dietary planning is to recommend a diet that provides adequate, but not excessive, levels of nutrients. It is important to note that when planning for individuals, the goal is to achieve recommended and adequate nutrient intakes using food-based guides. However, for group planning, this chapter presents a new approach, one based on considering the entire distribution of usual nutrient intakes, rather than focusing on the mean intake of a group.

While reading this chapter, keep in mind the following important points: First, the Dietary Reference Intakes (DRIs) apply to healthy people and do not pertain to those who are sick or malnourished or whose special circumstances may alter their nutrient needs. Second, an individual's exact requirement for a specific nutrient is generally unknown. The DRIs are intended to help practitioners arrive at a reasonable estimate of the nutrient level required to provide adequacy and prevent adverse effects of excess intake. Third, using the DRIs for assessment and planning is most effective when conducted as a cyclical activity that comprises assessment, planning, implementation, and reassessment.

When assessing and planning diets, it is important to be mindful of the limitations in the data that underpin the DRIs and their application, which include the following:

- The Estimated Average Requirements (EARs) may be based on data from a limited number of individuals.
- For most nutrients, the precise variation in requirements is not known but is approximated.
- In the absence of evidence to the contrary, variation in individual requirements is assumed to follow a normal distribution.
- The EAR is often extrapolated from one population group to another.
- The degree of uncertainty associated with the EAR has not been specified.

The appropriate application of the DRIs represents a significant departure from

---

BOX 1   Definitions Associated with Assessing and Planning Nutrient Intakes

Distribution of requirements: The distribution that reflects the individual-to-individual variability in requirements. Variability exists because not all individuals in a group have the same requirements for a nutrient, even if the individuals belong to the same life stage and gender group.

Probability of inadequacy: The outcome of a calculation that compares an individual's usual (long-term) intake to the distribution of requirements for people of the same life stage and gender group; used to determine the probability that the individual's intake does not meet his or her requirement.

Probability of adequacy: 100 percent minus the probability of inadequacy.

Prevalence of inadequacy: The percentage of a group with intakes that fall below requirements.

---

how nutrition assessment and planning were carried out using the former Recommended Dietary Allowances (RDAs) and Recommended Nutrient Intakes (RNIs). Although many practitioners may have regarded the use of RDAs and RNIs as a way to determine "exact" assessments of intake, this presumed level of accuracy was actually misleading. Dietary assessment is not an exact science. In fact, it generally has always involved a process that included a "best estimate" of an individual or group's intake. The new DRIs, however, afford an opportunity to substantially improve the accuracy of dietary assessment because they allow practitioners to calculate the probability of inadequacy for an individual and the prevalence of inadequacy within a group and to plan for a low probability of inadequacy while minimizing potential risk of excess (see Box 1). These concepts are explained in greater detail later in this chapter, beginning with a short review of the statistical foundation underlying the concept of a distribution.

STATISTICAL FOUNDATION

The DRIs and their applications are based on the statistical concept of a distribution. A distribution is an arrangement of data values showing their frequency of occurrence throughout the range of the various possible values. One of the most common distributions is a "normal" distribution, which is a symmetrical bell-shaped curve that has most of the values clustered in the center of the distribution and a few values falling out in the tails (see Figure 1).

Important measures that describe a distribution are the mean, median, and standard deviation.

- The mean is the average of the data values. It is calculated by adding all the data values and then dividing by the number of data values.
- The median is the data value that occurs right in the middle of the distribution. It is the point at which half the data values are below and half the data values are above. The median is also referred to as the 50th percentile. In a symmetrical/normal distribution, the mean and median occur in the same place.
- The standard deviation (SD) is a measure of how much, on average, each individual data value differs from the mean. The smaller the SD, the less each data value varies from the mean. The larger the spread of data values, the larger SD becomes.
- The variance is another measure of how much individual data values differ from the mean. It is equivalent to the square of the standard deviation (SD^2).

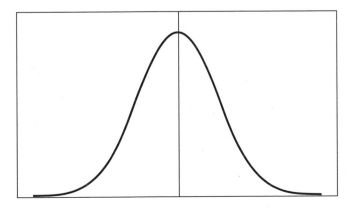

FIGURE 1 *Schematic of a normal distribution.*

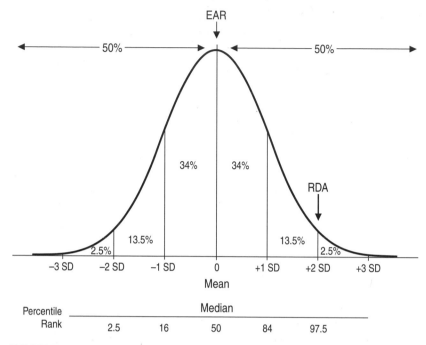

FIGURE 2 Normal requirement distribution of hypothetical nutrient showing percentile rank and placement of EAR and RDA on the distribution.

One important use of the normal distribution is the way it can be used to convert scores into percentile ranks, or probabilities. The "z-score" is a standard score that changes values into SD units (i.e., the score is now so many SDs above or below the mean). This score can be related directly to the normal distribution and the associated percentage probability of nutrient adequacy or inadequacy, as seen in Figure 2.

By making use of this property of the normal distribution, the probability (or prevalence) of adequacy or inadequacy can be estimated. For example, a z-score of +1.50 is associated with a probability of adequacy of 93 percent. A z-score of −1.00 is associated with a probability of adequacy of 15 percent. Table 1 lists a selection of z-scores and their associated probabilities. It should be noted that not all data will form a normal distribution. For example, a "skewed" distribution is one where the curve has one tail longer than the other end. If the data do not form a normal distribution, then the properties of the normal distribution do not apply.

TABLE 1 Probability of Adequacy for Selected Z-Scores

z-score	Probability of Adequacy
2.00	0.98
1.65	0.95
1.50	0.93
1.25	0.90
1.00	0.85
0.86	0.80
0.68	0.75
0.50	0.70
0.00	0.50
−0.50	0.30
−0.85	0.20
−1.00	0.15

Applying the DRIs Makes Use of Two Distributions

In applying the DRIs, two distributions are used simultaneously. The first is the distribution of requirements. The second is the distribution of intakes.

REQUIREMENT DISTRIBUTION

The distribution of requirements is the distribution upon which the DRIs (specifically the EAR and RDA) are based. This distribution reflects the variability in requirements between individuals. Variability exists because not all individuals have the same requirement for a nutrient. For nutrients where requirements are normally distributed, the EAR is located at the mean/median of the distribution. The RDA is located at 2 standard deviations above the mean, the level at which 97.5 percent of requirements should be met.

INTAKE DISTRIBUTION

The distribution of intakes is obtained from observed or reported nutrient intakes gathered through dietary assessment methods such as 24-hour recalls. A 24-hour recall is a detailed description of all foods and beverages consumed in the previous 24-hour period. Nutrient intake from supplements should also be collected. When more than one 24-hour recall is collected, intake data can reflect the day-to-day variability within an individual that occurs because different foods are eaten on different days.

When working with individuals, this variability is taken into account in the formulas used for assessment. When working with groups, statistical procedures should be used to adjust the distribution of observed intakes by partially removing the day-to-day variability in individual intakes so that the adjusted distribution more closely reflects a usual intake distribution.

Usual intake is an important concept in application of the DRIs. Usual intake is the average intake over a long period of time. It is seldom possible to accurately measure long-term usual intake due to day-to-day variation in intakes as well as measurement errors. Therefore, mean observed intakes (over at least two non-consecutive days or three consecutive days) are used to estimate usual intake.

Overlap of the Requirement Distribution and the Intake Distribution

The requirement and intake distributions can overlap to varying degrees. In some cases, the two distributions will barely intersect, if at all (see Figure 3, Panel A), and in others there may be a lot of overlap between intakes and requirements (see Figure 3, Panel B).

In applying the DRIs to assessment, the distribution of intakes is compared to the distribution of requirements and inferences are made about the degree of adequacy. In dietary planning, efforts are made to ensure that the distribution of intakes is adequate relative to the distribution of requirements.

WORKING WITH INDIVIDUALS

How to Assess the Nutrient Intakes of an Individual

The goal of assessing an individual's nutrient intake is to determine if that intake is meeting the person's nutrient requirements. Assessment of dietary adequacy for an individual is difficult because of the imprecision involved in estimating an individual's usual intake and the lack of knowledge of an individual's actual nutrient requirements. Interpreting nutrient intake data in relation to the DRIs can enhance the assessment of an individual's diet; however, the information obtained must be interpreted cautiously because an individual's true usual intake and true requirements must be estimated, and assessment of dietary adequacy is only one component of a nutritional status assessment. Ideally, intake data are combined with clinical, biochemical, or anthropometric information to provide a valid assessment of nutritional status.

Recognizing the inherent limitations and variability in dietary intakes and requirements is a major step forward in nutrition. The reports on using the DRIs for assessment and planning have provided a method with which one can

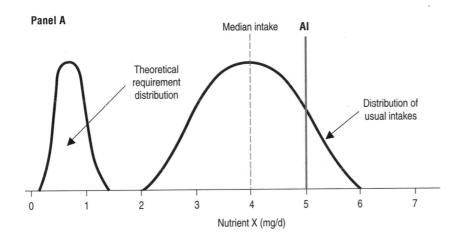

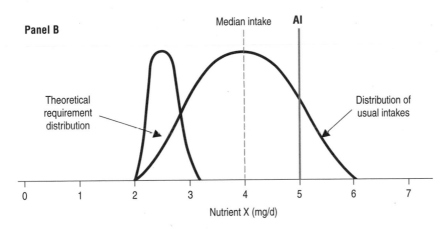

FIGURE 3 Overlap of requirement and intake distributions varies.

estimate the degree of confidence that an individual's intake meets his or her requirement. There are also equations that have been developed to estimate the degree of confidence that an individual's intake is above the AI, and below the Tolerable Upper Intake Level (UL).

It is important to keep in mind that the DRIs are estimates based on available data, and that even when an EAR, RDA, and UL for a nutrient are provided for a life stage and gender group, there is considerable uncertainty about these values. Because information on both dietary intakes and requirements are estimated, it is very difficult to exactly determine whether an individual's diet meets his or her individual requirement, even with the statistical approaches described in this chapter. Thus, assessment of dietary intakes should be used as only one part of a nutritional assessment, and the results must be kept in context. Nutrient intake data should always be considered in combination with other information, such as anthropometric measurements, biochemical indices, diagnoses, clinical status, and other factors. Dietary adequacy should be assessed and diet plans formulated based on the totality of evidence, and not on dietary intake data alone.

ESTIMATING AN INDIVIDUAL'S USUAL INTAKE AND REQUIREMENT

To conduct a dietary assessment, information is needed on both dietary intakes and dietary requirements. Information on dietary intake of individuals is usually gathered through food records or dietary recalls, and the requirement estimate is provided through the DRI process. In all cases the individual's usual intake and true requirement can only be approximated.

Estimation of Usual Intake

Obtaining accurate information on dietary intakes is challenging for a number of reasons, including the accuracy of dietary assessment techniques, as well as the challenges related to variability in intakes. The strongest methods for dietary assessment of nutrient adequacy are 24-hour recalls, diet records, or quantitative diet histories. Even so, the literature indicates that a sizeable proportion of individuals systematically misreport their dietary intakes, with the tendency toward underreporting (particularly for energy and percentage of energy from fat). It is unclear how this affects the accuracy of self-reported intakes of nutrients. Well-accepted, validated methods to statistically correct for the effects of underreporting are presently lacking.

There is also large day-to-day variation within a given individual's intake due to factors such as variation in appetite, food choices, day of the week, and season. The result is that the calculation of dietary intake from one or even several days of intake may give an inaccurate estimate of that individual's usual nutrient intake, especially if food choices vary greatly from one day to the next. Thus, observed dietary intake is probably not the same as the long-term usual intake of an individual. However, the observed mean intake is still the best available estimate of dietary intake, and can still be used providing that it is recognized there is an amount of variability associated with that best estimate.

Estimation of Requirement

It is nearly impossible to determine what an individual's exact requirement for a nutrient is, unless that individual has participated in a requirement study.

Therefore, the fall-back assumption is that the individual's requirement will be close to the average, in which case the EAR is the best estimate for an individual's unobservable requirement. It is important to note that there is variation in nutrient requirements between different individuals, and this needs to be taken into account when conducting an assessment.

Using a Qualitative Approach to Assess an Individual's Nutrient Intake

Many users of the DRIs may find a qualitative assessment of an individual's nutrient intakes to be useful. When conducting this type of descriptive assessment, it is important to keep in mind the limitations associated with the estimation of both intakes and requirements.

For nutrients with an EAR and RDA:

- Observed mean intake below the EAR very likely needs to be improved (because the probability of adequacy is 50 percent or less).
- Observed mean intake between the EAR and the RDA probably needs to be improved (because the probability of adequacy is more than 50 percent but less than 97.5 percent).
- Intakes below the RDA cannot be assumed to be inadequate because the RDA by definition exceeds the actual requirements of all but 2–3 percent of the population; many with intakes below the RDA may be meeting their individual requirements.
- The likelihood of nutrient inadequacy increases as usual intake falls further below the RDA.
- Only if intakes have been observed for a large number of days and are at or above the RDA should one have a high level of confidence that the intake is adequate.

For nutrients with an Adequate Intake (AI):

- If observed mean intake equals or exceeds the AI, it can be concluded that the diet is almost certainly adequate.
- If, however, observed mean intake falls below the AI, no estimate can be made about the probability of nutrient inadequacy.
- Professional judgment, based on additional types of information about the individual, should be exercised when interpreting intakes below the AI.

For nutrients with a UL:

- Observed mean intake less than the UL is likely to be safe.
- Observed mean intake equal to or greater than the UL may indicate a potential risk of adverse effects. The higher the intake in comparison to the UL, the greater the potential risk.

For nutrients with an Acceptable Macronutrient Distribution Range (AMDR):

- Observed mean intake between the lower and upper bound of the AMDR is within the acceptable range.
- Observed mean intake below the lower bound or above the upper bound of the AMDR may heighten concern for possible adverse consequences.

For energy:

- Body mass index (BMI) should be used to assess the adequacy of energy intake, rather than a comparison to the Estimated Energy Requirement (EER).

Using a Quantitative Approach to Assess an Individual's Nutrient Intake

An approach has been developed that statistically estimates the level of confidence that an individual's usual intake is above an individual's requirement, or below the UL. The equations developed for the assessment of individuals are based on the principles of hypothesis testing and levels of confidence based on a normal distribution curve.

The equations proposed here are not applicable to all nutrients because they assume a normal distribution of daily intakes and requirements. For nutrients for which a distribution is skewed (such as iron requirements of menstruating women, or dietary intakes of vitamin A, vitamin B_{12}, vitamin C, and vitamin E), a different methodology needs to be developed. For these nutrients, individual assessment should continue to place emphasis on other types of information available.

Nutrients with an EAR

For nutrients with an EAR, a z-score is calculated using the following equation:

$$z\text{-}score = \frac{\text{mean observed intake} - \text{EAR}}{\sqrt{[(\text{SD of requirement})^2 + (\text{within-person SD})^2 / \text{ number of days of intake records}]}}$$

The use of this equation requires the following information:

- Mean observed intake: The mean nutrient intake of an individual is the best estimate of an individual's usual intake.
- EAR: The EAR is the best estimate of an individual's requirement for a nutrient.
- SD (standard deviation) of requirement: This is the variation in requirements between individuals. It is calculated as the coefficient of variation (CV) times the EAR (see Appendix H).
- Within-person SD of intake: The variation in day-to-day nutrient intake within the individual is an indicator of how much observed intake may deviate from usual intake. (This has been estimated in the original DRI reports by using CSFII data; see Appendix I.)
- The number of days of intake records or recalls.

As illustrated in Box 2, the equation solves for a z-score on the normal distribution curve. Some z-scores and their associated probabilities are listed in Table 1. The larger the z-score, the larger the probability associated with that value. The numerator of the equation is the difference between the estimated intake and the estimated requirement. It can intuitively be seen that the higher an intake is compared to the requirement, the larger the numerator will be. The denominator of the equation is the term that incorporates all the variability. Thus, as the variability gets smaller, the z-score will get larger. Note that an increase in the number of days of records will lead to a decrease in the amount of variability.

NUTRIENTS WITH AN AI

For nutrients with an AI it is not possible to estimate the requirement of individuals. The AI represents an intake (not a requirement) that is likely to exceed the actual requirements of almost all individuals in a life stage and gender group. In fact, the AI may even be higher than an RDA (if it was possible to calculate one).

When trying to compare an individual's intake to his or her requirement, the AI is not very useful because it is in excess of the median requirement, perhaps by a very large margin. Therefore, when intakes are compared to the AI, all that can be concluded is whether the intake is above the AI or not. It is possible to determine the confidence with which one can conclude that usual intake exceeds the AI using the following equation:

BOX 2 Example: Using the Quantitative Approach for Individual Assessment for a Nutrient with an EAR

Suppose a 40-year-old woman had a magnesium intake of 320 mg/day, based on 3 days of dietary records. The question is whether this observed mean intake of 320 mg/day indicates that her usual magnesium intake is adequate.

To determine the probability that her usual intake meets her requirement, the following data are used:

- The mean observed intake for this woman is 320 mg/day.
- The EAR for magnesium for women 31–50 years is 265 mg/day
- The SD of the requirement distribution for magnesium is 10 percent of the EAR (Appendix H), therefore 26.5 mg/day.
- The within-person SD (day-to-day variability) in magnesium intake for women this age is estimated to be 86 mg/day (Appendix I).
- There are 3 days of dietary records.

Solving for the z-score yields:

$$\text{z-score} = \frac{320 - 265}{\sqrt{[(26.5)^2 + (86)^2 / 3]}} = \frac{55}{56} = 0.98 \approx 1.0$$

Table 1 lists a selection of and their associated probabilities. Looking up a z-score of 1.0, it can be seen that 85% probability of correctly concluding that this intake is adequate for a woman in this age category.

$$\text{z-score} = \frac{\text{mean observed intake} - \text{AI}}{\text{within-person SD} / \sqrt{\text{number of days of intake records}}}$$

The use of this equation requires the following information:

- Mean Observed Intake: The individual's mean observed intake
- AI: The AI for a similar life stage and gender group

- Within-person SD of intake: The variation in day-to-day nutrient intake within the individual is an indicator of how much observed intake may deviate from usual intake (see Appendix I)
- The number of days of intake records or recalls

Solving for the equation gives the confidence with which one can conclude that usual intake is greater than the AI. If an individual's intake equals or exceeds the AI, it can be concluded that the diet is almost certainly adequate. However, if the calculation does not result in the conclusion that there is a high probability that the usual intake is larger than the AI, it cannot be inferred that intake is inadequate. Professional judgment, based on additional types of information about the individual, should be exercised when interpreting intakes below the AI.

NUTRIENTS WITH A UL

The UL can be used to assess the likelihood that an individual may be at risk of adverse effects from high intakes of that nutrient. An equation has been determined to assess the probability that usual intake is below the UL given the mean observed intake. This equation is useful because even when mean observed intake is less than the UL, it cannot always be concluded with the desired amount of accuracy that usual intake is also below the UL (due to the variability associated with observed intake). This is particularly the case when the observed mean intake is a value close to that of the UL (as could be the case when considering intake from food plus supplements).

When using a UL to assess a person's nutrient intake, it is important to know whether the UL applies to intake from all sources or just from specific sources, such as supplements, fortified foods, or pharmacological preparations. The equation is as follows:

$$z\text{-score} = \frac{\text{mean observed intake} - \text{UL}}{\text{within-person SD} / \sqrt{\text{number of days of intake records}}}$$

The use of this equation requires the following information:

- Mean Observed Intake: The individual's mean observed intake (from applicable sources)
- UL: The UL for a similar life stage and gender group
- The within-person SD of intake: The variation in day-to-day nutrient intake within the individual is an indicator of how much observed intake may deviate from usual intake (see Appendix I)
- The number of days of intake records or recalls

Solving for the equation yields the confidence with which one can conclude that usual intake is less than the UL. Intakes less than the UL are likely to be safe; and intakes equal to or greater than the UL may indicate a potential risk of adverse effects. The higher the intake in comparison to the UL, the greater the potential risk.

The consequences associated with nutrient excess vary for different nutrients. It should also be noted that the UL does not apply to individuals who are consuming high intakes of nutrient on the advice of a physician who is monitoring the nutritional status of the individual.

NUTRIENTS WITH AN AMDR

The AMDRs represent intakes of macronutrients that minimize the potential for chronic disease over the long term, permit essential nutrients to be consumed at adequate levels, and are associated with adequate energy intake and physical activity to maintain energy balance. To estimate the degree of confidence that an individual's diet falls within the AMDR, the equations developed for the AI and the UL can be used. The equation for the AI can be used to determine the degree of confidence that intake is above the lower bound of the AMDR, and the equation for the UL can be used to determine the degree of confidence that intake is below the upper bound of the AMDR.

Practically, observed mean intake between the lower and upper bounds of the AMDR is within the acceptable range. Observed mean intake below the lower bound or above the upper bound of the AMDR may heighten concern for possible adverse consequences.

ENERGY

Theoretically, the usual energy intake of an individual could be compared with his or her requirement to maintain current weight with a certain level of physical activity, as estimated using the EER equations. However, by definition, the EER provides an estimate that is the midpoint of the range within which the energy expenditure of an individual could vary, and the individual's actual expenditure could be considerably above or below this estimated midpoint. Accordingly, comparing an individual's intake with the calculated average expenditure is essentially meaningless because of the difficulty in interpreting the result.

In contrast, BMI provides a useful indicator of the adequacy of usual energy intake in relation to usual energy expenditure. A BMI within the normal range of 18.5 up to 25 kg/m^2 (for adults) indicates that energy intake is adequate relative to expenditure. A BMI below the normal range indicates inadequate energy intake, whereas a BMI above the normal range is indicative of excessive energy intake.

Quantitative vs. Qualitative Approaches to Dietary Assessment of Individuals

Box 2 provides a brief example of a quantitative assessment for a nutrient (magnesium) with an EAR. A qualitative assessment could be done using the same mean intake of 320 mg/day. This value is higher than the EAR (265 mg/day) and equal to the RDA (320 mg/day). Thus, it would be assumed that the woman's intake was almost certainly adequate, when in fact there is only 85 percent confidence that this intake is adequate.

The shortcoming of the qualitative method is that it does not incorporate any variability at all. If the variability in magnesium intake was even larger than 86 mg/day, the probability that an intake of 320 mg is adequate for this woman would be even lower than 85 percent, but the result of the qualitative assessment would not change at all.

For this reason it is strongly encouraged that the statistical method be the method of choice when assessing nutrient adequacy, because even an intake that looks as though it is at the upper end of the distribution (e.g., at or above the RDA) may have an unacceptably low probability of being adequate depending on the amount of variability associated with the estimated intake.

Using the DRIs to Plan an Individual's Diet

The goal for individual planning is to ensure that the diet, as eaten, has an acceptably low risk of nutrient inadequacy while simultaneously minimizing the risk of nutrient excess. More simply put, the goal is to plan an individual's intake that will result in a low risk of that person not meeting his or her requirements.

For nutrients that have an RDA, this value should be used as a guide for planning. For nutrients with an AI, the AI should be used. The EAR should not be used for planning an individual's nutrient intake because, by definition, a diet that provides the EAR of a nutrient has a 50 percent likelihood of not meeting an individual's requirement.

Planning diets for individuals involves two steps: First, appropriate nutrient intake goals must be set, taking into account the various factors that may affect a person's nutrient needs. For example, a person who smokes may have greater needs for vitamin C. Second, the diet developed should be one that the individual can afford and will want to consume. Food-based education tools such as the United States Department of Agriculture's (USDA's) Food Guide Pyramid and Canada's Food Guide are commonly used by practitioners to teach individuals how to plan healthful diets that are adequate in nutrients.

Dietary planning involves using the DRIs to set goals for what intakes should be. When planning for nutrients such as vitamins, minerals, and protein, a low

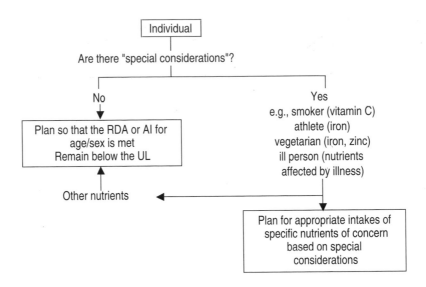

FIGURE 4 *Decision tree for planning diets of individuals.*

risk of inadequacy is planned for by meeting the RDA or AI, and a low risk of excess is planned by remaining below the UL.

In some cases it may be appropriate to use a target other than the RDA for individuals since the DRIs apply only to the apparently healthy population. Special guidance should be provided for those with greatly increased or decreased needs. Although the RDA or AI may serve as the basis for such guidance, qualified health care personnel should make the necessary adaptations for specific situations. Figure 4 is a flow chart that describes decisions that need to be made during the planning process.

PLANNING NUTRIENT INTAKES FOR AN INDIVIDUAL USING THE RDA

The RDA may be used for planning nutrient intakes that result in an acceptably low probability of inadequacy for an individual. The RDA is intended to encompass the normal biological variation in the nutrient requirements of individuals. It is set at a level that meets or exceeds the actual nutrient requirements of 97–98 percent of individuals in a given life stage and gender group. This level of intake, at which there is a 2–3 percent probability of an individual not meeting his or her requirement, has traditionally been adopted as the appropriate reference for planning intakes for individuals.

There are neither adverse effects nor documented benefits associated with exceeding the RDA, provided that intake remains below the UL. When counseling an individual, a practitioner must consider whether there is any recognizable benefit to increasing an individual's current intake level. The likelihood of the benefit must be weighed against the cost, monetary and otherwise, likely to be incurred by increasing the intake level.

If intake levels other than the RDA are chosen, they should be explicitly justified. For example, for women between the ages of 19 and 30 years, the RDA for iron is 18 mg/day, which was set to cover the needs of women with the highest menstrual blood losses. A particular woman might feel that her menstrual losses are light and, accordingly, she may be willing to accept a 10 percent risk of not meeting her requirement and thus would have an intake goal of only 13 mg/day (see Part III, "Iron"; Part IV, "Appendix G").

The EAR is not recommended for planning nutrient intakes of individuals. Despite the fact that the EAR is the best estimate of an individual's requirement, by definition, half the individuals in a group have requirements that are higher than the EAR. Accordingly, an intake at the level of the EAR is associated with a probability of inadequacy of 50 percent and is not suitable as a goal for planning. As intake increases above the EAR, the probability of inadequacy decreases and reaches 2–3 percent with intakes at the RDA.

Planning Nutrient Intakes for an Individual Using the AI

When scientific evidence is not sufficient to set an EAR and thus calculate an RDA for a particular nutrient, an AI is usually developed. Under these circumstances, the AI is the recommended target for planning the nutrient intakes of individuals. Although greater uncertainty exists in determining the probability of inadequacy for a nutrient that has an AI instead of an RDA, the AI provides a useful basis for planning. Intake at the level of the AI is likely to meet or exceed an individual's requirement, although the possibility still exists that it could fail to meet the requirements of some individuals. The probability of inadequacy associated with a failure to achieve the AI is unknown.

Planning Nutrient Intakes for an Individual Using the UL

The UL can be used to plan intakes that have a low probability of adverse effects resulting from excessive consumption. The UL is not a recommended level of intake, but rather an amount that can be biologically tolerated with no apparent risk of adverse effects by almost all healthy people. Thus, the goal for planning an individual's diet is to not exceed the UL. It is important to note that for many nutrients the UL applies to intake from all sources, whereas for some it may only apply to intake from certain sources, such as supplements, fortificants, and pharmacological preparations. (The profiles of individual nutrients found in Part III provide this information.)

For most nutrients, intakes at or above the UL would rarely be attained from unfortified food alone.

Planning Nutrient Intakes for an Individual Using the AMDR

In addition to meeting the RDA or AI, and remaining below the UL, an individual's intake of macronutrients should be planned so that carbohydrate, fat, and protein are within their respective acceptable ranges.

Planning Energy Intakes for an Individual

The underlying objective of planning for energy is similar to planning for other nutrients: to attain an acceptably low risk of inadequacy and of excess. However, the approach to planning for energy differs substantially from planning for other nutrients. When planning for individuals for nutrients such as vitamins and minerals, there are no adverse effects to consuming an intake above an individual requirement, provided intake remains below the UL. The situation for energy is quite different because for individuals who consume energy above their requirements and needs over long periods of time, weight gain will occur. This difference is reflected in the fact that there is no RDA for energy, as it would be inappropriate to recommend an intake that exceeded the requirement for a large number of individuals. Thus, the requirement for energy is expressed as an EER.

As explained in Part II, an EER is based on energy expenditure and is defined as the average dietary energy intake required to maintain current body weight and activity level (and to allow for growth or milk production, as appropriate) in healthy, normal-weight individuals of specified age, sex, height, weight, and physical activity level (PAL) that is consistent with good health.

The best way to plan for energy intake of individuals is to consider their body weight or BMI. When body weight is stable in normal-weight individuals (BMI of 18.5 kg/m^2 up to 25 kg/m^2), the energy requirement is equal to total energy expenditure and is also the usual intake.

The prediction equations to calculate an EER can be used as a starting point for planning (see Part II, "Energy"). They are only a starting point because energy expenditures vary from one individual to another even though their characteristics may be similar. The EER is the midpoint of a range of energy requirements. By definition, the EER would be expected to underestimate the true energy expenditure 50 percent of the time and to overestimate it 50 percent of the time. These errors in estimation would eventually lead to a gain or loss in body weight, which would be undesirable when the goal is to maintain a healthy weight. Body weight should be monitored and the amount of energy in the diet adjusted up or down from the EER as required to maintain an appropriate body weight. Additionally, self-reported energy intake should not be relied on to determine a person's energy needs, since underreporting of intakes is a serious and pervasive problem.

Developing Dietary Plans for an Individual

Once appropriate nutrient intake goals have been identified for the individual, these must be translated into a dietary plan that is acceptable to the individual. This is most frequently accomplished using nutrient-based food guidance systems such as national food guides.

Special Considerations

Factors such as nutrient bioavailability and physiological, lifestyle, and health characteristics may alter nutrient requirements and lead to the need for adjustments in DRI values when planning dietary intakes. Table 2 summarizes some common special considerations.

TABLE 2 Common Reasons for Adjustment in DRI Values When Planning Dietary Intake

Consideration	Nutrient	Adjustment
Recommended consumption from synthetic sources	Folic acid for women of childbearing age	It is recommended that all women capable of becoming pregnant take 400 µg folic acid every day from fortified foods, supplements, or both, in addition to the amount of food folate found in a healthful diet.
	Vitamin B_{12} for those older than 50 years of age	It is advisable for those older than 50 years to meet the RDA mainly by consuming foods fortified with vitamin B_{12} or a supplement containing vitamin B_{12}.
Smoking	Vitamin C	The requirement for smokers is increased by 35 mg/day.
Bioavailability in vegetarian diets	Iron	The requirement for iron is 1.8 times higher for vegetarians due to the lower bioavailability of iron from a vegetarian diet.
	Zinc	The requirement for zinc may be as much as 50 percent greater for vegetarians, particularly for strict vegetarians whose major food staples are grains and legumes.
Age of menstruation	Iron (it is assumed that girls younger than 14 years do not menstruate and that girls 14 years and older do menstruate)	If menstruation occurs prior to age 14, an additional amount (about 2.5 mg/day) would be needed to cover menstrual blood losses. Conversely, girls ages 14 and above who are not yet menstruating can subtract 2.5 mg from the RDA for this age group.
Athletes engaged in regular intense exercise	Iron	Average requirements for iron may range from 30 to 70 percent above those for normally active individuals.
Recommendation set according to reference weight	Protein	Recommendation is set in g/kg/day. RDA for adults is 0.80 g/kg/day.
Recommendation set per 1,000 kcal	Fiber	Recommendation is 14 g/1,000 kcal.

KEY POINTS FOR WORKING WITH INDIVIDUALS

ASSESSING NUTRIENT INTAKES

✓ The goal of assessing an individual's nutrient intake is to determine if that intake is meeting his or her nutrient requirements.

✓ Assessment requires using the individual's observed or reported mean intake as an estimate of usual intake and using the EAR of the appropriate life stage and gender group as an estimate of the individual's requirement.

✓ For nutrients with an EAR, a statistical equation can be applied to assess the likelihood of adequacy. This equation yields a z-score that allows a practitioner to determine a probability value that reflects the degree of confidence that the person's usual intake meets his or her requirement.

✓ For nutrients with an AI, a statistical equation can be applied to determine whether usual intake is at or above the AI, in which case intake is deemed adequate. Intakes below the AI cannot be assessed.

✓ For nutrients with a UL, a statistical equation can be applied to determine whether usual intake falls below the UL, in which case the person is assessed as having a low risk of adverse effects related to excessive intake.

✓ The RDA should not be used for assessing an individual's intake.

✓ In all cases, individual assessments should be cautiously interpreted, preferably in combination with other information on factors that can affect nutritional status, such as anthropometric data, biochemical measurements, dietary patterns, lifestyle habits, and the presence of disease.

PLANNING NUTRIENT INTAKES

✓ The goal of planning nutrient intakes for individuals is to achieve a low probability of inadequacy while not exceeding the UL for each nutrient.

✓ Planning diets for individuals involves two steps: First, appropriate nutrient goals must be set, taking into account the various factors that may affect a person's nutrient needs. Second, the diet developed should be one that the individual can afford and will want to consume.

✓ For nutrients with an EAR and an RDA, the probability of inadequacy is 50 percent at the EAR and 2–3 percent at the RDA. Thus, the RDA is often used as a guide for planning for individuals. If an RDA, is not available, the AI should be used as a guide for planning nutrient intake.

✓ For nutrients with a UL, this value should be used as the level not to exceed.

✓ An individual's intake of macronutrients should be planned so that carbohydrate, fat, and protein are within their respective AMDRs.

✓ The best way to plan for energy intake of individuals is to consider the healthfulness of their body weight or BMI.

WORKING WITH GROUPS

Although some nutrition professionals primarily work with individuals, others need to be able to assess and plan the nutrient intakes of groups. Examples of such groups include nursing home residents, research study participants, and children attending residential schools. This section describes ways to assess and plan nutrient intakes of groups.

How to Assess the Nutrient Intakes of a Group

The goal of assessing the nutrient intakes of groups is to determine the prevalence of inadequate (or excessive) nutrient intakes within a particular group of individuals (see Box 1 for definitions). Within any given group, even a homogeneous group such as individuals in the same life stage and gender group, variability will exist among the different individuals' nutrient needs and nutrient intakes. To accurately determine the proportion of a group that has a usual intake of a nutrient that is less than their requirement, information on both the distribution of usual intakes and the distribution of requirements in the group is needed.

Several characteristics of dietary intake data make estimating the distribution of usual intakes for a group challenging. When single 24-hour recalls or diet records are obtained from members of a group, the variability of the nutrient intakes will reflect both differences between individuals as well as differences within individuals (i.e., on any given day, a particular individual could eat much more or much less of a nutrient than usual).

To obtain a distribution of usual intakes for a group, the distribution of observed intakes (i.e., the intake obtained from a single 24-hour recall) must

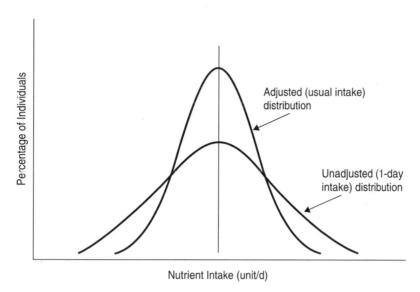

FIGURE 5 Comparison of 1-day and usual intakes.

be statistically adjusted to remove the effects of within-person variability, so that the distribution reflects only between-person variability. To do this, at least two 24-hour recalls or diet records obtained on nonconsecutive days (or at least three days of data from consecutive days) are needed from a representative subsample of the group. When this adjustment is performed, the intake distribution narrows (i.e., the tails of the distribution draw closer to the center). If intake distributions are not properly adjusted, the prevalence of nutrient inadequacy will be incorrectly estimated and is usually overestimated (see Figure 5).

Several methods to obtain usual intake distributions are available. The National Research Council (NRC) and Iowa State University have both developed software programs for adjusting intake distributions. Further information is available at http://cssm.iastate.edu/software/side.html. Although these methods will adjust for variability in day-to-day intakes, they do not make up for inaccuracies in reported or observed intakes.

The summary below explains how the DRIs are appropriately used in the assessment of a group's nutrient intakes. Further explanation of the approach and the methods used are provided in the sections that follow:

- For nutrients with an EAR, the EAR can be used to estimate the prevalence of inadequate intakes using the probability approach or a shortcut derived from the probability approach called the EAR cut-point method.
- The RDA is inappropriate for assessing nutrient intakes of groups because the RDA is the intake level that exceeds the requirements of a large proportion of individuals in a group. Consequently, estimating the prevalence of nutrient inadequacy in a group by determining the proportion of individuals with intakes below the RDA leads to an overestimation of the true prevalence of inadequacy.
- For nutrients without an EAR, the AI is instead used. Groups with mean or median intakes at or above the AI can generally be assumed to have a low prevalence of inadequate intakes.
- For nutrients with a UL, this value can be used to estimate the proportion of a group at potential risk of adverse effects from excessive nutrient intake.
- For nutrients with an AMDR, the proportion of the group that falls below, within, and above the AMDR can be used to assess population adherence to the recommendations and to determine the proportion of the population that is outside the range. If significant proportions of the population fall outside the range, concern could be heightened for possible adverse consequences.
- For energy, the distribution of BMI within a group can be assessed, and the proportions of the group with BMIs below, within, and above the desirable range would reflect the proportions with inadequate, adequate, and excessive energy intakes.

USING THE PROBABILITY APPROACH TO ASSESS PREVALENCE OF NUTRIENT INADEQUACY IN A GROUP

The probability approach is a statistical method that involves determining the probability of inadequacy of the usual intake level for each person in the group and then averaging these individual probabilities across the group to obtain an estimate of the group's prevalence of inadequacy. This method depends on two key assumptions: that intakes and requirements are independent and thus no correlation exists between usual intakes and requirements (this is thought to be true for most nutrients, although it is not known to be true for energy) and that the distribution of requirements for the nutrient in question is known. This method then uses statistical equations to estimate the prevalence of inadequacy.

Case studies one and two at the end of the chapter illustrate the use of the probability approach. Practically, this approach will most likely be used only when the EAR cut-point method cannot be used.

Using the EAR Cut-Point Method to Assess Prevalence of Nutrient Inadequacy in a Group

The EAR cut-point method is a shortcut derived from the probability approach. When certain conditions are satisfied, the proportion of the group with intakes below the EAR will be similar to the proportion that does not meet their requirement. The conditions (assumptions) that must be satisfied to use the EAR cut-point method are:

- *Intakes and requirements must not be correlated:* This is thought to be true for most nutrients, but is known *not* to be true for energy, as individuals with higher energy requirements have higher energy intakes.
- *The distribution of requirements must be symmetrical:* This is thought to be true for most nutrients, but is known not to be true for iron for menstruating women. Blood (and therefore iron) losses during menstrual flow greatly vary among women, and some women have unusually high losses. As a result, the distribution of iron requirements for this life stage and gender group is skewed rather than symmetrical, and the EAR cut-point method cannot be used to assess the prevalence of inadequacy. Instead, the probability approach should be used, as shown in case study two.
- *The distribution of intakes must be more variable than the distribution of requirements.* Stated another way, the SD of the intake distribution is greater than the SD of the requirement distribution. This is thought to be true among groups of free-living individuals. Note, however, that the assumption that intakes are more variable than requirements might not hold for groups of similar individuals who were fed similar diets (e.g., prison inmates). If the assumption is not met, the probability method can be used instead of the EAR cut-point method.

The reasons that the EAR cut-point method can approximate the prevalence of inadequacy in a group as determined by the full probability method are explained below and illustrated in the third case study at the end of the chapter.

1. Although the probability of inadequacy exceeds 50 percent when usual intakes are below the EAR, not everyone with an intake below the EAR fails to meet his or her own requirement: Some individuals with lower-than-average requirements will have adequate intakes (their usual intake, although below the EAR, exceeds their own requirement).

2. Similarly, although the probability of inadequacy is less than 50 percent when usual intakes are above the EAR, not everyone with intakes above the EAR meets their own requirement. Some individuals with higher-than-average

requirements will have inadequate intakes (their usual intake, although above the EAR, is below their own requirement).

3. When the requirement distribution is symmetrical, when intakes are more variable than requirements, and when intakes and requirements are independent, the proportion of the group described in item 1 cancels out the proportion described in item 2. The prevalence of inadequacy in the group can thus be approximated by the proportion with usual intakes below the EAR. See Box 3 for an example.

THE RDA IS INAPPROPRIATE FOR ASSESSING GROUP NUTRIENT INTAKES

It is not appropriate to use the RDA to assess nutrient intakes of groups. In the past, the RDA, or the RNI in Canada, has been used incorrectly to make inferences about nutrient inadequacy in groups by using the RDA as a cut-point or comparing mean or median intakes with the RDA.

The RDA should not be used as a cut-point because it overestimates the requirements of 97.5 percent of the population. The mean or median intake of a group should not be compared with the RDA to assess nutrient adequacy in a group because the prevalence of inadequacy depends on the distribution of usual intakes, and this is not taken into account when only the mean or median is used. For example, as shown in Box 3, women 51 to 70 years of age had a median dietary vitamin B_6 intake of 1.51 mg/day in the Third National Health and Nutrition Examination Survey (NHANES III, 1988–1994). Comparing this median intake with the RDA for this group, 1.5 mg/day, might lead one to believe that inadequate vitamin B_6 intake is not a problem. However, appropriate analysis of the data relative to the EAR reveals that the prevalence of inadequacy in this group is actually greater than 25 percent.

USING THE AI TO ASSESS A GROUP'S NUTRIENT INTAKES

The AI has limited uses in assessing the nutrient intakes of groups. When an AI is set for a nutrient, it means that there was insufficient evidence to establish the distribution of requirements and thereby determine an EAR. For this reason, it is simply not possible to determine the proportion of a group with intakes below requirements. Accordingly, only limited inferences can be made about the adequacy of group intakes. If the median or mean intake of a group is at or above the AI, it can be assumed that the prevalence of inadequate intakes in the group is low.

If group median or mean intake is below the AI, nothing can be concluded about the prevalence of inadequacy. Again, this occurs because we do not know the requirement distribution, and whether its upper end (if it could be deter-

---

BOX 3 Assessing Group Nutrient Intakes—The RDA Is Inappropriate

The EAR for vitamin B_6 for women aged 51–70 years is 1.3 mg /day and the RDA is 1.5 mg/day. Shown below is a distribution of dietary vitamin B_6 intakes for a group of women 51–70 years of age. The distribution has been adjusted for individual variability using the method developed by the National Research Council. The data are from NHANES III.

Selected Percentiles of Dietary Vitamin B_6 Intake, Women 51-70 Years of Age, NHANES III

Percentile	5th	10th	15th	25th	50th	75th	85th	90th	95th
Vitamin B_6 intake (mg/day)	0.92	1.02	1.11	1.24	1.51	1.90	2.13	2.31	2.65

Comparing the median intake of 1.51 mg/day to the RDA of 1.5 mg/day for this group might lead one to believe that inadequate vitamin B_6 intake is not a problem. However, comparison of the distribution of usual intakes to the EAR cut-point shows that the EAR value of 1.3 mg/day falls somewhere between the 25th percentile and the 50th percentile of usual intakes. Thus, it can be concluded that greater than 25 percent of usual intakes are below the EAR cut-point and the prevalence of inadequacy in this group is estimated to be greater than 25 percent (but less than 50 percent).

---

mined) is relatively close to the AI or falls well below it. It follows from the above discussion that individuals with intakes below the AI cannot be assessed as having inadequate intakes. Although the proportion of a group with usual intakes below the AI could be determined, great care should be taken to avoid implying that this proportion does not meet their requirements (i.e., the AI should not be used as a cut-point in the way that the EAR may be).

USING THE UL TO ASSESS A GROUP'S NUTRIENT INTAKES

The UL can be used to estimate the proportion of a group with intakes above the UL and, therefore, at potential risk of adverse health effects from excess nutrient intake. The method for applying the UL is similar to the EAR cut-point method in that the proportion of the group with intakes above the UL is determined.

Because ULs for nutrients are based on different sources of intake, the appropriate usual intake distribution must be used in the assessment. For some nutrients, such as fluoride, phosphorus, and vitamin C, the distribution of usual intakes would need to include intake from all sources. For others, such as magnesium, folate, niacin, and vitamin E, only the distribution of usual intakes from synthetic sources added to foods and from supplements (and in the case of magnesium, medications) would be needed.

Another issue to consider when interpreting the proportion of a group with intakes above the UL is that there is considerable uncertainty with regard to some of the ULs for children. In many cases, these ULs were established based on extrapolation from the ULs for adults or infants, and thus for some nutrients, this resulted in very small margins or an overlap between the adult RDA and the UL for young children. Surveys in the United States have revealed that young children have a high prevalence of intakes above the UL for nutrients such as vitamin A and zinc; however, few studies have been conducted in children to assess the effects of such intakes.

USING THE AMDR TO ASSESS A GROUP'S NUTRIENT INTAKE

By determining the proportion of the group that falls below, within, and above the AMDR, it is possible to assess population adherence to the recommendations and to determine the proportion of the population that is outside the range. If significant proportions of the population fall outside the range, concern could be heightened for possible adverse consequences.

ASSESSING THE ENERGY ADEQUACY OF A GROUP'S DIET

The probability approach and the EAR cut-point method do not work for assessing energy adequacy. This is because empirical evidence indicates a strong correlation between energy intake and energy requirement. This correlation most likely reflects either the regulation of energy intake to meet needs or the adjustment of energy expenditure to be consistent with intakes. Therefore, the use of BMI as a biological indicator is preferable. The distribution of BMI within a population group can be assessed, and the proportions of the group with BMIs below, within, and above the desirable range would reflect the proportions with inadequate, adequate, and excessive energy intakes.

How to Plan for the Nutrient Intakes of a Group

The goal of planning nutrient intakes for groups is to achieve usual intakes in the group that meet the requirements of most individuals, but that are not excessive. This can be challenging because the amount and selection of foods that group individuals eat will vary, even if the same meal is offered. Situations where group planning occurs include residential schools, prisons, military garrisons, hospitals, nursing homes, child nutrition programs, and food assistance programs.

When planning for groups, a practitioner should aim for a low prevalence of inadequate intakes. In the past, this may have involved considering the average intake of the group and comparing it with the RDA, which was inappropriate because even if a group's average intake meets the RDA, the prevalence of inadequacy is likely to be unacceptably high. This is because the variability in nutrient intakes among group members usually exceeds the variability in the requirements of group members, and it is the variability in requirements that is used to set the RDA.

Instead, the new DRIs present an approach to planning that involves consideration of the entire distribution of usual nutrient intakes within a group, rather than just the average intake of the group. The goal is that the distribution of usual nutrient intakes that results from the plan will have a low prevalence of inadequate or excessive intake, as defined by the proportion of individuals in the group with usual intakes less than the EAR or greater than the UL. An important caveat: By focusing explicitly on the distribution of nutrient intakes of a group as the goal of group planning, the framework presented here is, in many respects, a new paradigm, and it should be tested before being implemented in large-scale group-feeding situations.

To apply the framework presented here, an acceptable prevalence of inadequacy must be defined (a critical step on the part of the planner) and the distribution of usual intakes in the group must be estimated. As previously stated, this is accomplished by determining the distribution of reported or observed intakes, and performing a statistical adjustment to estimate the distribution of usual intakes. A target (desired) usual intake distribution can then be determined by positioning the distribution of usual intakes relative to the EAR to achieve the desired prevalence of inadequacy.

Because the goal of planning is to achieve a target distribution of usual intakes, assessment must occur (see "Probability Approach" and "EAR Cut-Point Method" earlier in the chapter). In most cases, planning group intakes is an ongoing process, in which planners set goals for usual intake, implement the plan, assess whether the goals have been achieved, and then accordingly modify their planning procedures.

Before describing how the different DRI values are appropriately used to plan intakes for groups, the next section explains the importance of a target usual intake distribution and how to estimate this distribution for nutrients with normal distributions and for nutrients with skewed distributions.

What Is a Target Usual Nutrient Intake Distribution?

Suppose a practitioner is interested in planning a group diet with a high probability of nutrient adequacy (e.g., such that the prevalence of inadequacy in the group is no more than 2–3 percent). Given this target, and assuming that the EAR cut-point method can be used in the assessment, the usual intake distribution of the group should be positioned so that only 2–3 percent of the individuals in the group have usual intakes less than the EAR.

To achieve this goal of a low prevalence of nutrient inadequacy, it may be necessary to modify the baseline usual nutrient intake distribution. The change may be as simple as a shift (up or down) of the entire baseline distribution or it may include changes in both the location and the shape of the distribution. In either case, the appropriate changes to the baseline usual nutrient intake distribution are intended to result in the desired distribution of usual intakes. This desired distribution is referred to as the target usual nutrient intake distribution.

The simplest approach to determining the target usual nutrient intake distribution is to shift the baseline distribution, with the assumption that there will be no change in its shape. This is illustrated for a hypothetical nutrient in Figure 6. Panel A shows the baseline usual intake distribution, in which the prevalence of inadequate intakes (the percentage of the group below the EAR) is about 30 percent. If the planning goal were to attain a prevalence of inadequacy of no more than 2–3 percent, the target usual nutrient intake distribution could be achieved by simply shifting the baseline usual intake distribution up, as shown in Panel B.

The appropriate shift (up or down) can be calculated as the additional (or decreased) amount of the nutrient that must be consumed to achieve the prevalence of usual intakes below the EAR that is the planning goal. For example, the EAR for zinc for girls aged 9 to 13 years is 7 mg/day. Current data from the National Health and Nutrition Examination Survey (NHANES III, 1988–1994) show that about 10 percent of the girls have usual intakes below the EAR. If the goal were to plan intakes so that only 2–3 percent fell below the EAR, intakes would have to be increased. When the intervention is designed to increase everyone's usual zinc intake, then the amount of the increase can be calculated as the difference between the current intake at the second to third percentile, which is 6.2 mg/day, and the desired intake at the second to third percentile, which is the EAR of 7 mg/day. This difference is 0.8 mg/day, which means that the distribution of usual intakes needs to shift up by 0.8 mg/day in order to have only 2–3 percent of the girls with intakes below the EAR.

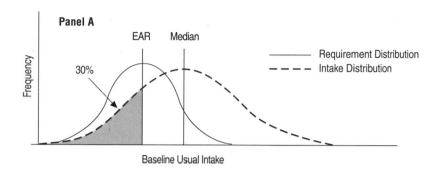

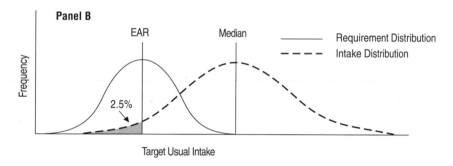

FIGURE 6 Concept of a target usual intake distribution. Panel A shows the baseline usual nutrient intake distribution with 30 percent prevalence of inadequate intakes. Panel B shows the effect of shifting the baseline distribution to attain the target usual nutrient intake distribution of 2–3 percent inadequate intakes.

How to Estimate the Target Intake Distribution for Groups with Normal Intake Distributions

To set a target usual nutrient intake distribution with a selected prevalence of inadequacy for a specific group, it is useful to examine a simple example depicting a normal distribution of usual intake.

When it is known that the usual intake distribution of the group being assessed approximates normality, as depicted in all panels of Figure 7, the position of the target usual nutrient intake distribution can be estimated very simply with a table of selected areas under the normal distribution. The median (midpoint) of the target usual intake distribution can be determined using the following equation:

$$\text{EAR} + (Z \times \text{SD}_{usual\ intake})$$

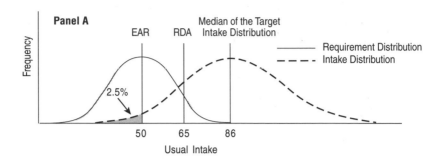

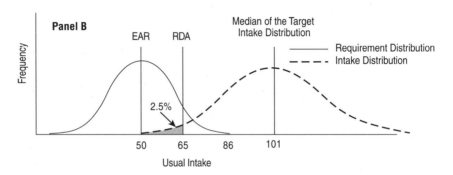

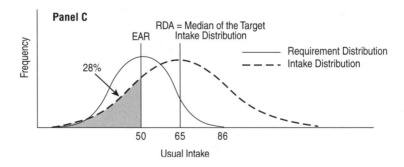

FIGURE 7 Target usual intake distributions. Panel A: Low group prevalence of inadequacy: 2.5 percent of the population has usual intake below the estimated average requirement. Panel B: Low individual risk of inadequacy: 2.5 percent of the population has usual intake below the RDA. Panel C: Higher group and individual risk of inadequacy: target median intake equals the RDA.

where Z comes from a table of areas under the curve of a normal distribution and $SD_{usual\ intake}$ is the standard deviation of the intake distribution. Table 3 reproduces part of a table of z-scores.

For example, as shown in Panel of A of Figure 7, when the EAR is 50 units and the $SD_{usual\ intake}$ is 18 units, a 2.5 percent prevalence of inadequacy (Z = 1.96 at 2.5 percent) would be expected when the median intake was 86 units (86 = 50 + [1.96 × 18]). On the other hand, if a 5 percent prevalence of inadequacy were chosen, the calculated median intake would be 80 (80 = 50 + [1.65 × 18]), a lower value since more of the group would have intakes below the EAR.

How to Estimate the Target Intake Distribution for Groups with Skewed Intake Distributions

The previous section described how to estimate a target distribution assuming a normal distribution of usual intakes within the group. However, in most cases, the usual intakes within a group are not normally distributed. Therefore, the $SD_{usual\ intake}$ cannot be used to identify the position of the target usual nutrient intake distribution. Instead, the necessary approach is similar in principle to the one in the previous section, although it does not depend on the SD of usual intake and a z-score. A practitioner would first specify the acceptable prevalence of inadequate intake, and then position the usual intake distribution so

TABLE 3 Setting the Target Median Intake[a] for Nutrients with Intake Distributions Approximating Normality: Selecting Z-Scores

Acceptable Group Risk of Inadequate Intakes (%)	Z-Score: Multiplier for the Standard Deviation of Intake
0.05	3.27
0.5	2.57
1.0	2.33
1.5	2.17
2.0	**2.05**
2.5	**1.96**
3.0	**1.88**
5.0	1.65
10.0	1.28
15.0	1.03
25.0	0.68
50.0	0.00

[a] Target median intake = EAR + Z × $SD_{usual\ intake}$ where EAR = Estimated Average Requirement, Z = statistical tool to determine areas under the normal distribution, SD = standard deviation of intake.

that the percentile of usual intake associated with this specified prevalence of inadequate intake equals the EAR.

Using the DRIs to Plan a Group's Nutrient Intakes

The summary below explains how DRIs are appropriately used in planning a group's nutrient intakes. Further details are provided in the sections that follow and in the case studies at the end of the chapter.

- For nutrients with an EAR and RDA, the EAR is used in conjunction with the usual nutrient intake distribution to plan for an acceptably low prevalence of inadequate intakes within the group. For most nutrients, the planning goal is to minimize the prevalence of intakes below the EAR. The RDA is not recommended for use in planning the nutrient intakes of groups.
- For nutrients without an EAR, the AI is used instead. The AI is used as the target for the mean, or median, intake of the group. The goal is to increase the group's mean or median intake to the level of the AI.
- For nutrients with a UL, this value is used to plan for an acceptably low prevalence of intakes at risk of being excessive.
- For nutrients with an AMDR, an additional goal of planning is to achieve a macronutrient distribution in which the intakes of most of the group fall within the AMDRs.
- For energy, the goal is for the group's mean intake to equal the EER. For energy, the estimated energy requirement of a reference individual or an average of estimated maintenance energy needs for the group members can be used in planning energy intake of groups.

USING THE EAR TO PLAN A GROUP'S NUTRIENT INTAKES

For nutrients that have an EAR, this value is used in conjunction with the usual nutrient intake distribution to plan for an acceptably low prevalence of inadequate intakes within the group. For most nutrients, the planning goal is to minimize the prevalence of intakes below the EAR.

USING THE AI TO PLAN A GROUP'S NUTRIENT INTAKES

Due to limitations in available data, the AIs for various nutrients are set using different criteria. For some nutrients, the AI is based on the observed mean or median intakes by groups that are maintaining health and nutritional status consistent with meeting requirements. In these cases, the AI is conceptually similar to the median of a target usual nutrient intake distribution. For other nutrients, the AI is the level of intake at which subjects in an experimental

TABLE 4 Method Used to Estimate Adequate Intake (AI) for Groups of Healthy Adults

Estimation Method	Nutrient
Experimental derivation	Biotin
	Calcium
	Choline
	Vitamin D
	Fiber, total
	Fluoride
	Potassium
	Sodium and chloride
Mean intake	Chromium
Median intake	Vitamin K
	Manganese
	Pantothenic acid
	n-6 Polyunsaturated fatty acids
	n-3 Polyunsaturated fatty acids
	Water, total

study met the criterion of adequacy. In these cases, the AI is not directly comparable to a target median intake.

Because of these differences in how the AI is set for different nutrients, the appropriate use of the AI in planning group intakes also varies. The AI can be used if the variability in the usual intake of the population being planned for is similar to the variability in intake of the healthy population that was used to set the AI. In this case, the appropriate use of the AI would be as the target median intake of the group.

However, if the AI is not based on a group mean or median intake of a healthy population, practitioners must recognize that there is a reduced level of confidence that achieving a mean or median intake at the AI will result in a low prevalence of inadequacy. In addition, the AI cannot be used to estimate the proportion of a group with inadequate intakes. Thus, regardless of how the AI has been estimated, it is not possible to use the AI to plan a target distribution of usual intakes with a known prevalence of inadequacy. Table 4 presents a summary of the nutrients for which AIs have been estimated and notes the cases in which these estimates reflect experimental derivation and observed mean and median intake of healthy groups. Practitioners who want to compare their target groups to the groups used to set the AIs can obtain this information in each of the individual nutrient profiles found in Part III.

Using the UL to Plan a Group's Nutrient Intakes

For nutrients that have a UL, the planning goal is to achieve an acceptably low prevalence of intakes above the UL.

Using the EER to Plan a Group's Diet

As is true for individuals, the underlying objective in planning the energy intake of a group is similar to planning intakes for other nutrients: to attain an acceptably low prevalence of inadequacy and potential excess. When planning the energy intakes of groups, the goal is for the group's mean intake to equal the EER. Because energy intake is related to energy requirement, it is assumed that people in the group with energy requirements above the EER will choose energy intakes that are above the EER, and those with requirements below the EER will choose intakes below the EER, so that the average intake will equal the EER.

The EAR cut-point approach should not be used for planning energy intakes, because it is expected, and desirable, for half of the group to have intakes below the EER.

There are two possible approaches to estimate energy intakes of groups. One can estimate energy requirements for the reference person or obtain an average of estimated maintenance energy needs for the group members. For example, to plan for a large group of men aged 19 through 30 years, one can estimate the EER for the reference male with a weight of 70 kg (154 lbs) and a height of 1.76 m (~ 5 ft 8 in) and who is considered low active, and use this number (~ 2,700 kcal) as the target for the group. This approach would require the assumption that all members of the group were similar to the reference person or that the reference person accurately represented the group's average values for age, height, weight, and activity level, and that these variables were symmetrically distributed.

The preferred approach would be to plan for an intake equal to the average energy expenditure for the group. For example, assuming that there is access to data on height, weight, age, and activity level, the energy expenditure for each individual in the group could be estimated. The average of these values would then be used as the planning goal for the maintenance of the group's current weight and activity level. As with other planning applications, assessing the plan for a group's energy intake, following its implementation, would lead to further refinements. In the case of energy, however, assessment would be based on monitoring body weight rather than on reported energy intake.

CASE STUDIES

Case Study One: Using the Probability Approach to Assess Intakes in a Group

Using a group of 650 adult men aged 19 to 30 years and a hypothetical nutrient with an EAR of 7 mg/day for this age and gender group illustrates the probability approach. Individuals in this group, even though they are similar in age and gender, differ in both their requirements for the nutrient and their usual intakes of the nutrient. At a conceptual level, determining the prevalence of inadequate nutrient intakes in the group would simply involve comparing each individual's usual nutrient intake with his individual requirement, and totaling the number of men with usual intakes below their individual requirements. For example, a man with a usual nutrient intake of 9 mg/day and a requirement of 10 mg/day would not meet his requirement and would be classified as inadequate, whereas another man with a usual nutrient intake of 9 mg/day and a requirement of 5 mg/day would exceed his requirement. In practice, however, we almost never know individuals' nutrient requirements. Instead, we may have information on the distribution of requirements for a small group of individuals who are similar in age and gender, and who took part in studies to determine nutrient requirements. From that information, we can determine the probability, or risk, that a given intake will be adequate or inadequate.

Knowledge of the distribution of requirements allows one to construct a risk curve that defines the probability that any given intake is inadequate, whether the requirement distribution is statistically normal or not. Figure 8 shows a risk curve for the example nutrient with an EAR of 7 mg/day. The requirement distribution for this nutrient is statistically normal, and the SD is ~ 1.5 mg/day. As described earlier, for nutrients with normal requirement distributions, 95 percent of individuals have requirements within ± 2 SD of the EAR. In this example, 95 percent of men aged 19 to 30 years would have requirements between 4 mg/day (7 mg/day minus twice the SD of 1.5 mg/day) and 10 mg/day (7 mg/day plus twice the SD of 1.5 mg/day). The probability of inadequacy associated with any intake can be determined by assessing where the intake level intersects the risk curve.

As illustrated in Figure 8, the probability of inadequacy at a usual intake at or below about 3 mg/day is associated with a probability of inadequacy of 1.0 (100 percent), meaning that virtually everyone with a usual intake in this range does not meet their own requirement. When usual intakes are at or above about 11 mg/day, the probability of inadequacy is zero, meaning that virtually everyone with a usual intake in this range would meet their own requirement. When usual intake is between 4 mg/day and 10 mg/day, the probability of inadequacy varies, and can be estimated by determining where the usual intake level intersects the risk curve:

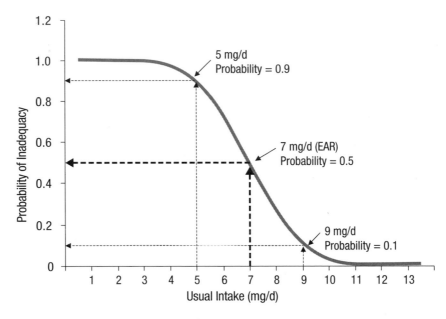

FIGURE 8 Risk curve. This risk curve is from a normal requirement distribution with a mean of 7 mg/day and a SD of 1.5 mg/day.

- It is relatively high at intakes that are just above the lower end of the distribution of requirements (about 0.9 or 90 percent at a usual intake of 5 mg/day in this example).
- By definition, the probability of inadequacy at the EAR is 0.5 or 50 percent (7 mg/day in this example).
- It is relatively low at intakes that are closer to the upper end of the distribution of requirements (about 0.1 or 10 percent at a usual intake of 9 mg/day in this example).

The information on the probability of inadequacy of different usual intake levels is used to estimate the prevalence of inadequate intakes in the group. This is done by determining the probability of inadequacy for each usual intake level in the group, and then computing the average for the group as a whole. Figure 9 and Table 5 illustrate this approach. Figure 9 shows the risk curve from Figure 8, as well as a usual intake distribution for the group of 650 men in the example (each "box" in the figure represents 10 men and there are 65 boxes). Table 5 shows the usual intake levels from the distribution shown in Figure 9, the associated probability of inadequacy, and the number of men at that intake level.

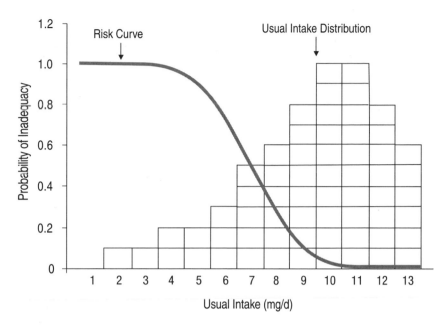

FIGURE 9 Comparison of the risk curve to a usual intake distribution. In this simplified usual intake distribution, each "box" represents 10 men aged 19 to 30 years. The prevalence of inadequate intakes in the group is estimated by determining the probability of inadequacy associated with each individual usual intake level, and then calculating the average probability.

To illustrate how Figure 9 and Table 5 work to determine the prevalence of inadequacy, consider men with intakes of 5 mg/day and 9 mg/day. Twenty men have usual intakes of 5 mg/day, and an intake of 5 mg/day intersects the risk curve at a probability of inadequacy of 0.90. Because each individual with a usual intake of 5 mg/day has a 90 percent (0.9) probability of being inadequate, one would expect 18 of 20 men (90 percent) to be inadequate. In contrast, 80 men have usual intakes of 9 mg/day, and an intake of 9 mg/day intersects the risk curve at a probability of inadequacy of 10 percent.

One would thus expect 8 men (10 percent of the 80 men with usual intakes of 9 mg/day) to be inadequate. The average probability of inadequacy is calculated by totaling the number of individuals likely to have inadequate intakes, and then dividing by the total number of men. (This is mathematically identical to adding up all the individual probabilities of inadequacy [i.e., 1.0 + 1.0 + 1.0 + . . . + 0 + 0 + 0] and dividing by the total number of men.) In this example, the group prevalence of inadequacy is approximately 20 percent.

TABLE 5 Using the Probability Approach to Estimate Group Prevalence of Inadequacy in a Group of 650 Adult Men Ages 19 to 30 Years for a Nutrient with an EAR of 7 mg/day

Usual Intake Level (mg/day)	Probability of Inadequacy	Number of People	Probability × Number[a]
2	1.0	10	10
3	1.0	10	10
4	0.97	20	19.4
5	0.90	20	18.0
6	0.73	30	21.9
7	0.50	50	25.0
8	0.27	60	16.2
9	0.10	80	8.0
10	0.03	100	3.0
11	0	100	0
12	0	80	0
13	0	60	0
14	0	30	0
Total		**650**	**131.5**
Average probability	= probability × number/total		
	= 131.5/650 = 0.20 (20 percent)		

[a] This represents the number of men expected to have inadequate intakes at each intake level.

Case Study Two: Using the Probability Approach to Assess Iron Intakes in a Group of Menstruating Women

The probability approach involves first determining the risk of inadequacy for each individual in the population, and then averaging the individual probabilities across the group. For iron, Appendix Tables G-5, G-6, and G-7 give the probability of inadequacy at various intakes. These tables may be used to calculate the risk of inadequacy for each individual, and then the estimated prevalence of inadequacy for a population. In addition, Appendix C of the original report titled, *Dietary Reference Intakes: Applications in Dietary Assessment* (2000), demonstrates how to carry out the necessary calculations to obtain a prevalence estimate for a group.

This case study presents a simplified estimate that could also be determined manually. The estimate is illustrated in Table 6 for a hypothetical group of 1,000 menstruating women not taking oral contraceptives and consuming a typical omnivorous diet. The first and second columns of this table are based on information in Appendix Tables G-4 and G-7. Intakes below 4.42 mg/day are assumed to have a 100 percent probability of inadequacy (risk = 1.0). Individuals with intakes above 18.23 mg/day are assumed to have a zero risk of inadequacy. For intakes between these two extremes, the risk of inadequacy is calculated as 100 minus the midpoint of the percentile of requirement. For example, intakes between 4.42 and 4.88 fall between the 2.5 and 5th percentile of requirement. The midpoint is 3.75, and the probability of inadequacy is 100 − 3.75 ≈ 96.3 percent, or a risk of 0.96. The appropriate risk of inadequacy is then multiplied by the number of women with intakes in that range. In this case study, only one woman had an intake between 4.42 and 4.87 mg/day, so the number of women with inadequate intake is 0.96 (1 × 0.96). In the next range (4.88 mg/day to 5.46 mg/day, or between the 5th and 10th percentiles) there were three women, with an associated number of women with inadequate intake of 2.79 (3 × 0.93). If this is done for each intake range, the total number of women with inadequate intakes can be determined. In this example, 165 of the 1,000 women have inadequate intakes, for an estimated prevalence of inad-

TABLE 6 Illustration of the Full Probability Approach to Estimate the Prevalence of Dietary Iron Inadequacy in a Group of 1,000 Menstruating Women (Not Using Oral Contraceptives and Following an Omnivorous Diet)

Percentiles of Requirement Distribution	Range of Usual Intake Associated with Requirement Percentiles (mg/day)	Probability of Inadequacy	Number of Women with Intake in Range	Number of Women with Inadequate Intake
< 2.5	< 4.42	1.0	1	1
2.5–5.0	4.42–4.88	0.96	1	0.96
5–10	4.89–5.45	0.93	3	2.79
10–20	5.46–6.22	0.85	10	8.5
20–30	6.23–6.87	0.75	15	11.25
30–40	6.88–7.46	0.65	20	13
40–50	7.47–8.07	0.55	23	12.65
50–60	8.08–8.76	0.45	27	12.15
60–70	8.77–9.63	0.35	50	17.5
70–80	9.64–10.82	0.25	150	37.5
80–90	10.83–13.05	0.15	200	30.0
90–95	13.06–15.49	0.08	175	14
95–97.5	15.50–18.23	0.04	125	5
> 97.5	> 18.23	0.0	200	0
Total			1,000	165

equacy of 16.5 percent. It is important to remember that this approach does not identify the specific women with inadequate intakes, but is rather a statistical calculation of the prevalence of inadequate intakes. Thus, it cannot be used to screen individuals at risk of inadequacy.

Note that the prevalence of nutrient inadequacy that is estimated by the full probability approach differs considerably from that estimated by the cut-point method (the proportion with intakes below the EAR). In this example, the EAR (median requirement) is 8.07 mg/day, and only 73 women have intakes below this amount. Thus, the cut-point method would lead to an estimated prevalence of inadequacy of 7.3 percent, which differs considerably from the estimate of 16.5 percent obtained by using the full probability approach. The reason for the discrepancy is that one of the conditions needed for the cut-point approach (a symmetrical requirement distribution) is not true for iron requirements of menstruating women.

Case Study Three: Using the EAR Cut-Point Method

The EAR cut-point method is illustrated in Figure 10, which shows a hypothetical joint distribution of usual intakes and individual requirements for a group of 60 individuals. This example is hypothetical because in practice we almost never have access to accurate data on either usual intakes of individuals or their individual requirements. Figure 10 includes a 45° dashed line labeled "Intake = Requirement." Individuals who fall to the right of and below this line have usual intakes that exceed their individual requirements (i.e., they have adequate intakes), whereas individuals who fall to the left of and above the line have usual intakes that do not meet their requirements (i.e., they have inadequate intakes). Determining the prevalence of inadequacy in this hypothetical situation is easy: one simply counts the number of individuals with usual intakes below their individual requirements. In this example, 13 individuals have intakes to the left of and above the "Intake = Requirement" line, so the group prevalence of inadequacy is 13/60, or 21.7 percent.

Figure 10 also shows the EAR (in this example, it is 4 mg/day) on both the requirement axis (the Y axis) and the usual intake axis (X axis). Focusing on the X axis, note that most individuals with usual intakes below the EAR have inadequate intakes (they are to the left of and above the "Intake = Requirement" line), but that some (who appear in the triangle labeled 1) have usual intakes that exceed their individual requirements. Similarly, although most individuals with usual intakes above the EAR meet their requirements (they are to the right of and below the "Intake = Requirement" line), some (who appear in the triangle labeled 2) do not.

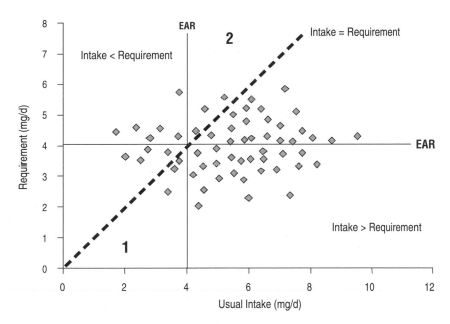

FIGURE 10 Joint distribution of requirements and usual intakes. Individuals with usual intakes below their individual requirements are found to the left of and above the dashed 45° line labeled Intake = Requirement. When assumptions for the EAR cut-point method are satisfied, this proportion of the group is mathematically similar to the proportion to the left of the vertical EAR line.

The assumptions required for use of the EAR cut-point method are satisfied in this example, as described below:

1. Requirement distribution is approximately symmetrical. In Figure 10, it can be seen that similar proportions of the group have requirements above and below the EAR of 4 mg/day (the number of individuals above the horizontal EAR line is similar to the number of individuals below).
2. Intakes and requirements are independent. Figure 10 shows that individuals with low requirements are just as likely as individuals with high requirements to have high (or low) usual intakes.
3. The usual intake distribution is more variable than the requirement distribution. In Figure 10, it can be seen that there is more variability in the intake distribution (it ranges from less than 2 mg/day to almost 10 mg/day) than in the requirement distribution (which ranges from about 2 mg/day to about 6 mg/day).

When the above conditions are met, the individuals in triangle 1 (with intakes below the EAR but above their own requirements) are similar in number to the individuals in triangle 2 (with intakes above the EAR and below their own requirements). These two triangles cancel one another out, and the number of individuals that do not meet their requirements (those found to the left of the 45° "Intake = Requirement" line) is thus mathematically similar to the number with usual intakes below the EAR.

The EAR cut-point method can also be applied to the example of 650 men described in the first case study, as the requirement distribution is symmetrical, intakes and requirements are independent, and the usual intake distribution is more variable than the requirement distribution. In this case, one would simply determine the number of men with intakes at or below the EAR of 7 mg/day. From Table 5, this would be 10 (2 mg/day) + 10 (3 mg/day) + 20 (4 mg/day) + 20 (5 mg/day) + 30 (6 mg/day) + 50 (7 mg/day), for a total of 140 men. Dividing this by the total group size of 650 yields the estimated prevalence of inadequacy of 21.5 percent, which is very similar to the estimate of 20 percent obtained using the full probability method.

In summary, the full probability method and a shortcut, known as the EAR cut-point method, can be used to estimate the prevalence of nutrient inadequacy in a group. Both methods require knowledge of the distribution of usual intakes for the group, and that intakes and requirements are independent. The EAR cut-point method has two additional requirements; namely, that the requirement distribution is symmetrical, and that the distribution of usual intakes is more variable than the distribution of requirements. If either of these two additional requirements is not met, the full probability method can be used instead, provided the requirement distribution is known.

Case Study Four: Planning Diets in an Assisted-Living Facility for Senior Citizens

An example of planning diets for institutionalized groups is menu planning for senior citizens who reside in an assisted-living facility. Menus planned for these institutions usually assume that the residents have no other sources of foods or nutrients, and thus the menus are designed to meet all nutrient needs of the residents. The goal of menu planning is to provide meals that provide adequate nutrients for a high proportion of the residents, or conversely, the prevalence of inadequate intakes is acceptably low among the residents.

The planner is developing a menu for an assisted living facility in which the residents are retired nuns aged 70 years and above. For this age group, the EAR for vitamin B_6 is 1.3 mg/day. Assume that no data can be located on the distribution of usual intakes of this group or a similar group, and that resources are not available to conduct a dietary survey in the institution. How could the planner proceed to determine the target intake distribution of vitamin B_6 needed to attain an acceptable prevalence of inadequacy?

STEP 1. DETERMINE AN ACCEPTABLY LOW PREVALENCE OF INADEQUACY

For vitamin B_6, the EAR was set at a level adequate to maintain plasma pyridoxal phosphate levels at 20 nmol/L. This plasma level is not accompanied by observable health risks, and thus allows a moderate safety margin to protect against the development of signs or symptoms of deficiency. This cut-off level was selected recognizing that its use may overestimate the B_6 requirement for health maintenance of more than half the group. For this reason, assume that the planner has determined that a 10 percent prevalence of inadequacy (i.e., 10 percent with intakes below the EAR) would be an acceptable planning goal.

STEP 2. DETERMINE THE TARGET USUAL NUTRIENT INTAKE DISTRIBUTION

Next, the planner needs to position the intake distribution so the nutrient intake goals are met. In this example, the planner decides that the prevalence of inadequacy in the group will be set at 10 percent, and as a result the usual intake distribution of the group should be positioned such that only 10 percent of the group has usual intakes less than the EAR.

Because data on the usual nutrient intake distributions of the residents are not available, other sources must be used to estimate the target usual nutrient intake distribution. Data on the distribution of usual dietary intakes of vitamin B_6 are available from several national surveys and thus are used. The adjusted percentiles for women are summarized in Table 7.

Assuming there are no changes in the shape of the distribution, the amount of the shift can be calculated as the additional amount of the nutrient that must be consumed to reduce the proportion of the group that is below the EAR. This is accomplished by determining the difference between the EAR and the intake at the acceptable prevalence of inadequacy (in this case, the 10th percentile of the usual intake distribution).

TABLE 7 Selected Percentiles of the Distributions of Usual Intake of Vitamin B_6 from Foods in Older Women

Study	n	\multicolumn{7}{c}{Percentile of Usual Intake Distribution of Vitamin B_6 (mg/day)}
		5th	10th	25th	50th	75th	90th	95th
Survey A	1,368	0.92	1.04	1.24	1.53	1.93	2.43	2.76
Survey B	221	0.76	0.88	1.11	1.41	1.76	2.12	2.35
Survey C	281	0.5	0.6	0.7	1.0	1.3	1.6	1.8

TABLE 8 Identification of the Target Median Intake^a of Vitamin B$_6$ to Obtain a 10 Percent Prevalence of Inadequacy in Older Women

Study	EAR (mg/day)	Intake at 10th Percentile (mg/day)	Difference (EAR – intake at 10th percentile)	Median Intake (mg/day)	Target Median Intake (mg/day)
Survey A	1.3	0.88	0.42	1.41	1.83
Survey B	1.3	1.04	0.26	1.53	1.79
Survey C	1.3	0.6	0.7	1.0	1.70

^{a} The target median intake is estimated by adding the difference between the Estimated Average Requirement (EAR) and the intake at the acceptable prevalence of inadequacy (in this case, 10 percent) to the observed median intake.

Examination of the data from the three surveys shows that estimated usual intakes of vitamin B$_6$ vary by as much as 30 percent among the surveys. As a result, the difference between the EAR of 1.3 mg and the intake at the 10th percentile varies, depending on which data are used. Table 8 shows that for Survey A the difference is 0.26 mg (1.3 mg – 1.04 mg = 0.26 mg); for Survey B, the difference is 0.42 mg (1.3 mg – 0.88 mg = 0.42 mg); and for Survey C, the difference is 0.7 mg (1.3 mg – 0.6 mg = 0.7 mg). In this example, the planner may have no reason to choose data from one particular survey as "more applicable" to the group than another, so he may estimate target usual nutrient intake distributions using all three data sets. Accordingly, the target intake distributions shift up by 0.26 mg, by 0.42 mg, and by 0.7 mg. using Survey A, B, or C. In each case the target usual nutrient intake distribution would lead to the accepted prevalence of inadequacy. Rather than choosing one set of survey data over another, the planner could simply average the summary measures described in the next section.

STEP 3. SELECT A SUMMARY MEASURE OF THE TARGET USUAL NUTRIENT INTAKE DISTRIBUTION TO USE IN PLANNING

After the planner has estimated a target usual intake distribution, then this information needs to be operationalized into a menu. In order to do this, the planner will first have to select a summary measure of the target usual nutrient intake distribution to use as a tool in planning the menu. The median of the target intake distribution is the most useful; it can be calculated as the median of the current intake distribution, plus (or minus) the amount that the distribution needs to shift to make it the target usual intake distribution.

In the current example, although the baseline intakes at the 10th percentile and the median differ among the three surveys, the estimates of the medians of the target usual intake distributions are quite similar, as shown in Table 8. Assuming that a 10 percent prevalence of intakes below the EAR was considered acceptable, a median intake for vitamin B_6 of 1.7 to 1.8 mg/day would be the planning goal. Accordingly, the menu would need to be planned so that vitamin B_6 intakes would be at this level.

Estimates of target nutrient intakes must be converted to estimates of foods to purchase, offer, and serve that will result in the usual intake distributions meeting the intake goals. This is not an easy task. Meals with an average nutrient content equal to the median of the target usual nutrient intake distribution may not meet the planning goals, as individuals in a group tend to consume less than what is offered and served to them. Thus, the planner might aim for a menu that offers a choice of meals with a nutrient content range that includes, or even exceeds, the median of the target usual nutrient intake distribution.

Step 4. Assess Implementation of the Plan

Ideally, after the menu had been planned and implemented, a survey would be conducted to assess intakes and determine whether the planning goal had been attained. This would then be used as the basis for further planning.

KEY POINTS FOR WORKING WITH GROUPS

Assessing Nutrient Intakes

✓ The goal of assessing nutrient intakes of groups is to determine the prevalence of inadequate (or excessive) nutrient intakes within a particular group of individuals.

✓ Assessment of groups should always be performed using intakes that have been adjusted to represent a usual intake distribution.

✓ The probability approach and the EAR cut-point method are two statistical methods of determining the prevalence of inadequacy in a group. The EAR cut-point method is a simpler method derived from the probability approach.

✓ For nutrients in which it is appropriate to do so, the EAR can be used as part of the EAR cut-point method to determine the prevalence of nutrient inadequacy within a group. Otherwise, the probability approach can be used.

✓ The AI has limited application in assessing a group's nutrient intakes. For nutrients with an appropriately estimated AI, groups with mean or median intakes at or above the AI can generally be assumed to have a low prevalence of inadequate intakes.

✓ The UL can be used to estimate the proportion of a group at potential risk of adverse effects from excessive nutrient intakes.

✓ The RDA should not be used in the assessment of a group's nutrient intakes. Comparing mean or median intake with the RDA is inappropriate.

✓ To assess the energy adequacy of an individual or group diet, information other than self-reported intakes should be used because underreporting of energy intake is a serious and pervasive problem. Body weight for height, BMI, or other anthropometric measures are suitable for use in assessing long-term energy intake.

PLANNING NUTRIENT INTAKES

✓ The goal of planning nutrient intakes for groups is to achieve usual intakes that meet the requirements of most individuals, but that are not excessive.

✓ The DRIs present an approach to planning that involves consideration of the entire distribution of usual nutrient intakes within a group.

✓ The basic steps in planning for groups are as follows: First the practitioner decides on an acceptable prevalence of inadequacy. The distribution of usual intakes in the group must then be estimated using the distribution of reported or observed intakes. Finally, a target usual intake distribution is determined by positioning the distribution of usual intakes relative to the EAR to achieve the desired prevalence of inadequacy.

✓ For nutrients with an EAR, the planning goal is to aim for an acceptably low prevalence of intakes below the EAR.

✓ The RDA is not recommended for use when planning nutrient intakes of groups.

✓ For nutrients with an AI, this value is used as the target for the mean or median intake when planning for groups.

✓ For nutrients with a UL, the planning goal is to achieve an acceptably low prevalence of intakes above the UL.

✓ When planning a group's energy intake, the goal is for the group's mean intake to equal the EER.

SUMMARY

The DRI values can be used by nutrition professionals to assess and plan the nutrient intakes of individuals and of groups. Table 9 summarizes the chapter discussions on the appropriate uses of each of the DRI values to achieve these goals.

TABLE 9 Using the DRIs to Assess and Plan the Nutrient Intakes of Individuals and Groups

	EAR	RDA	AI	UL
When Assessing Diets				
For individuals:	Usual intake below the EAR likely needs to be improved. The probability of adequacy is 50 percent or less.	Not recommended for use when assessing nutrient intakes of individuals.	Usual intake at or above the AI has a low probability of inadequacy.	Usual intake above the UL may place an individual at risk of adverse effects.
For groups:	Used as part of the EAR cut-point method to determine the prevalence of nutrient inadequacy within a group.	Not used when assessing nutrient intakes of groups.	Limited application. Groups with mean or median intakes at or above the AI can generally be assumed to have a low prevalence of inadequate intakes.	Used to estimate the proportion of a group at potential risk of adverse effects from excessive nutrient intake.
When Planning Diets				
For individuals:	Intake at EAR has 50 percent probability of not meeting requirement.	Low probability of inadequate intake at RDA. Therefore, often used as a guide.	Intakes at AI will likely meet or exceed an individual's requirement.	Low probability of adverse effects from excessive consumption so average intake should not exceed the UL.
For groups:	Aim for an acceptably low prevalence of intakes below the EAR.	Not used when planning the nutrient intakes of groups.	Use as a target for the mean or median intake.	Aim for an acceptably low prevalence of intakes above the UL.

PART II
ENERGY, MACRONUTRIENTS,
WATER, AND
PHYSICAL ACTIVITY

Part II of this publication takes information from the DRI reports titled *Dietary Reference Intakes for Energy, Carbohydrate, Fiber, Fat, Fatty Acids, Cholesterol, Protein, and Amino Acids* (2002/2005) and *Dietary Reference Intakes for Water, Potassium, Sodium, Chloride, and Sulfate* (2005) and presents nutrient reference values for carbohydrates, fiber, fatty acids, protein, amino acids, and water, as well as recommendations for energy, fat, cholesterol, and physical activity.

"Macronutrients, Healthful Diets, and Physical Activity" begins with a review of the available data regarding the relationships of carbohydrates, fiber, fat, fatty acids, cholesterol, protein, and amino acids, collectively known as macronutrients, and physical activity and energy to major chronic diseases. It will introduce the term Acceptable Macronutrient Distribution Range (AMDR), which is a range of intake for a particular energy source that is associated with reduced risk of chronic disease. AMDRs are set for fat, carbohydrate, protein, and *n*-6 and *n*-3 polyunsaturated fatty acids.

"Energy" introduces the term Estimated Energy Requirement (EER), which is defined as the average dietary energy intake that is predicted to maintain energy balance in a healthy individual of a defined age, gender, height, weight, and level of physical activity consistent with good health. "Physical Activity" provides recommendations for levels of physical activity associated with a normal body mass index and reduced risk of chronic disease. The remaining chapters discuss data on carbohydrates (sugars and starches), fiber, fats and fatty acids, cholesterol, protein and amino acids, and water. In these chapters, AIs are provided for *Total Fiber*, linoleic acid and α-linolenic acid, and water, and EARs and RDAs are provided for carbohydrate, and protein. No ULs were set for any of the macronutrients or for water.

TABLE 1 Acceptable Macronutrient Distribution Ranges

Macronutrient	AMDR (as percent of energy)[a]		
	Children 1–3 y	Children 4–18 y	Adults
Fat	30–40	25–35	20–35
n-6 polyunsaturated fatty acids[b] (linoleic acid)	5–10	5–10	5–10
n-3 polyunsaturated fatty acids[b] (α-linolenic acid)	0.6–1.2	0.6–1.2	0.6–1.2
Carbohydrate	45–65	45–65	45–65
Protein	5–20	10–30	10–35

Additional Macronutrient Recommendations

Macronutrient	Recommendation
Dietary cholesterol	As low as possible while consuming a nutritionally adequate diet
Trans fatty acids	As low as possible while consuming a nutritionally adequate diet
Saturated fatty acids	As low as possible while consuming a nutritionally adequate diet
Added sugars	Limit to a maximal intake of no more than 25 percent total energy[c]

[a] **AMDR** = Acceptable Macronutrient Distribution Range. This is the percent of energy intake that is associated with reduced risk of chronic disease, yet provides adequate amounts of essential nutrients.

[b] Approximately 10 percent of the total can come from longer-chain *n*-3 or *n*-6 fatty acids.

[c] Not a recommended intake. A daily intake of added sugars that individuals should aim for to achieve a healthful diet was not set.

MACRONUTRIENTS, HEALTHFUL DIETS, AND PHYSICAL ACTIVITY

U nlike vitamins and minerals, fats, carbohydrates, and proteins can substitute for one another to some extent in order to meet the body's energy needs. Thus, for a certain level of energy intake, increasing the
proportion of one macronutrient necessitates decreasing the proportion of one
or both of the other macronutrients. Acceptable ranges of intake for each of
these energy sources were set based on a growing body of evidence that has
shown that macronutrients play a role in the risk of chronic disease.

These ranges, termed Acceptable Macronutrient Distribution Ranges
(AMDRs), are defined as a range of intake for a particular energy source that is
associated with reduced risk of chronic diseases (e.g., coronary heart disease
[CHD], obesity, diabetes, and/or cancer) while providing adequate intakes of
essential nutrients. These ranges are also based on adequate energy intake and
physical activity to maintain energy balance. The AMDR of a macronutrient is
expressed as a percentage of total energy intake because its requirement, in a
classical sense, is not independent of other energy fuel sources or of the total
energy requirement of the individual. Each must be expressed in terms relative
to the other. A key feature of each AMDR is that it has a lower and upper
boundary. If an individual consumes below or above this range, there is a potential for increasing risk of chronic diseases shown to affect long-term health,
as well as increasing the risk of insufficient intakes of essential nutrients.

For example, with regard to carbohydrate and fat, studies have shown a
connection between low-fat and, therefore, high-carbohydrate diets and decreased high density lipoprotein (HDL) cholesterol in the bloodstream, an indicator associated with increased risk of CHD. Conversely, diets too high in fat
may result in increased energy and saturated fat intake, and therefore lead to
increased risk of obesity and its complications, such as CHD.

In this chapter, AMDRs for carbohydrate, fat, fatty acids (n-6 and n-3 polyunsaturated), and protein are discussed. Recommendations for cholesterol,
trans fatty acids, saturated fatty acids, and added sugars are also provided (see
Table 1).

Finally, the chapter reviews the available data regarding the relationships between major chronic diseases that have been linked with consumption of dietary macronutrients (carbohydrate, fiber, fat, fatty acids, cholesterol, protein, and amino acids) and physical activity.

ACCEPTABLE MACRONUTRIENT DISTRIBUTION RANGES (AMDRs)

Many causal relationships among over- or underconsumption of macronutrients, physical inactivity, and chronic disease have been proposed. When the diet is modified for one energy-yielding nutrient, it invariably changes the intake of other nutrients, which makes it extremely difficult to have adequate substantiating evidence for providing clear and specific nutritional guidance.

However, based on the evidence to suggest a role in chronic disease, as well as information to ensure sufficient intakes of other essential nutrients, Acceptable Macronutrient Distribution Ranges (AMDRs) have been established. An AMDR is defined as a range of intakes for a particular energy source that is associated with reduced risk of chronic disease while providing adequate intakes of essential nutrients. The AMDR of a macronutrient is expressed as a percentage of total energy intake because its requirement is not independent of other energy fuel sources or of the total energy requirement of the individual.

A key feature of each AMDR is that it has a lower and upper boundary. Intakes that fall above or below this range appear to increase the risk of chronic disease and may result in the inadequate consumption of essential nutrients. AMDRs have been set for carbohydrate, protein, fat, and *n*-6 and *n*-3 polyunsaturated fatty acids based on evidence from intervention trials, with support of epidemiological evidence. Recommendations have been made for limiting cholesterol, *trans* fatty acids, saturated fatty acids, and added sugars (see Table 1).

An AMDR was not set for fiber or monounsaturated fatty acids. An AMDR was not set for fiber because it is an insignificant contributor to total energy intake; no known adverse effects associated with its consumption were available. Monounsaturated fatty acids are not essential in the diet, and the evidence relating low and high intakes of monounsaturated fatty acids to chronic disease is limited. Practical limits on intakes of monounsaturated fatty acids will be imposed by AMDRs for total fat and other types of fatty acids.

Total Fat and Carbohydrate

Basis for Adult AMDRs for Total Fat and Carbohydrate

These AMDRs were estimated based on evidence indicating a risk for coronary heart disease (CHD) with diets high in carbohydrate and low in fat and on evidence for increased risk for obesity and its complications (including CHD) at high intakes of fat.

Intakes of low-fat, high-carbohydrate diets, compared with higher fat intakes, can induce a lipoprotein pattern called the atherogenic lipoprotein phenotype (characterized by high triglycerides, low HDL cholesterol, and small low density lipoprotein [LDL] cholesterol particles), which is associated with high risk of CHD, particularly in sedentary people who tend to be overweight. On the other hand, when fat intake is high, many individuals consume additional energy, and therefore gain additional weight. Weight gain on high-fat diets can be detrimental to individuals already susceptible to obesity and can worsen the metabolic consequences of obesity, particularly the risk of CHD. Moreover, high-fat diets are usually accompanied by increased intakes of saturated fatty acids, which can raise LDL cholesterol levels, further increasing risk of CHD. Diets containing energy from fat and carbohydrate in the recommended ranges minimize the risks of diabetes, obesity, and CHD. In addition, these ranges allow adequate consumption of essential nutrients and moderate saturated fat intake. Diets containing less than the minimum AMDR for carbohydrate are highly unlikely to meet the AI for fiber.

Basis for AMDRs for Children for Total Fat and Carbohydrate

The AMDR for carbohydrate for children is the same as for adults. Children have a higher fat oxidation rate than adults, and low-fat diets can lead to reduced intake of certain micronutrients, including fat-soluble vitamins. Conversely, high-fat intakes during childhood may set the stage for CHD and obesity, although the evidence for this is tenuous.

Because the evidence is less clear on whether low- or high-fat intakes during childhood can lead to increased risk of chronic diseases later in life, the estimated AMDRs for children are primarily based on a transition from high-fat intakes during infancy to the lower adult AMDR. During childhood, the amount of saturated fat in the diet should be as low as possible without compromising nutritional adequacy.

Protein

Basis for AMDR for Children and Adults

There is no evidence suggesting that the AMDR for protein should be at levels below the adult Recommended Dietary Allowance (RDA) for protein (see Part II, "Protein"), which is about 10 percent of energy for adults. In addition, there were insufficient data to suggest a UL for protein (see Part II, "Protein") and insufficient data to suggest an upper range or boundary for an AMDR for protein. All of the AMDRs were set, in part, to complement the AMDRs for fat and carbohydrate.

n-6 Polyunsaturated Fatty Acids

BASIS FOR AMDR FOR CHILDREN AND ADULTS

Based on usual median intakes of energy reported in the U.S. Continuing Survey of Food Intakes by Individuals (CSFII 1994–1996, 1998), it is estimated that a lower boundary level of 5 percent of energy from linoleic acid would be needed to meet the Adequate Intake (AI) (see Part II, "Dietary Fat: Total Fat and Fatty Acids"). The upper boundary for linoleic acid of 10 percent of energy intake is based on the following information:

- In North America, individual dietary intakes rarely exceed 10 percent of energy from linoleic acid.
- Epidemiological evidence for the safety of intakes greater than 10 percent of energy are generally lacking.
- High intakes of linoleic acid create a pro-oxidant state that may predispose to several chronic diseases, such as CHD and cancer. Human studies demonstrate that enrichment of lipoproteins and cell membranes with *n*-6 polyunsaturated fatty acids contributes to a pro-oxidant state.

n-3 Polyunsaturated Fatty Acids

BASIS FOR AMDR FOR CHILDREN AND ADULTS

Based on usual median intakes of energy report in CSFII (1994–1996, 1998), it is estimated that a lower boundary level of 0.6 percent of energy from α-linolenic acid would be needed to meet the AI (see Part II, "Dietary Fat: Total Fat and Fatty Acids"). The upper boundary corresponds to the highest α-linolenic acid intakes from foods consumed by individuals in the United States and Canada. Data supporting the benefit of even higher intakes of α-linolenic acid were not considered strong enough to warrant an upper boundary greater than 1.2 percent of energy.

A growing body of evidence suggests that higher intakes of α-linolenic acid, eicosapentaenoic acid (EPA), and docosahexaenoic acid (DHA) may afford some degree of protection against CHD. However, it is impossible to estimate an AMDR for all *n*-3 fatty acids because the physiological potency of EPA and DHA is much greater than that of α-linolenic acid. Up to 10 percent of the AMDR for *n*-3 fatty acids can be consumed as EPA and/or DHA.

ADDITIONAL MACRONUTRIENT RECOMMENDATIONS

Saturated Fatty Acids, *Trans* Fatty Acids, and Cholesterol

BASIS FOR RECOMMENDATIONS

There are no known risks of chronic disease associated with consuming diets very low in saturated fatty acids, *trans* fatty acids, or cholesterol. Since certain micronutrients are found mainly in animal foods (which are typically high in saturated fats and cholesterol), it is possible that diets low in saturated fat and cholesterol may contain low levels of micronutrients, such as iron and zinc. Furthermore, analysis of nutritionally adequate menus indicates that there is a minimum amount of saturated fat that can be consumed so that adequate levels of linoleic and α-linolenic acids are provided.

A substantial body of evidence suggests that saturated fatty acids, *trans* fatty acids, and cholesterol raise blood total and LDL cholesterol levels, which in turn increases risk of CHD. Because there is a positive linear trend between intake of each of these fats and risk of CHD, even very low intakes of each may increase risk. It is thus recommended that intakes of saturated fatty acids, *trans* fatty acids, and cholesterol remain as low as possible while a nutritionally adequate diet is consumed.

Added Sugars

BASIS FOR RECOMMENDATIONS

It has been shown the increasing intakes of added sugars can result in decreased intakes of certain micronutrients in United States subpopulations. This can occur because of the abundance of added sugars in energy-dense, nutrient-poor foods in a diet. As such, it is suggested that adults and children consume no more than 25 percent of energy from added sugars to ensure sufficient consumption of essential micronutrients. Note that a daily intake of added sugars that individuals should aim for to achieve a healthy diet was not set. Foods containing added sugars and few micronutrients include soft drinks, fruit drinks, cakes, cookies, and candies.

The impact of total sugar intake on the intake of micronutrients does not appear to be as great as for added sugars. Total sugars include both the added sugars and the naturally occurring sugars found in fruits, milk, and dairy products.

TABLE 2 Relationship of Macronutrients and Physical Activity to Chronic Disease

	Energy	Fat	Protein
Cancer	• Animal studies suggest that energy restriction may inhibit cell proliferation and tumor growth. • Increased childhood energy intakes have been associated with increased cancer mortality. • Excess energy contributes to obesity, which may increase risk of certain cancers.	• High fat intakes have been implicated in development of certain cancers, although evidence is mixed. • Epidemiological studies have shown an inverse relationship between fish consumption and risk of breast and colorectal cancer, possibly due to protective effects of *n*-3 fatty acids.	• No clear role for total protein has yet emerged.
Heart Disease	• Excess energy contributes to obesity, which increases risk of heart disease.	• Increased saturated fat intake can increase total and LDL blood cholesterol levels. • Increasing intakes of *trans* fatty acids and cholesterol increase total and LDL blood cholesterol levels, although there is wide interindividual variation in serum cholesterol response to dietary cholesterol. • Monounsaturated and polyunsaturated fatty acids decrease total and LDL blood cholesterol levels. • High intakes of *n*-6 and *n*-3 polyunsaturated fats are associated with decreased risk of heart disease.	• Independent effects of protein on heart disease mortality have not been shown. • Soy-based protein may reduce blood cholesterol, but the evidence is mixed.

Carbohydrate	Fiber	Physical Activity
• Several case-control studies have shown increased risk of colorectal cancer in people with high intakes of sugar-rich foods. • High vegetable and fruit intake and avoidance of foods with highly refined sugars have been negatively correlated to risk of colon cancer.	• High fiber diets may protect against colorectal cancer, though the evidence is conflicting. • Fiber may protect against hormone-related cancers including prostate, endometrial, and ovarian cancer. • Certain cereal foods may protect against some types and stages of breast cancer.	• Regular exercise has been negatively correlated with risk of colon cancer. • Numerous epidemiological studies suggest that regular physical activity decreases risk of breast cancer. • Exercise may help compensate for potential cancer-promoting effects of excess energy intake. • Exercise may bolster the immune system.
• High carbohydrate (low fat) intakes tend to increase plasma triacylglycerol and decrease plasma HDL cholesterol levels. These effects are more extreme if the source is monosaccharides, especially fructose.	• Dietary fiber, particularly naturally occurring viscous fiber, reduces total and LDL cholesterol levels. • Reduced rates of heart disease have been observed in individuals consuming high fiber diets. • Dietary fiber intake has been shown to be negatively associated with hypertension in men.	• Numerous studies have shown an inverse relationship between exercise and heart disease mortality. • Regular exercise increases HDL cholesterol; decreases triacylglycerol, blood pressure, and risk of cardiac arrhythmias; enhances fibrinolysis, glucose effectiveness, and insulin sensitivity; and lessens platelet adherence.

continued

TABLE 2 Continued

	Energy	Fat	Protein
Dental Caries			
Type II Diabetes Mellitus	• Excess energy contributes to obesity, which may increase risk of Type II diabetes. • Obesity, particularly abdominal obesity, is a risk factor for Type II diabetes.	• Some studies show a correlation between high fat intakes and insulin resistance, but it is not clear whether the association is due to fat or to obesity.	
Obesity	• Excess energy intake causes obesity.	• Available data on whether diets high in total fat increase the risk for obesity are conflicting; this may be partly due to underreporting of food intake, notably fat intake.	• Available data on whether diets high in protein are associated with obesity are mixed: some have shown a positive association with protein intake and body fatness, others have demonstrated weight loss.
Bone Health			• The relationship between protein intake and bone health is very controversial with some studies showing bone loss and osteoporosis in relationship to high intakes and others showing no association in the presence of adequate calcium intakes.

Carbohydrate	Fiber	Physical Activity
• Sugars play a role in development of dental caries (as do fluoride, oral hygiene and frequency of food intake).		
• While there is little evidence that total carbohydrate is associated with Type II diabetes, there may be increased risk when the glycemic index of a meal, rather than total carbohydrate, is considered.	• Viscous soluble fibers may attenuate the insulin response and thus protect against Type II diabetes.	• Increased physical activity levels improve insulin sensitivity in people with Type II diabetes. • Physical activity can reduce risk of Type II diabetes and can reduce total and abdominal obesity, which are risk factors for Type II diabetes.
• Published reports have produced conflicting results about the existence of a direct link between high sugar intakes and obesity; this may be partly due to underreporting of food intake.	• Intervention studies suggest that high fiber diets may assist in weight loss, although evidence overall is mixed.	• Physical inactivity is a major risk factor for development of obesity.
		• Physical activity increases bone mass in children and adolescents and maintains bone mass in adults. • Physical activity enhances muscle strength, coordination, and flexibility, which may prevent falls and fractures in elderly adults.

RELATIONSHIP TO CHRONIC DISEASE

During the past 40 years, a growing body of evidence has accumulated regarding the risk of chronic disease and consumption of energy and the macronutrients, specifically dietary fats, carbohydrate, protein, and fiber. Because most diets are composed of a variety of foods that provide varying amounts of macronutrients, research to determine causal relationships is somewhat limited. Research linking chronic diseases with dietary macronutrients and physical activity is summarized in Table 2.

KEY POINTS FOR MACRONUTRIENTS, HEALTHFUL DIETS, AND PHYSICAL ACTIVITY

✓ Fats, carbohydrates, and proteins can substitute for one another to some extent to meet the body's energy needs.

✓ Acceptable Macronutrient Distribution Ranges (AMDRs) were set for some macronutrients based on evidence that consumption above or below these ranges may be associated with nutrient inadequacy and increased risk of developing chronic diseases, including coronary heart disease, obesity, diabetes, and/or cancer.

✓ An AMDR is defined as a range of intakes for a particular energy source that is associated with reduced risk of chronic disease while providing adequate intakes of essential nutrients.

✓ The AMDR for a macronutrient is expressed as a percentage of total energy intake because its requirement is not independent of other energy fuel sources or of the total energy requirement of the individual.

✓ To meet the body's daily nutritional needs while minimizing risk for chronic disease, adults should consume 45–65 percent of their total calories from carbohydrates, 20–35 percent from fat, and 10–35 percent from protein. The acceptable ranges for children are similar to those for adults, except that infants and younger children need a somewhat higher proportion of fat in their diets.

✓ These ranges may be more useful and flexible for dietary planning than single values recommended in the past.

✓ AMDRs were not set for fiber or monounsaturated fatty acids.

✓ Over- and underconsumption of macronutrients as well as physical inactivity and energy imbalance have been linked to major chronic diseases such as cancer, obesity, coronary heart disease, dental caries, and Type II diabetes, and to skeletal health.

TABLE 1 Equations to Estimate Energy Requirement

Infants and Young Children

Estimated Energy Requirement (kcal/day) = Total Energy Expenditure + Energy Deposition

0–3 months	EER^a = (89 × weight [kg] −100) + 175
4–6 months	EER = (89 × weight [kg] −100) + 56
7–12 months	EER = (89 × weight [kg] −100) + 22
13–35 months	EER = (89 × weight [kg] −100) + 20

Children and Adolescents 3–18 years

Estimated Energy Requirement (kcal/day) = Total Energy Expenditure + Energy Deposition

Boys

3–8 years	EER = 88.5 – (61.9 × age [y]) + PA^b × [(26.7 × weight [kg]) + (903 × height [m])] + 20
9–18 years	EER = 88.5 – (61.9 × age [y]) + PA × [(26.7 × weight [kg]) + (903 × height [m])] + 25

Girls

3–8 years	EER = 135.3 – (30.8 × age [y]) + PA × [(10.0 × weight [kg]) + (934 × height [m])] + 20
9–18 years	EER = 135.3 – (30.8 × age [y]) + PA × [(10.0 × weight [kg]) + (934 × height [m])] + 25

Adults 19 years and older

Estimated Energy Requirement (kcal/day) = Total Energy Expenditure

Men	EER = 662 – (9.53 × age [y]) + PA × [(15.91 × weight [kg]) + (539.6 × height [m])]
Women	EER = 354 – (6.91 × age [y]) + PA × [(9.36 × weight [kg]) + (726 × height [m])]

Pregnancy

Estimated Energy Requirement (kcal/day) = Nonpregnant EER + Pregnancy Energy Deposition

1st trimester	EER = Nonpregnant EER + 0
2nd trimester	EER = Nonpregnant EER + 340
3rd trimester	EER = Nonpregnant EER + 452

Lactation

Estimated Energy Requirement (kcal/day) = Nonpregnant EER + Milk Energy Output – Weight Loss

0–6 months postpartum	EER = Nonpregnant EER + 500 – 170
7–12 months postpartum	EER = Nonpregnant EER + 400 – 0

NOTE: These equations provide an estimate of energy requirement. Relative body weight (i.e., loss, stable, gain) is the preferred indicator of energy adequacy.

^{a} **EER** = Estimated Energy Requirement.

^{b} **PA** = Physical Activity Coefficient (see Table 2).

ENERGY

Energy is required to sustain the body's various functions, including respiration, circulation, physical work, metabolism, and protein synthesis. This energy is supplied by carbohydrates, proteins, fats, and alcohol in the diet. A person's energy balance depends on his or her dietary energy intake and energy expenditure. Numerous factors affect energy expenditure and requirements, including age, body composition, gender, and physical activity level. An imbalance between energy intake and expenditure results in the gain or loss of body components, mainly in the form of fat, and determines changes in body weight.

The Estimated Energy Requirement (EER) is defined as the average dietary energy intake that is predicted to maintain energy balance in a healthy adult of a defined age, gender, weight, height, and a level of physical activity that is consistent with good health. A person's body weight is a readily monitored indicator of the adequacy or inadequacy of habitual energy intake.

To calculate the EER, prediction equations for normal-weight individuals (body mass index [BMI] of 18.5 kg/m^2 up to 25 kg/m^2) were developed using data on total daily energy expenditure as measured by the doubly labeled water (DLW) technique. Equations can be found in Table 1. In children and in pregnant and lactating women, the EER accounts for the needs associated with growth, deposition of tissues, and the secretion of milk at rates that are consistent with good health. The EER does not represent the exact dietary energy intake needed to maintain energy balance for a specific individual; instead it reflects the average needs for those with specified characteristics.

Although EERs can be estimated for four levels of activity from the equations provided in Table 2, the active Physical Activity Level (PAL) is recommended to maintain health. Thus, energy requirements are defined as the amounts of energy that need to be consumed by an individual to sustain a stable body weight in the range desired for good health (BMI of 18.5 kg/m^2 up to 25 kg/m^2), while maintaining a lifestyle that includes adequate levels of physical activity.

There is no Recommended Dietary Allowance (RDA) for energy because energy intakes above the EER would be expected to result in weight gain. Similarly, the Tolerable Upper Intake Level (UL) concept does not apply to energy because any intake above a person's energy requirement would lead to weight gain and likely increased risk of morbidity.

TABLE 2 Physical Activity Coefficients (PA Values) for Use in EER Equations

	Sedentary (PAL[a] 1.0–1.39)	Low Active (PAL 1.4–1.59)	Active (PAL 1.6–1.89)	Very Active (PAL 1.9–2.5)
	Typical daily living activities (e.g., household tasks, walking to the bus)	Typical daily living activities PLUS 30–60 minutes of daily moderate activity (e.g., walking at 5–7 km/h)	Typical daily living activities PLUS at least 60 minutes of daily moderate activity	Typical daily living activities PLUS at least 60 minutes of daily moderate activity PLUS an additional 60 minutes of vigorous activity or 120 minutes of moderate activity
Boys 3–18 y	1.00	1.13	1.26	1.42
Girls 3–18 y	1.00	1.16	1.31	1.56
Men 19 y +	1.00	1.11	1.25	1.48
Women 19 y +	1.00	1.12	1.27	1.45

[a] PAL = Physical Activity Level.

When energy intake is lower than energy needs, the body adapts by reducing voluntary physical activity, reducing growth rates (in children), and mobilizing energy reserves, primarily adipose tissue, which in turn leads to weight loss. In adults, an abnormally low BMI is associated with decreased work capacity and limited voluntary physical activity.

When energy intake is higher than energy needs, weight gain occurs and consequently chronic disease risk increases, including risk of Type II diabetes, hypertension, coronary heart disease (CHD), stroke, gallbladder disease, osteoarthritis, and some types of cancer.

ENERGY AND THE BODY

Function

Energy is required to sustain the body's various functions, including respiration, circulation, metabolism, physical work, and protein synthesis.

Background Information

Energy in foods is released in the body through the oxidation of various organic substances, primarily carbohydrates, fats, and amino acids, yielding the chemical energy required to sustain metabolism, nerve transmission, respiration, circulation, physical work, and other bodily functions. The heat produced during oxidation is used to maintain body temperature.

Carbohydrate, fat, protein, and alcohol provide all of the energy supplied by foods and are generally referred to as macronutrients (in contrast to vitamins and elements, which are referred to as micronutrients). The amount of energy released by the oxidation of macronutrients is shown in Table 3.

ENERGY VERSUS NUTRIENTS

For many nutrients, a Recommended Dietary Allowance (RDA) is calculated by adding two standard deviations (SD) to the median amounts that are sufficient to meet a specific criterion of adequacy in order to meet the needs of nearly all healthy individuals (see Part I, "Introduction to the Dietary Reference Intakes"). However, this is not the case with energy because excess energy cannot be eliminated and is eventually deposited in the form of body fat. This reserve provides a means to maintain metabolism during periods of limited food intake, but it can also result in obesity. Therefore, it seems logical to base estimated energy intake on the amounts of energy that need to be consumed to maintain energy balance in adults who maintain desirable body weights, also taking into account the increments in energy expenditure elicited by their habitual level of activity.

There is another fundamental difference between the requirements for energy and those for nutrients. A person's body weight is a readily monitored indicator of the adequacy or inadequacy of habitual energy intake. A compara-

TABLE 3 Energy Provided by Macronutrients

Macronutrient	Kcal/g[a]
Carbohydrate	4
Fat	9
Protein	4
Alcohol[b]	7

[a] These values for carbohydrate, fat, protein, and alcohol are known as Atwater Factors. Atwater, a pioneer in the study of nutrients and metabolism, proposed the use of these values. They are often used in nutrient labeling and diet formulation.

[b] The alcohol (ethanol) content of beverages is usually described in terms of percent by volume. One mL of alcohol weighs 0.789 g and provides 5.6 kcal/mL.

bly obvious and individualized indicator of inadequate or excessive intake is not usually evident for other nutrients.

Body Mass Index

Body mass index, or BMI, is defined as weight in kilograms divided by the square of height in meters. A growing body of literature supports the use of BMI as a predictor of the impact of body weight on morbidity and mortality risks. The National Institutes of Health (NIH) and the World Health Organization (WHO) have defined BMI cutoffs for adults over 19 years of age, regardless of age and gender: underweight is defined as a BMI of less than 18.5 kg/m², overweight as a BMI from 25 up to 30 kg/m², and obese as a BMI of 30 kg/m² or higher. A healthy or desirable BMI is considered to be from 18.5 kg/m² up to 25 kg/m². This range of BMI is used in deriving the equations for estimating the energy requirement.

Components of Energy Expenditure

Basal and resting metabolism: The basal metabolic rate (BMR) reflects the energy needed to sustain the metabolic activities of cells and tissues, plus the energy needed to maintain blood circulation, respiration, and gastrointestinal and renal function while awake, in a fasting state, and resting comfortably (i.e., the basal cost of living). BMR includes the energy expenditure associated with remaining awake, reflecting the fact that the sleeping metabolic rate (SMR) during the morning is some 5–10 percent lower than BMR during the morning hours.

BMR is commonly extrapolated to 24 hours and is then called basal energy expenditure (BEE), expressed as kcal per 24 hours. Resting metabolic rate (RMR) reflects energy expenditure under resting conditions and tends to be somewhat higher (10–20 percent) than under basal conditions, due to the increases in energy expenditure caused by recent food intake (i.e., by the thermic effect of food) or by the delayed effect of recently completed physical activity.

Basal, resting, and sleeping energy expenditures are related to body size, being most closely correlated with the size of fat-free mass (FFM), which is the weight of the body less the weight of its fat mass. The size of the FFM generally explains 70–80 percent of the variance in RMR among individuals. However, RMR is also affected by age, gender, nutritional state, inherited variations, and differences in the endocrine state.

Thermic effect of food: The thermic effect of food (TEF) refers to the increased energy expenditure caused by food consumption, including its digestion, transport, metabolization, and storage. The intensity and duration of meal-induced

TEF are primarily determined by the amount and composition of the foods consumed, mainly due to the metabolic costs of handling and storing ingested nutrients. The increments in energy expenditure during digestion above baseline rates, divided by the energy content of the food consumed, vary from 5 to 10 percent for carbohydrate, 0 to 5 percent for fat, and 20 to 30 percent for protein. The high TEF for protein reflects the relatively high metabolic cost involved in processing the amino acids. The TEF for a mixed diet is 10 percent of the food's energy content.

Thermoregulation: This is the process by which mammals regulate their body temperature within narrow limits. Because most people can adjust their clothing and environment to maintain comfort, the additional energy cost of thermoregulation rarely has an appreciable effect on total energy expenditure.

Physical activity: The energy expended for physical activity varies greatly among individuals and from day to day. In sedentary people, about two-thirds of total energy expenditure (TEE) goes to sustain basal metabolism over 24 hours (the BEE), while one-third is used for physical activity. In very active people, 24-hour TEE can rise to twice as much as BEE, while even higher total expenditures can occur among heavy laborers and some athletes.

In addition to the immediate energy cost of individual activities, exercise induces a small increase in energy expenditure that persists for some time after an activity has been completed. The body's excess post-exercise oxygen consumption (EPOC) depends on exercise intensity and duration and has been estimated at some 15 percent of the increment in expenditure that occurs during the activity.

Physical activity level: The ratio of total to basal daily energy expenditure (TEE:BEE) is known as the Physical Activity Level (PAL). PAL categories are defined as sedentary (PAL $\geq 1.0 < 1.4$), low active (PAL $\geq 1.4 < 1.6$), active (PAL $\geq 1.6 < 1.9$), and very active (PAL $\geq 1.9 < 2.5$). In this publication, PAL is used to describe and account for physical activity habits (see Part II, "Physical Activity").

Total energy expenditure: Total energy expenditure (TEE) is the sum of the basal energy expenditure, the thermic effect of food, physical activity, thermoregulation, and the energy expended in depositing new tissues and in producing milk. With the emergence of information on TEE by the doubly labeled water method, it has become possible to determine the energy expenditure of infants, children, and adults in free-living conditions. It refers to energy expended during the oxidation of energy-yielding nutrients to water and carbon dioxide.

DETERMINING DRIS

Estimated Energy Requirement

The Estimated Energy Requirement (EER) is defined as the average dietary energy intake that is predicted to maintain energy balance in a healthy adult of a defined age, gender, weight, height, and a level of physical activity that is consistent with good health. There is no RDA for energy because energy intakes above the EER would be expected to result in weight gain.

To calculate the EER for adults, prediction equations for normal-weight individuals (BMI of 18.5–25 kg/m^2) were developed using data on total daily energy expenditure as measured by the DLW technique (see Table 1). In children and in pregnant or lactating women, the prediction equations for the EER account for the additional needs associated with the deposition of tissues or the secretion of milk at rates that are consistent with good health.

Criteria for Determining Energy Requirements, by Life Stage Group

Life stage group	Criterion
0 through 6 mo	Energy expenditure plus energy deposition
7 through 12 mo	Energy expenditure plus energy deposition
1 through 18 y	Energy expenditure plus energy deposition
> 18 y	Energy expenditure
Pregnancy	
14 through 18 y	Adolescent female EER plus change in TEE plus pregnancy energy deposition
19 through 50 y	Adult female EER plus change in TEE plus pregnancy energy deposition
Lactation	
14 through 18 y	Adolescent female EER plus milk energy output minus weight loss
19 through 50 y	Adult female EER plus milk energy output minus weight loss

Factors That Affect Energy Expenditure and Requirements

Body composition and body size: Although body size and weight exert apparent effects on energy expenditure, it is disputed whether differences in body composition quantitatively affect energy expenditure. It is unlikely that body composition markedly affects energy expenditure at rest or the energy costs of physical activity in adults with BMIs of 18.5–25 kg/m². In adults with higher percentages of body fat, mechanical hindrances can increase the energy expenditure associated with certain activities.

The proportion of fat-free mass (FFM) is the major parameter in determining the rate of energy expenditure under fasting basal metabolic rate (BMR) and resting metabolic rate (RMR) conditions. RMR/kg of weight or RMR/kg of FFM falls as mass increases because the contributions made by the most metabolically active tissues (the brain, liver, and heart) decline as body size increases.

Findings from different studies suggest that low energy expenditure is a risk factor for weight gain in a subgroup of people susceptible to excess weight gain, but not in all susceptible people and not in those with a normal level of risk. These data are consistent with the general view that obesity is a multifactorial problem.

Physical activity: The increased energy expenditure that occurs during physical activity accounts for the largest part of the effect of activity on overall energy expenditure. Physical activity also affects energy expenditure in the post-exercise period, depending on exercise intensity and duration, environmental temperatures, one's state of hydration, and the degree of trauma to the body. This effect lasts for as many as 24 hours following exercise.

Spontaneous non-exercise activity reportedly accounts for 100–700 kcal/day. Sitting without fidgeting or sitting with fidgeting raises energy expenditure by 4 or 54 percent, respectively, compared with lying down. Standing while motionless or standing while fidgeting raises energy expenditure by 13 or 94 percent, respectively.

Gender: There are substantial data on the effects of gender on energy expenditure throughout the lifespan. Gender differences in BMR are due to the greater level of body fat in women and to differences in the relationship between RMR and FFM.

Growth: Energy requirements in infants and children include the energy associated with the deposition of tissues at rates consistent with good health. The energy cost of growth as a percentage of total energy requirements decreases from around 35 percent at age 1 month to 3 percent at age 12 months. It remains low until the adolescent growth spurt, when it then increases to about 4 percent. The timing of the adolescent growth spurt, which typically lasts 2 to 3 years, is also very variable, with the onset typically occurring between ages 10 and 13 years in the majority of children.

Older age: All three major components of energy expenditure (RMR, TEF, and energy expenditure of physical activity [EEPA]), decrease with aging. There is an average 1–2 percent decline per decade in men who maintain constant weight. The suggested breakpoint for a more rapid decline appears to occur at approximately age 40 years in men and age 50 years in women. For women, this may be due to an accelerated loss of FFM during menopause. PAL has been shown to progressively decrease with age and is lower in elderly adults compared to young adults.

Genetics: Individual energy requirements substantially vary due to combinations of differences in body size and composition; differences in RMR independent of body composition; differences in TEF; and differences in physical activity and EEPA. All of these determinants of energy requirement are potentially influenced by genetics, with cultural factors also contributing to variability.

Ethnicity: Data from studies of adults and children indicate that the BMR is usually lower in African Americans than Caucasians. Currently, insufficient data exist to create accurate prediction equations of BMRs for African American adults. In this publication, the general prediction equations in Table 1 are used for all races, recognizing their potential to overestimate BMR in some groups such as African Americans.

Environment: There is a modest 2–5 percent increase in sedentary TEE at low-normal environmental temperatures (20–28°C, or 68–82°F) compared with high-normal temperatures (28–30°C, or 82–86°F). However, in setting energy requirements, no specific allowance was made for environmental temperatures. The TEE values used to predict energy requirements can be considered values that have been averaged for the environmental temperatures of different seasons. High altitude also increases BMR and TEE due to the hypobaric hypoxia. However, it is unclear at which heights the effect becomes prominent.

Adaptation and accommodation: Adaptation implies the maintenance of essentially unchanged functional capacity in spite of some alteration in a steady-state condition, and it involves changes in body composition that occur over an extended period of time. The term adaptation describes the normal physiological responses of humans to different environmental conditions. An example of adaptation is the increase in hemoglobin concentration that occurs when individuals live at high altitudes.

Accommodation refers to relatively short-term adjustments that are made to maintain adequate functional capacity under altered steady-state conditions. The term accommodation characterizes an adaptive response that allows survival but results in some consequences on health or physiological function. The most common example of accommodation is a decrease in growth velocity in children. By reducing growth rate, children's bodies are able to save energy and may subsist for prolonged periods of time on marginal energy intakes, although this could be at the cost of eventually becoming stunted. The estimation of energy requirements from energy expenditure implicitly assumes that the efficiency of energy use is more or less uniform across all individuals, an assumption that is supported by experimental data.

The UL

The Tolerable Upper Intake Level (UL) is the highest daily nutrient intake that is likely to pose no risk of adverse effects for almost all people. The UL concept does not apply to energy because intake above an individual's energy requirements would lead to weight gain and likely increased risk of morbidity.

EFFECTS OF UNDERNUTRITION

Undernutrition is still a common health concern in many parts of the world, particularly in children. When energy intake does not match energy needs due to insufficient dietary intake, excessive intestinal losses, or a combination thereof, several mechanisms of adaptation come into play. A reduction in voluntary physical activity is a rapid means to reduce energy output. In children, a reduction in growth rate is another mechanism to reduce energy needs. However, if this condition persists in children, low growth weight results in short stature and low weight-for-age, a condition known as stunting. A chronic energy deficit elicits the mobilization of energy reserves, primarily adipose tissue, which leads to changes in body weight and body composition over time.

In children, the effects of chronic undernutrition include decreased school performance, delayed bone age, and an increased susceptibility to infections. In adults, an abnormally low BMI is associated with decreased work capacity and limited voluntary physical activity.

ADVERSE EFFECTS OF OVERCONSUMPTION

Two major adverse effects result from the overconsumption of energy:

- *Adaptation to high levels of energy intake*: When people are given a diet providing a fixed, but limited, amount of excess energy, they initially gain weight. However, over a period of several weeks, their energy expenditure will increase, mostly because of their increased body size. As such, their body weight will eventually stabilize at a higher weight level.

Reducing energy intake will produce the opposite effect. For most individuals, it is likely that the main mechanism for maintaining body weight is controlling food intake rather than adjusting physical activity.

- *Increased risk of chronic disease*: A BMI of ≥ 25 kg/m^2 is associated with an increased risk of premature mortality. In addition, as BMI increases beyond 25 kg/m^2, morbidity risk increases for Type II diabetes, hypertension, coronary heart disease (CHD), stroke, gallbladder disease, osteoarthritis, and some types of cancer. Because some studies suggest that disease risk begins to rise at lower BMI levels, some investigators have recommended aiming for a BMI of 22 kg/m^2 at the end of adolescence. This level would allow for some weight gain in mid-life without surpassing the 25 kg/m^2 threshold.

For the above reasons, energy intakes associated with adverse risks are defined as those that cause weight gain in individuals with body weights that fall within the healthy range (BMI of 18.5–25 kg/m^2) and overweight individuals (BMI of 25–30 kg/m^2). In the case of obese individuals who need to lose weight to improve their health, energy intakes that cause adverse risks are those that are higher than intakes needed to lose weight without causing negative health consequences.

KEY POINTS FOR ENERGY

✓   Energy is required to sustain the body's various functions, including respiration, circulation, metabolism, physical work, and protein synthesis.

✓   A person's energy balance depends on his or her dietary energy intake and total energy expenditure, which includes the basal energy expenditure, the thermic effect of food, physical activity, thermoregulation, and the energy expended in depositing new tissues and in producing milk.

✓   Imbalances between energy intake and expenditure result in the gain or loss of body components, mainly in the form of fat. These gains or losses determine changes in body weight.

✓   The EER is the average dietary energy intake that is predicted to maintain energy balance in a healthy adult of a defined age, gender, weight, height, and a level of physical activity that is consistent with good health.

✓   In children and in pregnant and lactating women, the EER accounts for the needs associated with growth, deposition of tissues, and the secretion of milk at rates that are consistent with good health.

✓ A person's body weight is a readily monitored indicator of the adequacy or inadequacy of habitual energy intake.

✓ Numerous factors affect energy expenditure and requirements, including age, body composition, gender, and ethnicity.

✓ There is no RDA for energy because energy intakes above the EER would be expected to result in weight gain.

✓ The UL concept does not apply to energy because any intake above a person's energy requirements would lead to undesirable weight gain.

✓ When energy intake is less than energy needs, the body adapts by mobilizing energy reserves, primarily adipose tissue.

✓ In adults, an abnormally low BMI is associated with decreased work capacity and limited voluntary physical activity.

✓ The overconsumption of energy leads to the adaptation to high levels of energy intake with weight gain and an increased risk of chronic diseases, including Type II diabetes, hypertension, CHD, stroke, gallbladder disease, osteoarthritis, and some types of cancer.

TABLE 1 Physical Activity Recommendations

ADULT

An average of 60 minutes per day of moderately intense physical activity (e.g., brisk walking or jogging at 3–4 mph) or shorter periods of more vigorous exertion (e.g., jogging for 30 minutes at 5.5 mph), in addition to activities identified with a sedentary lifestyle, was associated with a normal BMI range and is the amount of physical activity recommended for normal-weight adults.

CHILDREN

An average of 60 minutes of moderately intense daily activity is also recommended for children.

PHYSICAL ACTIVITY

Physical activity promotes health and vigor, and the lack of it is now a recognized risk factor for several chronic diseases. Observational and experimental studies of humans and animals have provided biologically plausible insights into the benefits of regular physical activity on the delayed progression of several chronic diseases, including cancer, cardiovascular disease, Type II diabetes, obesity, and skeletal conditions. In addition, acute or chronic aerobic exercise may be related to favorable changes in anxiety, depression, stress reactivity, mood, self-esteem, and cognitive functioning.

Cross-sectional data from a doubly labeled water (DLW) database were used to define a recommended level of physical activity based on the physical activity level (PAL) that is associated with a normal body mass index (BMI) of 18.5–25 kg/m². An average of 60 minutes per day of moderately intense physical activity (e.g., brisk walking or jogging at 3–4 mph) or shorter periods of more vigorous exertion (e.g., jogging for 30 minutes at 5.5 mph), in addition to activities identified with a sedentary lifestyle, is the amount of physical activity recommended for normal-weight adults. An average of 60 minutes of moderately intense daily activity is also recommended for children. This amount of physical activity leads to an "active" lifestyle. Because the Dietary Reference Intakes are for the general healthy population, recommended levels of physical activity for weight loss of obese individuals are not provided.

Historically, most individuals have unconsciously balanced their dietary energy intake and total energy expenditure due to occupation-related energy expenditure. However, occupational physical activity has significantly declined over the years. According to the *1996 Surgeon General's Report* on physical activity and health, more than 60 percent of American adults were not regularly physically active and 25 percent were not active at all. This trend in decreased activity by adults is similar to trends seen in children who are less active both in and out of school. Physical activity and fitness objectives of the U.S. government's Healthy People 2010 seek to increase the proportion of Americans who engage in daily physical activity to improve health, fitness, and quality of life. Similar recommendations to increase physical activity have been proposed in Canada.

Excessive physical activity can lead to overuse injuries, dehydration and hyperthermia, hypothermia, cardiac events, and female athlete triad (loss of menses, osteopenia, and premature osteoporosis). To prevent adverse effects, previously sedentary people are advised to use caution when beginning a new activity routine.

DETERMINING RECOMMENDATIONS

Cross-sectional data from a DLW database were used to define a recommended level of physical activity for adults and children, based on the PAL associated with a normal BMI in the healthy range of 18.5 kg/m^2 up to 25 kg/m^2. PAL is the ratio of total energy expenditure (TEE) to basal energy expenditure (BEE). The data PAL categories were defined as sedentary (PAL $\geq 1.0 < 1.4$), low active (PAL $\geq 1.4 < 1.6$), active (PAL $\geq 1.6 < 1.9$), and very active (PAL $\geq 1.9 < 2.5$).

Because an average of 60 minutes per day of moderate-intensity physical activities (or shorter periods of more vigorous exertion) provides a PAL that is associated with a normal BMI range, this is the amount of activity that is recommended for normal-weight individuals. For children, the physical activity recommendation is also an average of 60 minutes of moderate-intensity daily activity. In terms of making a realistic physical activity recommendation for busy individuals to maintain their weight, it is important to recognize that exercise and activity recommendations consider "accumulated" physical activity.

Box 1 provides examples of various physical activities at different intensities. Additional examples of activity, along with instructions for keeping a weekly activity log, can be found in *Dietary Reference Intakes for Energy, Carbohydrate, Fiber, Fat, Fatty Acids, Cholesterol, Protein, and Amino Acids* (2002/2005).

Special Considerations

Pregnant women: For women who have been previously physically active, continuing physical activities during pregnancy and postpartum can be advantageous. However, excessive or improper activity can be injurious to the woman and fetus.

Appropriate physical fitness during pregnancy improves glucose tolerance and insulin action, improves emotional well-being, and helps prevent excessive weight gain. Fitness promotes a faster delivery, and the resumption of physical activity after pregnancy is important for restoring normal body weight. A full description of the benefits and hazards of exercise for the pregnant woman and fetus is beyond the scope of this publication. Women should consult with their physicians on how to safely exercise during pregnancy.

Physical Activity Level and Energy Balance

Increasing or maintaining an active lifestyle provides an important means for individuals to balance their energy intake with their total energy expenditure.

BOX 1 Examples of Various Physical Activities

Mild (ΔPAL/hr: 0.05–0.10)[a]

Billiards
Canoeing (Leisurely)
Dancing (Ballroom)
Golf (with Cart)
Horseback Riding (Walking)
Loading/Unloading Car
Playing
Taking out Trash
Walking (2 mph)
Walking the Dog
Watering Plants

Moderate (ΔPAL/hr: 0.13–0.22)

Calisthenics (No Weight)
Cycling (Leisurely)
Gardening (No Lifting)
Golf (without Cart)
Household Tasks, Moderate Effort
Mopping
Mowing Lawn (Power Mower)
Raking Lawn
Swimming (Slow)
Vacuuming
Walking (3–4 mph)

Vigorous (ΔPAL/hr: 0.23–0.63)

Chopping Wood
Climbing Hills (No Load up to 5-kg Load)
Cycling (Moderately)
Dancing (Aerobic, Ballet, Ballroom, Fast)
Jogging (10-Minute Miles)
Rope Skipping
Surfing
Swimming
Tennis

[a] ΔPAL/hr is the increase in PAL caused by the activity.

Changing one's usual activity level can have a major impact on total energy expenditure and energy balance. The ultimate indicator of this energy balance is body weight, as seen through its maintenance or change.

Energy intake and the energy expenditure of physical activity are controllable variables that impact energy balance, in contrast to other uncontrollable variables that include age, height, and gender. During exercise, energy expenditure can increase far beyond resting rates, and the increased energy expenditure induced by a workout can persist for hours, if not a day or longer. Furthermore, exercise does not necessarily boost appetite or intake in direct proportion to activity-related changes in energy expenditure.

HEALTHFUL EFFECTS OF PHYSICAL ACTIVITY

Observational and experimental studies of humans and animals provide biologically plausible insights into the benefits of regular physical activity on the delayed progression of several chronic diseases, including cancer, cardiovascular disease, Type II diabetes, obesity, and skeletal conditions. In addition, acute or chronic aerobic exercise may be related to favorable changes in anxiety, depression, stress reactivity, mood, self-esteem, and cognitive functioning.

It is difficult to determine a quantifiable recommendation for physical activity based on reduced risk of chronic disease. However, meeting the physical activity recommendation of 60 minutes per day offers additional benefits in reducing the risk of chronic disease; for example, by favorably altering blood lipid profiles, changing body composition by decreasing body fat, and increasing muscle mass, or both.

Endurance (Aerobic) Exercise

Traditionally, the types of activities recommended for cardiovascular fitness are those of a prolonged endurance nature, such as bicycling, hiking, jogging, and swimming. Because of the energy demands associated with these prolonged mild to moderate intensity endurance activities, they have the potential to decrease body fat mass and preserve fat-free mass, thus changing body composition.

Resistance Exercise and General Physical Fitness

Although resistance training exercises have not yet been shown to have the same effects as endurance activities on the risks of chronic disease, their effects on muscle strength are an indication to include them in exercise prescriptions, in addition to activities that promote cardiovascular fitness and flexibility. Exercises that strengthen the muscles, bones, and joints stimulate muscular and skeletal development in children, as well as assist in balance and locomotion in the elderly, thereby minimizing the incidence of falls and associated complications of trauma and bed rest.

EXCESSIVE PHYSICAL ACTIVITY

Excessive physical activity can lead to the following adverse effects:

- *Overuse injuries*: Too much or improper physical exercise can cause overuse injuries to muscles, bones, and joints, as well as injuries caused by accidents. In addition, pre-existing conditions can be aggravated by the initiation of a physical activity program. Activity-related injuries are often avoidable but do occur and need to be resolved in the interest of long-term general health and short-term physical fitness.
- *Dehydration and hyperthermia*: Exercise may cause dehydration, which can be aggravated by environmental conditions that increase fluid losses, such as heat, humidity, and lack of wind. People should consume water before, during (if possible), and after exercise.
- *Hypothermia*: Hypothermia can result from water exposure and heat loss during winter sports. Poor choice of clothing during skiing, accidental water immersion due to a capsized boat, weather changes, or physical exhaustion may lead to the inability to generate adequate body heat to maintain core body temperature, which can lead to death, even when temperatures are above freezing.
- *Cardiac events*: Although regular physical activity promotes cardiovascular fitness, heavy physical exertion can trigger the development of arrhythmias or myocardial infarctions or, in some instances, can lead to sudden death.
- *Female athlete triad*: Athletic women who undereat or overtrain can develop a condition, or cluster of conditions, called the "female athlete triad." In this triad, disordered eating and chronic energy deficits can lead to loss of menses, osteopenia, and premature osteoporosis, increasing the risk of hip, spine, and forearm fractures.

Prevention of Adverse Effects

Previously sedentary people are advised to begin a new activity routine with caution. The following people should seek medical evaluation, as well as clinical exercise testing, clearance, and advice prior to starting an exercise program: men over age 40 years, women over age 50 years, people with pre-existing medical conditions, and people with known or suspected risk factors or symptoms of cardiovascular and other chronic diseases (physical inactivity being a risk factor). For those with cardiovascular risk or orthopedic problems, physical activity should be undertaken with professional supervision. For all individuals, easy exercise should be performed regularly before more vigorous activities are conducted.

KEY POINTS FOR PHYSICAL ACTIVITY

✓   Lack of physical activity and obesity are now recognized risk factors for several chronic diseases.

✓   Observational and experimental studies of humans and animals provide biologically plausible insights into the benefits of regular physical activity on the delayed progression of several chronic diseases, including cancer, cardiovascular disease, Type II diabetes, obesity, and skeletal conditions.

✓   Acute or chronic aerobic exercise may be related to favorable changes in anxiety, depression, stress reactivity, mood, self-esteem, and cognitive functioning.

✓   Changing one's usual activity level can have a major impact on total energy expenditure and energy balance.

✓   In addition to activities that characterize a sedentary lifestyle, an average of 60 minutes per day of moderate-intensity physical activities (e.g., brisk walking or jogging at 3–4 mph) or shorter periods of more vigorous exertion (e.g., jogging for 30 minutes at 5.5 mph) is the amount of physical activity recommended for normal-weight adults. For children, the physical activity recommendation is also an average of 60 minutes of moderate-intensity daily activity.

✓   More than 60 percent of American adults are not regularly physically active and 25 percent are not active at all. Similar trends are seen in children.

✓   Excessive physical activity can lead to overuse injuries, dehydration and hyperthermia, hypothermia, cardiac events, and female athlete triad (loss of menses, osteopenia, and premature osteoporosis).

✓   Previously sedentary people are advised to begin a new activity routine with caution to prevent adverse effects.

TABLE 1 Dietary Reference Intakes for Dietary Carbohydrates: Sugars and Starches by Life Stage Group

	DRI values (g/day)		
	EAR[a]	RDA[b]	AI[c]
Life stage group[d]			
0 through 6 mo			60
7 though 12 mo			95
1 through 3 y	100	130	
4 through 8 y	100	130	
9 through 13 y	100	130	
14 through 18 y	100	130	
19 through 30 y	100	130	
31 through 50 y	100	130	
51 through 70 y	100	130	
> 70 y	100	130	
Pregnancy			
All ages	135	175	
Lactation			
All ages	160	210	

[a] **EAR** = Estimated Average Requirement. An EAR is the average daily nutrient intake level estimated to meet the requirements of half of the healthy individuals in a group.

[b] **RDA** = Recommended Dietary Allowance. An RDA is the average daily dietary intake level sufficient to meet the nutrient requirements of nearly all (97–98 percent) healthy individuals in a group.

[c] **AI** = Adequate Intake. If sufficient scientific evidence is not available to establish an EAR, and thus calculate an RDA, an AI is usually developed. For healthy breast-fed infants, the AI is the mean intake. The AI for other life stage and gender groups is believed to cover the needs of all healthy individuals in the group, but a lack of data or uncertainty in the data prevents being able to specify with confidence the percentage of individuals covered by this intake.

[d] All groups except Pregnancy and Lactation represent males and females.

DIETARY CARBOHYDRATES: SUGARS AND STARCHES

T he primary role of carbohydrates (i.e., sugars and starches) is to provide energy to all of the cells in the body. Carbohydrates are divided into several categories: monosaccharides, disaccharides, oligosaccharides, polysaccharides, and sugar alcohols.

The requirements for carbohydrates are based on the average minimum amount of glucose that is utilized by the brain. Evidence was insufficient to set a Tolerable Upper Intake Level (UL) for carbohydrates. However, a maximal intake level of 25 percent or less of total calories from added sugars is suggested. This suggestion is based on trends indicating that people with diets at or above this level of added sugars are more likely to have poorer intakes of important essential nutrients. DRI values are listed by life stage group in Table 1.

Nondiet soft drinks are the leading source of added sugars in U.S. diets, followed by sugars and sweets, sweetened grains, fruit ades, sweetened dairy products, and breakfast cereals and other grains.

Most carbohydrates occur as starches in food. Grains and certain vegetables are major contributors. Other sources include corn, tapioca, flour, cereals, popcorn, pasta, rice, potatoes, and crackers. Fruits and darkly colored vegetables contain little or no starch.

The amount of dietary carbohydrate that confers optimal health in humans is unknown. A significant body of data suggests that more slowly absorbed starchy foods that are less processed, or have been processed in traditional ways, may have health advantages over those that are rapidly digested and absorbed.

CARBOHYDRATE AND THE BODY

Function

The primary role of carbohydrates (i.e., sugars and starches) is to provide energy to the cells in the body. The only cells that have an absolute requirement for glucose are those in the central nervous system (i.e., the brain) and those cells that depend upon anaerobic glycolysis, such as red blood cells. Normally, the brain uses glucose almost exclusively for its energy needs.

Classification of Dietary Carbohydrates

Carbohydrates are classified by their number of sugar units: monosaccharides, such as glucose or fructose, consist of one sugar unit; disaccharides, such as sucrose, lactose, and maltose, consist of two sugar units; oligosaccharides, such as raffinose and stachyose, contain 3 to 10 sugar units and may be produced by the breakdown of polysaccharides; and polysaccharides, such as starch and glycogen, contain more than 10 sugar units and are the storage forms of carbohydrates in plants and animals, respectively. Sugar alcohols, such as sorbitol and mannitol, are alcohol forms of glucose and fructose, respectively.

SUGARS AND ADDED SUGARS

The term "sugars" is traditionally used to describe the monosaccharides and disaccharides. Monosaccharides include glucose, galactose, and fructose. Disaccharides include sucrose, lactose, maltose, and trehalose. Sugars are used to sweeten or preserve foods and to give them certain functional attributes, such as viscosity, texture, body, and browning capacity.

"Added sugars" are defined as sugars and syrups that are added to foods during processing or preparation. They do not include naturally occurring sugars, such as lactose in milk or fructose in fruits. Major food sources of added sugars include soft drinks, cakes, cookies, pies, fruit ades, fruit punch, dairy desserts, and candy. Specifically, added sugars include white sugar, brown sugar, raw sugar, corn syrup, corn-syrup solids, high-fructose corn syrup, malt syrup, maple syrup, pancake syrup, fructose sweetener, liquid fructose, honey, molasses, anhydrous dextrose, and crystal dextrose.

Although added sugars are not chemically different from naturally occurring sugars, many foods and beverages that are major sources of added sugars have lower micronutrient densities compared with foods and beverages that are major sources of naturally occurring sugars.

STARCHES

Starch is a carbohydrate polymer found in grains, legumes, and tubers. It is a polysaccharide composed of less than 1,000 to many thousands of α-linked glucose units and its two forms are amylase and amylopectin. Amylose is the linear form of starch, while amylopectin consists of linear and branched glucose polymers. In general, amylose starches are compact, have low solubility, and are less rapidly digested. Amylopectin starches are more rapidly digested, presumably because of their more open-branched structure.

Absorption, Metabolism, and Storage

The breakdown of starch begins in the mouth, where enzymes act on the linkages of amylase and amylopectin. The digestion of these linkages continues in the intestine, where more enzymes are released, breaking amylase and amylopectin into shorter glucose chains of varying lengths. Specific enzymes that are bound to the intestinal brush border membrane hydrolyze the glucose chains into monosaccharides, which are then absorbed into the bloodstream via active transport or facilitated diffusion mechanisms. Other sugars are also hydrolyzed to monosaccharide units before absorption.

Once absorbed, sugars (glucose, galactose, and fructose) are transported throughout the body to cells as a source of energy. Glucose is the major fuel used by most of the body's cells. Blood glucose concentration is highly regulated by the release of insulin, and the uptake of glucose by adipocytes and muscle cells is dependent on the binding of insulin to a membrane-bound insulin receptor.

Galactose and fructose are taken up by the liver (when blood circulates past it) where they are metabolized. Galactose is mostly converted to glycogen for storage. Fructose is transformed into intermediary metabolites or converted to a precursor for glycogen synthesis. When blood glucose is high and cellular energy demand is low, glucose can be converted to glycogen for storage (in skeletal muscle and liver), a process called glycogenesis. Glycogenesis is activated in the skeletal muscle by a rise in insulin concentration that occurs after the consumption of carbohydrate. It is activated in the liver by an increase in circulating monosaccharide or insulin concentrations.

Glycogen is present in the muscle for storage and utilization and in the liver for storage, export, and the maintenance of blood glucose concentrations. When blood glucose levels become too low, glycogenolysis occurs, which is the release of glucose from glycogen stores in the liver. Following glycogenolysis, the body can export glucose from the liver to maintain normal blood glucose concentrations and be used by other tissues. Muscle glycogen is mainly used in the muscle.

Gluconeogenesis, the production of glucose from a noncarbohydrate source (amino acids or glycerol), can occur during fasting (or in the absence of dietary carbohydrate), thus allowing the liver to continue to release glucose to maintain adequate blood glucose concentrations.

Glycemic Index

A significant body of data suggests that more slowly absorbed starchy foods that are less processed, or have been processed in traditional ways, may have health advantages over those that are rapidly digested and absorbed. The former have been classified as having a low glycemic index (GI) and reduce the diet's glycemic load. GI is a measure of the increase in blood glucose in the two hours after eating a given amount (e.g., 50 g) of a carbohydrate relative to its response to a reference carbohydrate (white bread or glucose). The glycemic load is an indicator of the glucose response or insulin demand that is induced by total carbohydrate intake. Dietary GI and glycemic load have relatively predictable effects on circulating glucose, hemoglobin A_{1c}, insulin, triacylglycerol, high density lipoprotein (HDL) cholesterol, and urinary C-peptide concentrations. As such, it is theoretically plausible to expect a low GI diet to reduce risk of Type II diabetes and cardiovascular disease. However, the sufficient evidence needed to recommend substantial dietary changes based on GI is not available.

DETERMINING DRIS

Determining Requirements

The requirements for carbohydrates are based on the average minimum amount of glucose that is utilized by the brain. Because brain size remains fairly constant after 1 year of age and approximates adult size, the EAR and RDA are identical for all age and gender groups after age 12 months, except pregnant and lactating women. The recommended amount also prevents ketosis, which is a rise in keto acid production in the liver to provide the brain with an alternative fuel in times of low glucose availability.

Criteria for Determining Carbohydrate Requirements, by Life Stage Group

Life stage group	Criterion
0 through 6 mo	Average content of human milk
7 through 12 mo	Average intake from human milk + complementary foods
1 through 18 y	Extrapolation from adult data
> 18 y	Brain glucose utilization
Pregnancy	
14 through 18 y	Adolescent female EAR plus fetal brain glucose utilization
19 through 50 y	Adult female EAR plus fetal brain glucose utilization
Lactation	
14 through 18 y	Adolescent female EAR plus average human milk content of carbohydrate
19 through 50 y	Adult female EAR plus average human milk content of carbohydrate

The AMDR

The AMDR for carbohydrates for both adults and children is 45–65 percent of total calories (see Part II, "Macronutrients, Healthful Diets, and Physical Activity").

The UL

The Tolerable Upper Intake Level (UL) is the highest level of daily nutrient intake that is likely to pose no risk of adverse effects for almost all people. Evidence was insufficient to set a UL for carbohydrates. However, a maximal intake level of 25 percent or less of total energy from added sugars is suggested, based on trends indicating that people with diets at or above this level of added sugars are more likely to have poorer intakes of important essential nutrients.

DIETARY SOURCES

Foods

According to U.S. Department of Agriculture food consumption survey data from 1994 to 1996, nondiet soft drinks were the leading source of added sugars in U.S. diets, accounting for one-third of added sugar intake. This was followed by sugars and sweets (16 percent), sweetened grains (13 percent), fruit ades and drinks (10 percent), sweetened dairy products (9 percent), and breakfast cereals and other grains (10 percent). Together, they account for 90 percent of the added sugars that are consumed in the United States.

Most carbohydrates occur as starches in food. Grains and certain vegetables are major contributors. Grain sources include corn, tapioca, flour, cereals, popcorn, pasta, rice, potatoes, and crackers. Fruits and darkly colored vegetables contain little or no starch.

INADEQUATE INTAKE AND DEFICIENCY

The amount of dietary carbohydrate that confers optimal health in humans is unknown. The ability of humans to endure weeks of starvation after endogenous glycogen supplies are exhausted is indicative of the body's ability to survive without an exogenous supply of glucose. However, adapting to a fat and protein fuel requires considerable metabolic adjustments.

In Western urban societies, one particular concern is the long-term effect of a diet so low in carbohydrate that it induces a chronically increased production of keto acids. Such a diet may lead to bone mineral loss, hypercholesterolemia, increased risk of urolithiasis, and impaired development and function of the central nervous system. It also may adversely affect a person's sense of well-being and fail to provide adequate glycogen stores. The latter is required for hypoglycemic emergencies and for maximal short-term power production by muscles.

ADVERSE EFFECTS OF OVERCONSUMPTION

Data are mixed on potential adverse effects of overconsuming carbohydrate (i.e., sugars and starches), which include dental caries, behavioral changes, cancer, risk of obesity, and risk of hyperlipidemia. For more information on the association between carbohydrates and chronic disease, see Part II, "Macronutrients, Healthful Diets, and Physical Activity."

KEY POINTS FOR DIETARY CARBOHYDRATES: SUGARS AND STARCHES

✓ Carbohydrates (sugars and starches) provide energy to the cells in the body.

✓ The requirements for carbohydrate are based on the average minimum amount of glucose that is utilized by the brain.

✓ Evidence was insufficient to set a UL for carbohydrates.

✓ A maximal intake level of 25 percent or less of total energy from added sugars is suggested, based on trends indicating that people with diets at or above this level of added sugars are more likely to have poorer intakes of important essential nutrients.

✓ Nondiet soft drinks are the leading source of added sugars in U.S. diets, followed by sugars and sweets, sweetened grains, fruit ades, sweetened dairy products, and breakfast cereals and other grains.

✓ Most carbohydrates occur as starches in food. Grains and certain vegetables are major contributors. Grain sources include corn, tapioca, flour, cereals, popcorn, pasta, rice, potatoes, and crackers.

✓ The amount of dietary carbohydrate that confers optimal health in humans is unknown.

✓ Of particular concern is the long-term effect of a diet so low in carbohydrate that it induces a chronically increased production of keto acids. Such a diet may lead to bone mineral loss, hypercholesterolemia, increased risk of urolithiasis, and impaired development and function of the central nervous system.

✓ Data are mixed on potential adverse effects of overconsuming carbohydrate.

TABLE 1 Dietary Reference Intakes for *Total Fiber*[a] by Life Stage Group

	DRI values (g/1,000 kcal) [g/day][b]	
	AI[c]	
	males	females
Life stage group		
0 through 6 mo	ND[d]	ND
7 through 12 mo	ND	ND
1 through 3 y	14 [19]	14 [19]
4 through 8 y	14 [25]	14 [25]
9 through 13 y	14 [31]	14 [26]
14 through 18 y	14 [38]	14 [26]
19 through 30 y	14 [38]	14 [25]
31 through 50 y	14 [38]	14 [25]
51 through 70 y	14 [30]	14 [21]
> 70 y	14 [30]	14 [21]
Pregnancy		
< 18 y		14 [28]
19 through 50 y		14 [28]
Lactation		
< 18 y		14 [29]
19 through 50 y		14 [29]

[a]*Total Fiber* is the combination of *Dietary Fiber*, the edible, nondigestible carbohydrate and lignin components as they exist naturally in plant foods, and *Functional Fiber*, which refers to isolated, extracted, or synthetic fiber that has proven health benefits.

[b] Values in parentheses are example of the total g/day of total fiber calculated from g/1,000 kcal multiplied by the median energy intake (kcal/1,000 kcal/day) from the Continuing Survey of Food Intakes by Individuals (CSFII 1994–1996, 1998).

[c] **AI** = Adequate Intake. If sufficient scientific evidence is not available to establish an Estimated Average Requirement (EAR), and thus calculate a Recommended Dietary Allowance (RDA), an AI is usually developed. For healthy breast-fed infants, the AI is the mean intake. The AI for other life stage and gender groups is believed to cover the needs of all healthy individuals in the group, but a lack of data or uncertainty in the data prevents being able to specify with confidence the percentage of individuals covered by this intake.

[d] **ND** = Not determined.

FIBER

The term *Dietary Fiber* describes the carbohydrates and lignin that are intrinsic and intact in plants and that are not digested and absorbed in the small intestine. *Functional Fiber* consists of isolated or purified carbohydrates that are not digested and absorbed in the small intestine and that confer beneficial physiological effects in humans. *Total Fiber* is the sum of *Dietary Fiber* and *Functional Fiber*. Fibers have different properties that result in different physiological effects, including laxation, attenuation of blood glucose levels, and normalization of serum cholesterol levels.

Since data were inadequate to determine an Estimated Average Requirement (EAR) and thus calculate a Recommended Dietary Allowance (RDA) for *Total Fiber,* an Adequate Intake (AI) was instead developed. The AIs for *Total Fiber* are based on the intake levels that have been observed to protect against coronary heart disease (CHD). The relationship of fiber intake to colon cancer is the subject of ongoing investigation and is currently unresolved. A Tolerable Upper Intake Level (UL) was not set for fiber. DRI values are listed by life stage group in Table 1.

Dietary Fiber is found in most fruits, vegetables, legumes, and grains. *Dietary* and *Functional Fibers* are not essential nutrients; therefore, inadequate intakes do not result in biochemical or clinical symptoms of a deficiency. As part of an overall healthy diet, a high intake of *Dietary Fiber* will not cause adverse effects in healthy people.

DEFINITIONS OF FIBER

Dietary Fiber, Functional Fiber, and Total Fiber

This publication defines *Total Fiber* as the combination of *Dietary Fiber*, the edible, nondigestible carbohydrate and lignin components as they exist naturally in plant foods, and *Functional Fiber*, which refers to isolated, extracted, or synthetic fiber that has proven health benefits. Nondigestible means that the material is not digested and absorbed in the human small intestine (see Box 1 for definitions). Fiber includes viscous forms that may lower serum cholesterol concentrations (e.g., oat bran, beans) and the bulking agents that improve laxation (e.g., wheat bran).

Dietary Fiber in foods is usually a mixture of the polysaccharides that are integral components of plant cell walls or intracellular structures. *Dietary Fiber*

BOX 1 Definitions of Fiber[a]

- *Dietary Fiber* consists of nondigestible carbohydrates and lignin that are intrinsic and intact in plants.
- *Functional Fiber* consists of isolated nondigestible carbohydrates that have beneficial physiological effects in humans.
- *Total Fiber* is the sum of *Dietary Fiber* and *Functional Fiber*.

---

[a] In the United States, dietary fiber is defined for regulatory purposes by a number of analytical methods that are accepted by the Association of Official Analytical Chemists International (AOAC). In Canada, a distinction is made between dietary fiber (defined as the endogenous components of plant material in the diet that are resistant to digestion by enzymes produced by man) and novel fibers, whose definition is similar to *functional fiber*. Novel fibers must be demonstrated to have beneficial effects to be considered as fiber for the purposes of labeling and claims.

---

sources contain other macronutrients (e.g., digestible carbohydrate and protein) normally found in foods. For example, cereal brans, which are obtained by grinding, are anatomical layers of the grain consisting of intact cells and substantial amounts of starch and protein. Other examples include plant nonstarch polysaccharides (e.g., cellulose, pectin, gums, and fibers in oat and wheat bran), plant carbohydrates (e.g., inulin, fructans), lignin, and some resistant starch.

Functional Fiber may be isolated or extracted using chemical, enzymatic, or aqueous steps, such as synthetically manufactured or naturally occurring isolated oligosaccharides and manufactured resistant starch. In order to be classified as a *Functional Fiber*, a substance must demonstrate a beneficial physiological effect. Potential *Functional Fibers* include isolated nondigestible plant (e.g., pectin and gums), animal (e.g., chitin and chitosan), or commercially produced (e.g., resistant starch, polydextrose) carbohydrates.

FIBER AND THE BODY

Function

Different fibers have different properties and thus varying functions. They aid in laxation and promote satiety, which may help reduce energy intake and therefore the risk of obesity. They can also attenuate blood glucose levels, normalize serum cholesterol levels, and reduce the risk of CHD. For example, viscous fibers can interfere with the absorption of dietary fat and cholesterol, as well as the enterohepatic recirculation of cholesterol and bile acids, which may result in reduced blood cholesterol concentrations and a reduced risk of CHD.

Absorption, Metabolism, and Excretion

Once consumed, *Dietary Fiber* and *Functional Fiber* pass relatively intact into the large intestine. Along the gastrointestinal tract, the properties of different fibers result in varying physiological effects:

Gastric emptying and satiety: Viscous fiber delays gastric emptying, thereby slowing the process of absorption in the small intestine. This can cause a feeling of fullness, as well as delayed digestion and absorption of nutrients, including energy. Delayed gastric emptying may also reduce postprandial blood glucose concentrations and potentially have a beneficial effect on insulin sensitivity.

Fermentation: Microflora in the colon can ferment fibers to carbon dioxide, methane, hydrogen, and short-chain fatty acids. Foods rich in hemicellulose and pectin, such as fruits and vegetables, contain *Dietary Fiber* that is more completely fermented than foods rich in celluloses, such as cereals. The consumption of *Dietary* and certain *Functional Fibers*, particularly those that are poorly fermented, is known to improve fecal bulk and laxation and ameliorate constipation.

Contribution of fiber to energy: When fiber is anaerobically fermented by micro-flora of the colon, the short-chain fatty acids that are produced are absorbed as an energy source. Although the exact yield of energy from fiber in humans remains unclear, current data indicate that the yield is between 1.5 and 2.5 kcal/g.

Physiological effects of isolated and synthetic fibers: Table 2 summarizes the beneficial physiological effects of certain isolated and synthetic fibers. Note that the discussion of these potential benefits should not be construed as endorsements of the fibers. For each fiber source listed, evidence relating to one of the three most commonly accepted benefits of fibers is presented: laxation, normalization of blood lipid levels, and attenuation of blood glucose responses.

DETERMINING DRIS

Determining Requirements

There is no biochemical assay that can be used to measure *Dietary Fiber* or *Functional Fiber* nutritional status. Blood fiber levels cannot be measured be-

TABLE 2 The Physiological Effects of Isolated and Synthetic Fibers

	Potential Effect on			
	Laxation	Normalization of Blood Lipid Levels	Attenuation of Blood Glucose Responses	Other Physiological Effects
Cellulose	Increases stool weight; may decrease transit time.	No effect on blood lipid levels or a slight increase in them.	Did not decrease postprandial glucose response.	—
Chitin and Chitosan	There was no evidence for a laxative effect in humans.	Numerous animal studies suggested that chitin and chitosan may decrease lipid absorption. However, this has not always been observed in controlled human studies. More research is needed.	No known reports in humans.	Some animal studies have shown that chitosan reduces fat absorption and may promote weight loss. However, human studies have found no effect of chitosan supplementation on weight.
Guar Gum	Little effect on fecal bulk or laxation.	Numerous studies have shown an 11–16 percent reduction in blood cholesterol levels with guar gum supplementation. In addition, guar gum has been shown to decrease triacylglycerol concentrations and blood pressure.	Viscous fibers, including guar gum, produced significant reductions in glycemic response in 33 of 50 studies.	—

TABLE 2 Continued

		Potential Effect on		
	Laxation	Normalization of Blood Lipid Levels	Attenuation of Blood Glucose Responses	Other Physiological Effects
Inulin, Oligofructose, and Fructooligo-saccharides	A few studies have shown a small increase in fecal bulk and stool frequency with ingestion of inulin or oligofructose.	Studies with inulin or oligofructose have provided mixed results.	Some, but not all, studies suggest that inulin and fructooligo-saccharides reduce fasting insulin concentrations or fasting blood glucose.	Numerous human studies show that the ingestion of fructooligo-saccharides increases fecal *Bifidbacteria*. This bacteria strain has been shown to have beneficial health effects in animals, but the potential benefits to humans are not well understood.
Oat Products and β-Glucans	Extracted β-glucans have minimal effects on fecal bulk. Oat bran increases stool weight by supplying rapidly fermented viscous fiber to the colon for bacterial growth.	In a large study of adults with multiple risk factors for heart disease, including high LDL cholesterol levels, oat cereal consumption was linked to a dose-dependent reduction in LDL cholesterol. Other research also suggests that oat products help lower LDL cholesterol.	Some research suggests that oat bran reduces postprandial rises in blood glucose levels.	—

continued

TABLE 2 Continued

	Potential Effect on			
	Laxation	Normalization of Blood Lipid Levels	Attenuation of Blood Glucose Responses	Other Physiological Effects
Pectin	A meta-analysis of about 100 studies showed that pectin is not an important fecal-bulking agent.	Pectin has been shown to lower cholesterol to varying degrees. There was some evidence that this effect was due to increased excretion of bile acids and cholesterol.	Viscous fibers, including pectin, have significantly reduced glycemic response in 33 of 50 studies.	—
Polydextrose	Polydextrose was shown to increase fecal mass and sometimes stool frequency. Findings on the effect of polydextrose on fecal bacterial production are mixed.	In one study, polydextrose lowered HDL (high density lipoprotein) cholesterol levels.	—	—
Psyllium	There is extensive literature on the laxative effect of psyllium, which is the active ingredient in some over the counter laxatives.	A number of studies have shown that psyllium lowers total and LDL cholesterol levels via the stimulation of bile acid production.	When added to a meal, psyllium has been shown to decrease the rise of postprandial glucose levels and to reduce the glycemic index of foods.	—

TABLE 2 Continued

	Potential Effect on			
	Laxation	Normalization of Blood Lipid Levels	Attenuation of Blood Glucose Responses	Other Physiological Effects
Resistant Dextrins	No evidence to support a laxative effect.	One study showed that resistant maltodextrin helps reduce blood cholesterol and triacylglycerol levels.	One animal study and two human studies suggest that resistant maltodextrins reduce fasting and postprandial blood glucose levels.	—
Resistant Starch	Increased fecal bulk due to increased starch intake has been reported. Because resistant starch is partly fermented in the colon, intake may lead to an increased production of short-chain fatty acids.	Several animal studies have shown that resistant starch lowers blood cholesterol and triacylglycerol levels. In humans, resistant starch does not appear to provide the cholesterol-lowering effects of viscous fiber, but rather acts more like nonviscous fiber.	In one study, adding resistant starch to bread at various levels was shown to reduce the glycemic index in a dose-dependent manner.	—

cause fiber is not absorbed. Therefore, the potential health benefits of fiber consumption have been considered in determining DRIs.

Since information was insufficient to determine an EAR and thus calculate an RDA, an AI was instead developed. The AIs for *Total Fiber* are based on the intake level observed to protect against CHD based on epidemiological, clinical, and mechanistic data. The reduction of risk of diabetes can be used as a secondary endpoint to support the recommended intake level. The relationship of fiber intake to colon cancer is the subject of ongoing investigation and is currently unresolved. Recommended intakes of *Total Fiber* may also help ameliorate constipation and diverticular disease, provide fuel for colonic cells, reduce blood glucose and lipid levels, and provide a source of nutrient-rich, low energy-dense foods that could contribute to satiety, although these benefits were not used as the basis for the AI.

There is no AI for fiber for healthy infants aged 0 to 6 months who are fed human milk because human milk does not contain *Dietary Fiber*. During the 7- to 12-month age period, solid food intake becomes more significant, and so *Dietary Fiber* intake may increase. However, there are no data on *Dietary Fiber* intake in this age group and no theoretical reason to establish an AI. There is also no information to indicate that fiber intake as a function of energy intake differs during the life cycle.

Criteria for Determining Fiber Requirements, by Life Stage Group

Life stage group	Criterion
0 through 6 mo	ND[a]
7 through 12 mo	ND
1 through 70 y	Intake level shown to provide the greatest protection against coronary heart disease (14 g/1,000 kcal) × median energy intake level from CSFII (1994-1996, 1998) (kcal/1,000 kcal/day)
Pregnancy and Lactation	Intake level shown to provide the greatest protection against coronary heart disease (14 g/1,000 kcal) × median energy intake level from CSFII (1994–1996, 1998) (kcal/1,000 kcal/day)

[a] Not determined.

The UL

The Tolerable Upper Intake Level (UL) is the highest daily nutrient intake that is likely to pose no risk of adverse effects for almost all people. Although occasional adverse gastrointestinal symptoms are observed when consuming some of the isolated or synthetic fibers, serious chronic adverse effects have not been observed. A UL was not set for *Dietary Fiber* or *Functional Fiber*. Due to the bulky nature of fibers, excess consumption is likely to be self-limited.

DIETARY SOURCES

Dietary Fiber is found in most fruits, vegetables, legumes, and grains. Nuts, legumes, and high-fiber grains typically contain fiber concentrations of more than 3 percent *Dietary Fiber*, or greater than 3 g/100 g of fresh weight. *Dietary Fiber* is present in the majority of fruits, vegetables, refined grains, and miscellaneous foods such as ketchup, olives, and soups, at concentrations of 1 to 3 percent or 1 g/100 g to 3 g/100 g of fresh weight.

Dietary Supplements

This information was not provided at the time the DRI values for fiber were set.

Bioavailability

Fiber is not absorbed by the body.

Dietary Interactions

Foods or diets that are rich in fiber may alter mineral metabolism, especially when phytate is present. Most studies that assess the effect of fiber intake on mineral status have looked at calcium, magnesium, iron, or zinc (see Table 3).

INADEQUATE INTAKE AND DEFICIENCY

Dietary and *Functional Fibers* are not essential nutrients, so inadequate intakes do not result in biochemical or clinical symptoms of a deficiency. A lack of these fibers in the diet, however, can cause inadequate fecal bulk and may detract from optimal health in a variety of ways depending on other factors, such as the rest of the diet and the stage of the life cycle.

TABLE 3 Potential Interactions of Dietary Fiber with Other Dietary Substances

Substance	Potential Interaction	Notes
FIBER AFFECTING OTHER SUBSTANCES		
Calcium	Decreased calcium absorption when ingested with *Dietary Fiber*	Some types of fiber have been shown to significantly increase fecal excretion of calcium. However, most human studies have reported no effect.
Magnesium	Decreased magnesium absorption when ingested with *Dietary Fiber*	Studies report no effect on magnesium balance or absorption.
Iron	Reduced iron absorption when ingested with *Dietary Fiber*	In one study, the addition of 12 g/day of bran to a meal decreased iron absorption by 51–74 percent, which was not explained by the presence of phytate. Other studies suggest that the effect of bran on iron absorption is due to phytate content rather than fiber.
Zinc	Reduced zinc absorption when ingested with *Dietary Fiber*	Most studies also include levels of phytate that are high enough to affect zinc absorption. Metabolic balance studies in adult males consuming 4 oat bran muffins daily show no changes in zinc balance.

ADVERSE EFFECTS OF CONSUMPTION

Although occasional adverse gastrointestinal symptoms were observed with the consumption of *Dietary* and *Functional Fibers*, serious chronic adverse effects have not been observed. The most potentially deleterious effects may arise from the interaction of fiber with other nutrients in the gastrointestinal tract. Additionally, the composition of *Dietary Fiber* varies, making it difficult to link a specific fiber with a particular adverse effect, especially when phytate is also present. It has been concluded that as part of an overall healthy diet, a high intake of *Dietary Fiber* will not cause adverse effects in healthy people. In addition, the bulky nature of fiber tends to make excess consumption self-limiting.

KEY POINTS FOR FIBER

✓ A new set of definitions for fiber has been developed for *Dietary Fiber, Functional Fiber,* and *Total Fiber*. The term *Dietary Fiber* describes the nondigestible carbohydrates and lignin that are intrinsic and intact in plants. *Functional Fiber* consists of the isolated nondigestible carbohydrates that have beneficial physiological effects in humans. *Total Fiber* is the sum of *Dietary Fiber* and *Functional Fiber*. Nondigestible means not digested and absorbed in the human small intestine.

✓ There is no biochemical assay that reflects *Dietary Fiber* or *Functional Fiber* nutritional status. Blood fiber levels cannot be measured because fiber is not absorbed.

✓ Since data were inadequate to determine an EAR and thus calculate an RDA for *Total Fiber*, an AI was instead developed.

✓ The AI for fiber is based on the median fiber intake level observed to achieve the lowest risk of CHD.

✓ A UL was not set for *Dietary Fiber* or *Functional Fiber*.

✓ *Dietary Fiber* is found in most fruits, vegetables, legumes, and grains.

✓ *Dietary* and *Functional Fibers* are not essential nutrients, therefore inadequate intakes do not result in biochemical or clinical symptoms of a deficiency.

✓ As part of an overall healthy diet, a high intake of *Dietary Fiber* will not cause adverse effects in healthy people.

TABLE 1 Dietary Reference Intakes for Dietary Fat: Total Fat and Fatty Acids by Life Stage Group

	DRI Values (g/day)		
	Total Fat/AI[a]	Linoleic Acid/AI	α-Linolenic Acid/AI
Life stage group			
Males and Female			
0 through 6 mo	31	4.4	0.5
7 through 12 mo	30	4.6	0.5
1 through 3 y	ND[b]	7	0.7
4 through 8 y	ND	10	0.9
Males			
9 through 13 y	ND	12	1.2
14 through 18 y	ND	16	1.6
19 through 30 y	ND	17	1.6
31 through 50 y	ND	17	1.6
51 through 70 y	ND	14	1.6
> 70 y	ND	14	1.6
Females			
9 through 13 y	ND	10	1.0
14 through 18 y	ND	11	1.1
19 through 30 y	ND	12	1.1
31 through 50 y	ND	12	1.1
51 through 70 y	ND	11	1.1
> 70 y	ND	11	1.1
Pregnancy			
All ages	ND	13	1.4
Lactation			
All ages	ND	13	1.3

[a] **AI** = Adequate Intake. If sufficient scientific evidence is not available to establish an EAR, and thus calculate an RDA, an AI is usually developed. For healthy breast-fed infants, the AI is the mean intake. The AI for other life stage and gender groups is believed to cover the needs of all healthy individuals in the group, but a lack of data or uncertainty in the data prevents being able to specify with confidence the percentage of individuals covered by this intake.

[b] **ND** = Not determined.

DIETARY FAT: TOTAL FAT AND FATTY ACIDS

A major source of energy for the body, fat also aids in the absorption of fat-soluble vitamins A, D, E, K, and other food components, such as carotenoids. Dietary fat consists mainly (98 percent) of triacylglycerol (which is made up of one glycerol molecule esterified with three fatty acid molecules) and small amounts of phospholipids and sterols. In this publication, total fat refers to all forms of triacylglycerol, regardless of fatty acid composition.

Neither an Estimated Average Requirement (EAR), and thus a Recommended Dietary Allowance (RDA), nor an Adequate Intake (AI) was set for total fat for individuals aged 1 year and older because data were insufficient to determine a defined intake level at which risk of inadequacy or prevention of chronic disease occurs. However, AIs were set for infants aged 0 through 12 months based on observed mean fat intake of infants who were principally fed human milk. Since there is no defined intake level of fat at which an adverse effect occurs, a Tolerable Upper Intake Level (UL) was not set for total fat. An Acceptable Macronutrient Distribution Range (AMDR) has been estimated for total fat at 20–35 percent of energy for adults and children ages 4 and older and 30–40 percent for children ages 1 through 3. Main food sources of total fat are butter, margarine, vegetable oils, visible fat on meat and poultry products, whole milk, egg yolk, nuts, and baked goods, such as cookies, doughnuts, pastries and cakes and various fried foods.

Fatty acids are the major constituents of triglycerides and fall into the following categories: saturated fatty acids, *cis* monounsaturated fatty acids, *cis* polyunsaturated fatty acids (*n*-6 fatty acids and *n*-3 fatty acids), and *trans* fatty acids.

Saturated fatty acids can be synthesized by the body, where they perform structural and metabolic functions. Neither an EAR (and thus an RDA) nor an AI was set for saturated fatty acids because they are not essential (meaning that they can be synthesized by the body) and have no known role in preventing chronic disease.

There is a positive linear trend between saturated fatty acid intake and total and low density lipoprotein (LDL) cholesterol levels and an increased risk of coronary heart disease (CHD). However, a UL was not set for saturated fatty acids because any incremental increase in intake increases the risk of CHD. It is recommended that individuals maintain their saturated fatty acid consumption as low as possible, while consuming a nutritionally adequate diet. Food sources of saturated fatty acids tend to be animal-based foods, including whole milk, cream, butter, cheese, and fatty meats. Coconut oil, palm oil, and palm kernel oil are also high in saturated fatty acids.

Monounsaturated fatty acids (*n*-9) can be synthesized by the body and confer no known independent health benefits. Neither an EAR (and thus an RDA) nor an AI was set. Evidence was insufficient to set a UL for *cis* monounsaturated fatty acids. Foods high in monounsaturated fatty acids include canola oil, olive oil, high-oleic sunflower oil, high-oleic safflower oil, and animal products, primarily meat fat. Animal products provide about 50 percent of dietary monounsaturated fatty acids.

Cis polyunsaturated acids include the *n*-6 fatty acids and *n*-3 fatty acids. The parent acid of the *n*-6 fatty acid series is linoleic acid, the only *n*-6 fatty acid that is an essential fatty acid (EFA), meaning that it cannot be made by the body and must be obtained through the diet. Linoleic acid acts as a precursor for arachidonic acid, which in turn serves as the precursor for eicosanoids (e.g., prostaglandins, thromboxanes, and leukotrienes). Alpha-linolenic (α-linolenic) acid, the parent acid of the *n*-3 fatty acid series is the only *n*-3 fatty acid that is an essential fatty acid meaning that it cannot be made by the body and must be obtained through the diet. The *n*-3 fatty acids play an important role as a structural membrane lipid, particularly in the nerve tissue and retina. The *n*-3 fatty acids also compete with the *n*-6 fatty acids for enzymes responsible for the production of the long-chain *n*-3 fatty acids and thereby influence the balance of *n*-3 and *n*-6 fatty acid-derived eicosanoids.

The AIs for linoleic acid are based on the median intake of linoleic acid by different life stage and gender groups in the United States, where the presence of *n*-6 polyunsaturated fatty acid deficiency is nonexistent in healthy individuals. Evidence was insufficient to set a UL for this and other *n*-6 polyunsaturated fatty acids. Foods rich in *n*-6 polyunsaturated fatty acids include nuts, seeds, and vegetable oils, such as sunflower, safflower, corn, and soybean oils.

The AIs for α-linolenic acid are based on the median intakes of α-linolenic acid in the United States, where the presence of *n*-3 polyunsaturated fatty acid deficiency is basically nonexistent in healthy individuals. Evidence was insufficient to set a UL for this and other *n*-3 fatty acids. Major food sources include certain vegetable oils and fish. Flaxseed, canola, and soybean oils contain high amounts of α-linolenic acid. Fatty fish, fish oils, and products fortified with fish oils contain longer chain *n*-3 fatty acids.

Trans fatty acids are not essential and confer no known health benefits. Therefore, no EAR (and thus an RDA) or AI was set. As with saturated fatty acids, there is a positive linear trend between *trans* fatty acid intake and LDL cholesterol concentration and therefore an increased risk of coronary heart diseases. It is recommended that individuals maintain their *trans* fatty acid consumption as low as possible without compromising the nutritional adequacy of their diet. Foods that contain *trans* fatty acids include traditional stick margarine and vegetable shortenings subjected to partial hydrogenation and various bakery products and fried foods prepared using partially hydrogenated oils. Milk, butter, and meats also contain trans fatty acids but at lower levels.

A lack of either of the two essential fatty acids (FFAs), linoleic or α-linolenic acid, will result in symptoms of deficiency that include scaly skin, dermatitis, and reduced growth. Such deficiency is very rare in healthy populations in the United States and Canada. Certain types of fatty acids, such as *trans* and saturated, have been shown to heighten the risk of heart disease in some people by boosting the level of LDL cholesterol in the bloodstream. DRI values are listed by life stage group in Table 1.

FAT, FATTY ACIDS, AND THE BODY

Background Information

Dietary fat consists mainly of triacylglycerol (98 percent) and small amounts of phospholipids and sterols. Triacylglycerols are made up of one glycerol molecule esterified with three fatty acid molecules. In this publication, total fat refers all to forms of triacylglycerol, regardless of fatty acid composition.

Fatty acids are hydrocarbon chains that contain a methyl (CH_3—) and a carboxyl (—COOH) end. Table 2 shows the major fatty acids found in the diet. Fatty acids vary in their carbon chain length and degree of unsaturation (the number of double bonds in the carbon chain) and can be classified as follows:

- saturated fatty acids
- *cis* monounsaturated fatty acids
- *cis* polyunsaturated fatty acids
  - *n*-6 fatty acids
  - *n*-3 fatty acids
- *trans* fatty acids

A very small amount of dietary fat occurs as phospholipids, a form of fat that contains one glycerol molecule that is esterified with two fatty acids and either inositol, choline, serine, or ethanolamine. In the body, phospholipids are mainly located in the cell membranes and the globule membranes of milk.

TABLE 2 Major Dietary Fatty Acids

Category of Fatty Acid	Specific Fatty Acids Found in the Diet
Saturated fatty acids	• caprylic acid, 8:0[a] • caproic acid, 10:0 • lauric acid, 12:0 • myristic acid, 14:0 • palmitic acid, 16:0 • stearic acid, 18:0
Cis monounsaturated fatty acids	• myristoleic acid, 14:1 n-7 • palmitoleic acid, 16:1 n-7 • oleic acid, 18:1 n-9 (account for 92% of monounsaturated dietary fatty acids) • cis-vaccenic acid, 18:1 n-7 • eicosenoic acid, 20:1 n-9 • erucic acid, 22:1 n-9
Cis polyunsaturated fatty acids n-6 polyunsaturated fatty acid	• linoleic acid,[b] 18:2 • γ-linoleic acid, 18:3 • dihomo-γ-linolenic acid, 20:3 • arachidonic acid, 20:4 • adrenic acid, 22:4 • docosapentaenoic acid, 22:5
n-3 polyunsaturated fatty acid	• α-linolenic acid,[b] 18:3 • eicosapentaenoic acid, 20:5 • docosapentaenoic acid, 22:5 • docosahexaenoic acid, 22:6
Trans fatty acid	• 9-trans, 18:1; 9-trans, 16:1; 9-cis,11-trans, 18:2; 9-trans,12-cis, 18:2; 9-cis,12-trans, 18:2

[a] The first value refers to chain length or number of carbon atoms and the second value refers to the number of double bonds.
[b] Linoleic acid and α-linolenic acid cannot be synthesized in the body and are therefore essential in the diet.

Function

A major source of energy for the body, fat aids in the absorption of fat-soluble vitamins A, D, E, K, and other food components, such as carotenoids. Fatty acids function in cell signaling and alter the expression of specific genes in-

TABLE 3 The Functions of Fat and Fatty Acids

Fat and Fatty Acids	Function
Total fat[a]	• Major source of energy • Aids in absorption of the fat-soluble vitamins and carotenoids
Saturated fatty acids	• Sources of energy • Structural components of cell membranes • Enable normal function of proteins
***Cis* monounsaturated fatty acids**	• Key components of membrane structural lipids, particularly nervous tissue myelin
***Cis* polyunsaturated fatty acids**	
n-6 polyunsaturated fatty acids	• Substrates for eicosanoid production, including prostaglandins • Precursors of arachidonic acid • Components of membrane structural lipids • Important in cell signaling pathways • Vital for normal epithelial cell function • Involved in the regulation of genes for proteins that regulate fatty acid synthesis
n-3 polyunsaturated fatty acids	• Precursors for synthesis of eicosapentaenoic acid (EPA) and docosahexaenoic acid (DHA). EPA is the precursor for *n*-3 eicosanoids
Phospholipids	• Major constituents of cell membranes

[a] Total fat refers to all forms of triacylglycerol, regardless of fatty acid composition.

volved in lipid and carbohydrate metabolism. Fatty acids, the major constituents of triglycerides, may also serve as precursors or ligands for receptors that are important regulators of adipogenesis, inflammation, insulin action, and neurological function. Table 3 summarizes the functions of fat and fatty acids.

Absorption, Metabolism, Storage, and Excretion

TOTAL FAT

In the intestine, dietary fat is emulsified with bile salts and phospholipids (secreted into the intestine by the liver), hydrolyzed by pancreatic enzymes, and almost completely absorbed. Following absorption, the fats are reassembled together with cholesterol, phospholipids, and apoproteins into chylomicrons, which enter the circulation through the thoracic duct. Chylomicrons come into contact with the enzyme lipoprotein lipase (LPL) (located on the surface of capillaries of muscle and adipose tissue) and LPL hydrolyzes the chylomicron triacylglycerol fatty acids. Most of the fatty acids released in this process are taken up by adipose tissue and re-esterfied into triacylglycerol for storage.

When fat is needed for fuel, free fatty acids from the liver and muscle are released into the circulation to be taken up by various tissues, where they are oxidized to provide energy. Muscle, which is the main site of fatty acid oxidation, uses both fatty acids and glucose for energy. Fatty acids released from fat tissue can also be oxidized by the liver.

As fatty acids are broken down through oxidation, carbon dioxide and water are released. Small amounts of ketone bodies are also produced and excreted in the urine. The cells of the skin and intestine also contain fatty acids. Thus, small quantities are lost when these cells are sloughed.

Saturated Fatty Acids

When absorbed along with fats containing appreciable amounts of unsaturated fatty acids, saturated fatty acids are absorbed almost completely by the small intestine. In general, the longer the chain length of the fatty acid, the lower the efficiency of absorption. Following absorption, long-chain saturated fatty acids are re-esterified along with other fatty acids into triacylglycerols and released in chylomicrons. Medium-chain saturated fatty acids are absorbed, bound to albumin, transported as free fatty acids in the portal circulation, and cleared by the liver. Oxidation of saturated fatty acids is similar to oxidation of other types of fatty acids (see "Total Fat" above).

A unique feature of saturated fatty acids is that they suppress expression of LDL receptors, thus raising blood LDL cholesterol levels. Like other fatty acids, saturated fatty acids tend to be completely oxidized to carbon dioxide and water. Saturated fatty acids also increase HDL cholesterol.

Cis Monounsaturated Fatty Acids

Absorption of cis monounsaturated fatty acids is in excess of 90 percent (based on oleic acid data) in adults and infants, and the pathways of digestion, absorption, metabolism, and excretion are similar to those of other fatty acids (see "Total Fat" above).

Cis-Polyunsaturated Fatty Acids

- n-6 *polyunsaturated fatty acids*: Digestion and absorption of *n*-6 fatty acids is efficient and occurs via the same pathways as those of other long-chain fatty acids (see "Total Fat" above). The parent fatty acid of the *n*-6 fatty acids series is linoleic acid. Humans can desaturate and elongate linoleic acid to form arachidonic acid. Arachidonic acid is the precursor to a number of eicosanoids (e.g., prostaglandins, thromboxanes, and leukotrienes) that are involved in platelet aggregation, hemodynamics, and coronary vascular tone. The *n*-6 fatty acids are almost completely absorbed and are either incorporated into tissue lipids, used in eicosanoid synthesis, or oxidized to carbon dioxide and water. Small amounts are lost via the sloughing of skin and other epithelial cells.
- n-3 *polyunsaturated fatty acids*: Digestion and absorption is similar to that of other long-chain fatty acids (see "Total Fat" above). The body cannot synthesize α-linolenic acid, the parent fatty acid of the *n*-3 series, and thus requires a dietary source of it. α-Linolenic acid is not known to have any specific functions other than to serve as a precursor for synthesis of eicosapentaenoic acid (EPA) and docosahexaenoic acid (DHA). The *n*-3 fatty acids are almost completely absorbed and are either incorporated into tissue lipids, used in eicosanoid synthesis, or oxidized to carbon dioxide and water. Small amounts are lost via sloughing of skin and other epithelial cells.

Trans Fatty Acids

As with other fatty acids, absorption is about 95 percent. *Trans* fatty acids are transported similarly to other dietary fatty acids and are distributed within the cholesteryl ester, triacylglycerol, and phospholipid fractions of lipoprotein. Available animal and human data indicate that the *trans* fatty acid content of tissues (except the brain) reflects diet content and that selective accumulation does not occur. *Trans* fatty acids are completely catabolized to carbon dioxide and water.

DETERMINING DRIS

Determining Requirements

Total Fat

Neither an EAR (and thus an RDA) nor an AI was set for total fat for individuals aged 1 year and older because data were insufficient to determine an intake level at which risk of inadequacy or prevention of chronic disease occurs. However, because of the importance of fat to provide the energy needed for growth, AIs were set for infants aged 0 through 12 months. These AIs were based on the observed mean fat intake of infants who were principally fed human milk (0–6 months) and human milk and complementary foods (7–12 months).

SATURATED FATTY ACIDS

Neither an EAR (and thus an RDA) nor an RDA was set for saturated fatty acids because they are not essential and have no known role in preventing chronic disease.

CIS MONOUNSATURATED FATTY ACIDS

Cis monounsaturated fatty acids (*n*-9) confer no known independent health benefits. Since these fatty acids are not required in the diet, neither an EAR (and thus an RDA) nor an AI was set.

CIS POLYUNSATURATED FATTY ACIDS

- n-6 *polyunsaturated fatty acids*: In the absence of adequate information on the amount of linoleic acid required to correct the symptoms of an *n*-6 polyunsaturated fatty acid deficiency, an EAR (and hence an RDA) could not be established. The AIs for linoleic acid are based on the median intake of linoleic acid by different life stage and gender groups in the United States, where the presence of *n*-6 polyunsaturated fatty acid deficiency is basically nonexistent in healthy individuals.
- n-3 *polyunsaturated fatty acids*: Because of the lack of evidence for determining a requirement in healthy individuals, an EAR (and thus an RDA) could not be established. The AIs for α-linolenic acid are based on the median intakes of α-linolenic acid in the United States where the presence of *n*-3 polyunsaturated fatty acid deficiency is basically nonexistent in healthy individuals.

TRANS FATTY ACIDS

Trans fatty acids confer no known health benefits. They are chemically classified as unsaturated fatty acids, but behave more like saturated fatty acids in the body. Therefore, no EAR (and thus RDA) or AI was set.

CONJUGATED LINOLEIC ACID

There are no known requirements for conjugated linoleic acid (CLA) in the body. Therefore, no EAR (and thus RDA) or AI was set.

Criteria for Determining Fat Requirements, by Life Stage Group

TOTAL FAT

Life stage group[a]	Criterion
0 through 6 mo	Average consumption of total fat from human milk
7 through 12 mo	Average consumption of total fat from human milk and complementary foods

LINOLEIC ACID

Life stage group	Criterion
0 through 6 mo	Average consumption of total n-6 fatty acids from human milk
7 through 12 mo	Average consumption of total n-6 fatty acids from human milk and complementary foods
1 through 18 y	Median intake from CSFII[b]
19 through 50 y	Median intake from CSFII for 19 to 30 y group
51 y and through 70 y	Median intake from CSFII
> 70 y	Median intake from CSFII for 51 through 70 y group
Pregnancy	Median intake from CSFII for all pregnant women
Lactation	Median intake from CSFII for all lactating women

ALPHA-LINOLENIC ACID

Life stage group	Criterion
0 through 6 mo	Average consumption of total n-3 fatty acids from human milk
7 through 12 mo	Average consumption of total n-3 fatty acids from human milk and complementary foods
1 through 18 y	Median intake from CSFII[b]
19 y and older	Median intake from CSFII for all adult age groups
Pregnancy	Median intake from CSFII for all pregnant women
Lactation	Median intake from CSFII for all lactating women

---

[a] A DRI value for total fat was not set for any life stage group other than infants.
[b] Continuing Survey of Food Intake by Individuals (1994–1996, 1998).

The AMDR

An AMDR has been estimated for total fat at 20–35 percent of energy for adults and children aged 4 and older and 30–40 percent for children ages 1 through 3. The AMDRs for *n*-6 polyunsaturated fatty acids (linoleic acid) and *n*-3 polyunsaturated fatty acids (α-linolenic acid) are 5–10 percent and 0.6–1.2 percent, respectively (see Part II, "Macronutrients, Healthful Diets, and Physical Activity").

The UL

TOTAL FAT

The Tolerable Upper Intake Level (UL) is the highest level of daily nutrient intake that is likely to pose no risk of adverse effects for almost all people. Since there is no defined intake level of total fat at which an adverse effect occurs, a UL was not set for total fat.

SATURATED FATTY ACIDS AND *TRANS* FATTY ACIDS

There is a positive linear trend between saturated fatty acid intake and total and LDL cholesterol levels and a positive linear trend between *trans* fatty acid and LDL cholesterol concentration. Any incremental increases in saturated and *trans* fatty acid intakes increase CHD risk, therefore a UL was not set for saturated or *trans* fatty acids. It is neither possible nor advisable to achieve zero percent of energy from saturated fatty acids or *trans* fatty acids in typical diets, since this would require extraordinary dietary changes that may lead to inadequate protein and micronutrient intake, as well as other undesirable effects. It is recommended that individuals maintain their saturated and *trans* fatty acid consumption as low as possible while following a nutritionally adequate diet.

CIS MONOUNSATURATED AND *CIS* POLYUNSATURATED FATTY ACIDS

Evidence was insufficient to set a UL for *cis* monounsaturated fatty acids, and *cis* polyunsaturated (*n*-6 and *n*-3) fatty acids.

DIETARY SOURCES

Foods

Dietary fat intake is primarily (98 percent) in the form of triacylglycerols and is derived from both animal- and plant-based products. The principal foods that contribute to fat intake are butter, margarine, vegetable oils, visible fat on meat and poultry products, whole milk, egg yolk, nuts, and baked goods, such as cookies, doughnuts, and cakes.

In general, animal fats have higher melting points and are solid at room temperature, which is a reflection of their high content of saturated fatty acids. Plant fats (oils) tend to have lower melting points and are liquid at room temperature because of their high content of unsaturated fatty acids. Exceptions to this rule are some tropical oils (e.g., coconut oil and palm kernel oil), which are high in saturated fat and solid at room temperature.

Trans fatty acids have physical properties that generally resemble saturated fatty acids, and their presence tends to harden fats. Food sources for the various fatty acids that are typically consumed in North American diets are listed in Table 4.

Dietary Supplements

This information was not provided at the time the DRI values for total fat and fatty acids were set.

INADEQUATE INTAKE AND DEFICIENCY

Total Fat

Inadequate intake of dietary fat may result in impaired growth and an increased risk of chronic disease. If fat intake, along with carbohydrate and protein intake, is too low to meet energy needs, an individual will be in negative energy balance. Depending on the severity and duration of the deficit, this may lead to malnutrition or starvation.

If the diet contains adequate energy, carbohydrate can replace fat as an energy source. However, fat restriction is of particular concern during infancy, childhood, and pregnancy, during which there are relatively high energy requirements for both energy expenditure and fetal development.

Imbalanced intake can also be of concern. Compared with higher fat diets, low-fat and high-carbohydrate diets may alter metabolism in a way that increases the risk of chronic diseases, such as coronary heart disease and diabetes. These changes include a reduction in high density lipoprotein (HDL) cholesterol concentration, an increase in serum triacylglycerol concentration, and higher responses in glucose and insulin concentrations following food consumption. This metabolic pattern has been associated with an increased risk of CHD and Type II diabetes, although strong evidence does not exist that low-fat diets actually predispose an individual to either CHD or diabetes.

Some populations that consume low-fat diets, and in which habitual energy intake is relatively high, have a low prevalence of these chronic diseases.

TABLE 4 Commonly Consumed Food Sources of Fatty Acids

Fatty Acid	Food Sources
Saturated fatty acids	Sources tend to be animal-based foods, including whole milk, cream, butter, cheese, and fatty meats such as pork and beef. Coconut, palm, and palm kernel oils also contain relatively high amounts of saturated fatty acids. Saturated fatty acids provide approximately 20–25 percent of energy in human milk.
Cis monounsaturated fatty acids	Animal products, primarily meat fat, provide about 50 percent of monounsaturated fatty acids in a typical North American diet. Oils that contain monounsaturated fatty acids include canola and olive oil. Monounsaturated fatty acids provide approximately 20 percent of energy in human milk.
Cis polyunsaturated fatty acids:	
n-6 polyunsaturated fatty acids	Nuts, seeds, and vegetable oils such as sunflower, safflower, corn, and soybean oils. γ-Linolenic acid is found in black currant seed oil and evening primrose oil. Arachidonic acid is found in small amounts in meat, poultry, and eggs.
n-3 polyunsaturated fatty acids	Major sources include certain vegetable oils and fish. Flaxseed, canola, and soybean contain high amounts of α-linolenic acid. Fatty fish are major dietary sources of EPA and DHA.
Trans fatty acids	Traditional stick margarine and vegetable shortenings subjected to partial hydrogenation, milk, butter, and meats. Pastries, fried foods, doughnuts, and french fries are also contributors of *trans* fatty acid intake. Human milk contains approximately 1–5 percent of total energy as *trans* fatty acids and, similarly, infant formulas contain approximately 1–3 percent.

Similarly, populations that consume high-fat diets (i.e., ≥ 40 percent of energy) and experience a low prevalence of chronic diseases often include people who engage in heavy physical labor, are lean, and have a low family history of chronic diseases.

Conversely, in sedentary populations, such as those in the United States and Canada where overweight and obesity are common, high-carbohydrate, low-fat diets induce changes in lipoprotein and glucose/insulin metabolism in ways that could raise the risk for chronic diseases. Available prospective studies have not concluded whether high-carbohydrate, low-fat diets present a health risk in the North American population.

n-6 Polyunsaturated Fatty Acids

Because adipose tissue lipids in free-living healthy adults contain about 10 percent of total fatty acids as linoleic acid, the biochemical and clinical signs of essential fatty acid deficiency do not appear during dietary fat restriction or malabsorption when they are accompanied by an energy deficit. In this situation, the release of linoleic acid and small amounts of arachidonic acid from adipose tissue reserves may prevent the development of essential fatty acid deficiency. However, during total parenteral nutrition (TPN) with dextrose solutions, insulin concentrations are high and mobilization of adipose tissue is prevented. This results in the characteristic signs of essential fatty acid deficiency.

When *n*-6 fatty acid intake is inadequate or absorption is impaired, tissue concentrations of arachidonic acid decrease, inhibition of the desaturation of oleic acid is reduced, and synthesis of eicosatrienoic acid from oleic acid increases. A lack of dietary *n*-6 polyunsaturated fatty acids is characterized by rough scaly skin, dermatitis, and an elevated eicosatrienoic acid:arachidonic acid (triene:tetraene) ratio.

n-3 Polyunsaturated Fatty Acids

A lack of α-linolenic acid in the diet can result in clinical symptoms of a deficiency (e.g., scaly dermatitis). Unlike essential fatty acid deficiency (of both *n*-6 and *n*-3 fatty acids), plasma eicosatrienoic acid (20:3 *n*-9) remains within normal ranges, and skin atrophy and scaly dermatitis are absent when the diet is only deficient in *n*-3 fatty acids.

Because of their function, growing evidence suggests that dietary *n*-3 polyunsaturated fatty acids (EPA and DHA) may reduce the risk of many chronic diseases including CHD, stroke, and diabetes. For example, *n*-3 fatty acids may reduce CHD risk through a variety of mechanisms, such as by preventing arrhythmias, reducing atherosclerosis, decreasing platelet aggregation and plasma triacylglycerol concentration, slightly increasing HDL concentration, modulating endothelial function, and decreasing proinflammatory eicosanoids.

ADVERSE EFFECTS OF OVERCONSUMPTION

As mentioned earlier, there is no defined level of fat intake at which an adverse effect, such as obesity, can occur. An AMDR for fat intake, however, has been estimated based on potential adverse effects occurring from consuming low-fat and high-fat diets (see Part II, "Macronutrients, Healthful Diets, and Physical Activity"). High-fat diets in excess of energy needs can cause obesity. Several studies have shown associations between high-fat intakes and an increased risk of CHD, cancer, and insulin resistance. However, the type of fatty acid consumed is very important in defining these associations. The potential adverse effects of overconsuming fatty acids are summarized in Table 5.

Special Considerations

Individuals sensitive to n-3 polyunsaturated fatty acids: People who take hypoglycemic medications should consume *n*-3 fatty acids with caution. Because *n*-3 fatty acids may excessively prolong bleeding time, DHA and EPA supplements should be taken with caution by people who take anticoagulants, including aspirin and warfarin.

Exercise: High-fat diets may result in a positive energy balance and therefore in weight gain under sedentary conditions. Active people can probably consume relatively high-fat diets while maintaining their body weight. Athletes may not be able to train as effectively on short-term (fewer than 6 days) high-fat diets as they could on high-carbohydrate diets. It is important to note that physical activity may account for a greater percentage of the variance in weight gain than does dietary fat.

Genetic factors: Some data indicate that genes may affect the relationship between diet and obesity. Some people with relatively high metabolic rates appear to be able to eat high-fat diets (44 percent of energy from fat) without becoming obese. Intervention studies have shown that people susceptible to weight gain and obesity appear to have an impaired ability to oxidize more fat after eating high-fat meals.

Alcohol: Significant alcohol intake (23 percent of energy) can depress fatty acid oxidation. If the energy derived from alcohol is not used, the excess is stored as fat.

TABLE 5 Potential Adverse Effects of Fatty Acid Overconsumption

Fatty Acid	Potential Adverse Effects of Overconsumption
Saturated fatty acids	In general, the higher the saturated fatty acid intake, the higher the serum total and LDL cholesterol concentrations. There is a positive linear relationship between serum total and LDL cholesterol concentrations and the risk of CHD or mortality from CHD.
Cis monounsaturated fatty acids	Overconsumption of energy related to a high-fat, high-monounsaturated fatty acid diet is one risk associated with excess monounsaturated fatty acid intake. High intakes can also cause an increased intake of saturated fatty acids, since many animal fats that contain one have the other.
Cis polyunsaturated fatty acids:	
n-6 polyunsaturated fatty acids	An AMDR was estimated based on the adverse effects from consuming a diet too high or low in n-6 polyunsaturated fatty acids (see Part II, "Macronutrients, Healthful Diets, and Physical Activity").
n-3 polyunsaturated fatty acids	Data on the effects of EPA and DHA intakes on bleeding times are mixed. Until more information is available, supplemental forms of EPA and DHA should be taken with caution. An AMDR was estimated based on the adverse effects from consuming a diet too high or low in n-3 polyunsaturated fatty acids (see Part II, "Macronutrients, Healthful Diets, and Physical Activity").
Trans fatty acids	There is a positive linear trend between trans fatty acid intake and LDL concentration, and therefore an increased risk of CHD. Recent data have shown a dose-dependent relationship between trans fatty acid intake and the LDL:HDL ratio. The combined results of numerous studies have indicated that the magnitude of this effect is greater for trans fatty acids, compared with saturated fatty acids.

Interaction of n-6 *and* n-3 *fatty acid metabolism:* Many studies, primarily in animals, have suggested that the balance between linoleic and α-linolenic acids is important in determining the amounts of arachidonic acid, eicosapentaenoic acid (EPA), and docosahexaenoic acid (DHA) in tissue lipids. An inappropriate ratio may involve too high an intake of either linoleic acid or α-linolenic acid, too little of one fatty acid, or a combination leading to an imbalance between the two. The ratio between the two is likely to be of most importance in diets that are low in or devoid of arachidonic acid, EPA, and DHA. The importance of this ratio is unknown in diets that are high in these three fatty acids.

n-6:n-3 *polyunsaturated fatty acid ratio:* The ratio of linoleic acid to α-linolenic acid in the diet is important because the two fatty acids compete for the same desaturase enzymes. Thus, a high ratio of linoleic acid to α-linolenic acid can inhibit the conversion of α-linolenic acid to DHA, while a low ratio will inhibit the desaturation of linoleic acid to arachidonic acid.

Although limited, the available data suggest that linoleic to α-linolenic acid ratios below 5:1 may be associated with impaired growth in infants. Based on limited studies, the linoleic to α-linolenic acid or total *n*-3 to *n*-6 fatty acid ratios of 5:1–10:1, 5:1–15:1, and 6:1–16:1 have been recommended for infant formulas. Based on limited studies, a reasonable linoleic to α-linolenic acid ratio of 5:1–10:1 has been recommended for adults.

KEY POINTS FOR FAT AND FATTY ACIDS

✓   A major source of energy for the body, fat aids in tissue development and the absorption of the fat-soluble vitamins A, D, E, K, and other food components, such as carotenoids.

✓   Dietary fat contains fatty acids that fall into the following categories: saturated fatty acids, *cis* monounsaturated fatty acids, *cis* polyunsaturated fatty acids (*n*-6 fatty acids and *n*-3 fatty acids), *trans* fatty acids, and conjugated linoleic acid.

✓   Neither an EAR (and thus RDA) nor an AI was set for total fat for individuals aged 1 year and older because data were insufficient to determine an intake level at which risk of inadequacy or prevention of chronic disease occurs. A UL was not set for total fat. AIs for total fat were set for infants aged 0 through 12 months based on observed mean fat intake of infants who were principally fed human milk.

✓   An AMDR has been estimated for total fat at 20–35 percent of energy for adults and children aged 4 and older and 30-40 percent for children ages 1 through 3.

✓ The main food sources of total fat are butter, margarine, vegetable oils, visible fat on meat and poultry products, whole milk, egg yolk, nuts, and baked goods.

✓ Neither an EAR (and thus RDA) nor an AI was set for *trans* or saturated fatty acids because they are not essential and have no known role in preventing chronic disease.

✓ There is a positive linear trend between both *trans* and saturated fatty acid intake and LDL cholesterol levels, and thus increased risk of CHD. A UL was not set for *trans* or saturated fatty acids because any incremental increase in intake increases the risk of CHD.

✓ It is recommended that individuals maintain their *trans* and saturated fatty acid intakes as low as possible while consuming a nutritionally adequate diet.

✓ Food sources of saturated fatty acids tend to be meats, bakery items, and full-fat dairy products. Foods that contain *trans* fatty acids include traditional stick margarine and vegetable shortenings that have been partially hydrogenated, with lower levels in meats and dairy products.

✓ *Cis* monounsaturated fatty acids can be synthesized by the body and confer no known health benefits. Since they are not required in the diet, neither an AI nor an RDA was set. There was insufficient evidence to set a UL.

✓ Animal products, primarily meat fat, provide about 50 percent of dietary *cis* monounsaturated fatty acids intake.

✓ Linoleic and α-linolenic fatty acids are essential, and therefore must be obtained from foods. AIs were set based on intake of healthy individuals. There was insufficient evidence to set a UL for *cis* polyunsaturated (*n*-6 and *n*-3) fatty acids.

✓ Foods rich in *n*-6 polyunsaturated fatty acids include nuts, seeds, certain vegetables, and vegetable oils, such as sunflower, safflower, corn, and soybean oils. Major food sources of α-linolenic fatty acids include certain vegetable oils (flaxseed, canola, and soybean oils) and fatty fish.

✓ High-fat diets in excess of energy needs can cause obesity. Several studies have shown associations between high-fat intakes and an increased risk of CHD, cancer, and insulin resistance. However, the type of fatty acid consumed is very important in defining these associations.

CHOLESTEROL

Cholesterol plays an important role in steroid hormone and bile acid biosynthesis. It also serves as an integral component of cell membranes. Most people absorb between 40 and 60 percent of ingested cholesterol. Such variability, which is probably due in part to genes, may contribute to the individual differences that occur in plasma cholesterol response to dietary cholesterol.

All tissues are capable of synthesizing enough cholesterol to meet their metabolic and structural needs. Consequently, there is no evidence for a biological requirement for dietary cholesterol. Neither an Estimated Average Requirement (EAR), and thus a Recommended Dietary Allowance (RDA), nor an Adequate Intake (AI) was set for cholesterol.

Much evidence indicates a positive linear trend between cholesterol intake and low density lipoprotein (LDL) cholesterol concentration, and therefore an increased risk of coronary heart disease (CHD). A Tolerable Upper Intake Level (UL) was not set for cholesterol because any incremental increase in cholesterol intake increases CHD risk. It is recommended that people maintain their dietary cholesterol intake as low as possible, while consuming a diet that is nutritionally adequate in all required nutrients.

High amounts of cholesterol are found in liver and egg yolk. The main adverse effect of dietary cholesterol is increased LDL cholesterol concentration, which could result in an increased risk for CHD.

CHOLESTEROL AND THE BODY

Function

Cholesterol is a sterol that is present in all animal tissues. Tissue cholesterol occurs primarily as free (unesterified) cholesterol, but is also bound covalently (via chemical bonds) to fatty acids as cholesterol esters and to certain proteins. Cholesterol is an integral component of cell membranes and serves as a precursor for hormones such as estrogen, testosterone, and aldosterone, as well as bile acids.

Absorption, Metabolism, Storage, and Excretion

Cholesterol in the body comes from two sources: endogenous and dietary. All cells can synthesize sufficient amounts of cholesterol for their metabolic and structural needs. Dietary cholesterol comes from foods of animal origin, such as eggs, meat, poultry, fish, and dairy products.

Dietary and endogenous cholesterol are absorbed in the proximal jejunum, primarily by passive diffusion. Cholesterol balance studies show a wide variation in the efficiency of intestinal cholesterol absorption (from 20 to 80 percent), with most people absorbing between 40 and 60 percent of ingested cholesterol. Such variability, which is probably due in part to genetic factors, may contribute to the differences seen among individuals in plasma cholesterol response to dietary cholesterol. In addition, cholesterol absorption may be reduced by decreased intestinal transit time.

In the body, cholesterol can be stored in the liver; secreted into the plasma in lipoproteins, primarily very low density lipoproteins (VLDL); oxidized and secreted as bile acids; or directly secreted into the bile. Free and esterified cholesterols circulate principally in LDL in the blood. The body tightly regulates cholesterol homeostasis by balancing intestinal absorption and endogenous synthesis with hepatic excretion and bile acids derived from hepatic cholesterol oxidation. Increased hepatic cholesterol delivery from the diet and other sources results in a complex mixture of metabolic effects that are generally directed at maintaining tissue and plasma cholesterol homeostasis. Observational studies have shown that increased dietary cholesterol intake leads to a net increase in plasma LDL cholesterol concentrations.

DETERMINING DRIS

Determining Requirements

All tissues are capable of synthesizing enough cholesterol to meet their metabolic and structural needs. Consequently, there is no evidence for a biological requirement for dietary cholesterol. Neither an Estimated Average Requirement (EAR), and thus a Recommended Dietary Allowance (RDA), nor an Adequate Intake (AI) was set for cholesterol. However, it is recommended that people maintain their dietary cholesterol intake as low as possible, while consuming a diet nutritionally adequate in all required nutrients.

The UL

The Tolerable Upper Intake Level (UL) is the highest level of daily nutrient intake that is likely to pose no risk of adverse effects for almost all people. Much evidence indicates a positive linear trend between cholesterol intake and LDL cholesterol concentration, and therefore an increased risk of CHD.

A UL was not set for cholesterol because any incremental increase in cholesterol intake increases CHD risk. Because cholesterol is unavoidable in ordinary non-vegan diets, eliminating cholesterol in the diet would require significant dietary changes. These changes require careful planning to ensure adequate intakes of proteins and certain micronutrients. Still, it is possible to eat a low-cholesterol, yet nutritionally adequate, diet.

DIETARY SOURCES

Foods

Foods of animal origin contain cholesterol. High amounts are found in liver and egg yolk. Moderate amounts are found in meats, some types of seafood, including shrimp, lobster, certain fish (such as salmon and sardines), and full-fat dairy products.

ADVERSE EFFECTS OF CONSUMPTION

The main adverse effect of dietary cholesterol is increased LDL cholesterol concentration, which could result in an increased risk for CHD. Serum HDL concentration also increases, although to a lesser extent, but the impact of such a diet-induced change in CHD risk is uncertain. Studies have shown that serum cholesterol concentrations increase with increased dietary cholesterol and that the relationship of blood cholesterol to the risk of CHD progressively increases. On average, an increase of 100 mg/day of dietary cholesterol is predicted to result in a 0.05–0.1 mmol/L increase in total serum cholesterol, of which approximately 80 percent is in the LDL fraction.

There is also increasing evidence that genetic factors underlie a substantial portion of the variation among individuals in response to dietary cholesterol. Although mixed, there is evidence that increases in serum cholesterol concentration due to dietary cholesterol are blunted by diets low in saturated fat, high in polyunsaturated fat, or both.

No consistent significant associations have been established between dietary cholesterol intake and cancer, including lung, breast, colon, and prostate cancers.

KEY POINTS FOR CHOLESTEROL

✓ Cholesterol plays an important role in steroid hormone and bile acid biosynthesis and serves as an integral component of cell membranes.

✓ Because all tissues are capable of synthesizing enough cholesterol to meet their metabolic and structural needs, there is no evidence for a biological requirement for dietary cholesterol.

✓ Neither an EAR, RDA, nor AI was set for cholesterol.

✓ Much evidence indicates a positive linear trend between cholesterol intake and LDL cholesterol concentration, and therefore increased risk of CHD.

✓ It is recommended that people maintain their dietary cholesterol intake as low as possible, while consuming a diet nutritionally adequate in all required nutrients.

✓ A UL was not set for cholesterol because any incremental increase in cholesterol intake increases CHD risk.

✓ High amounts of cholesterol are found in liver and egg yolk. Meats, some types of seafood, including shrimp, lobster, and certain fish, as well as full-fat dairy products contain moderate amounts of cholesterol.

✓ The main adverse effect of dietary cholesterol is increased LDL cholesterol concentration, which could result in an increased risk of CHD.

TABLE 1 Dietary Reference Intakes for Total Protein by Life Stage Group[a]

	DRI values (g/kg/day)				
	EAR[b]		RDA[c]		AI[d]
	males	females	males	females	
Life stage group					
0 through 6 mo					1.52 (9.1)
7 through 12 mo	1.0	1.0	1.2 (11)[e]	1.2 (11)	
1 through 3 y	0.87	0.87	1.05 (13)	1.05 (13)	
4 through 8 y	0.76	0.76	0.95 (19)	0.95 (19)	
9 through 13 y	0.76	0.76	0.95 (34)	0.95 (34)	
14 through 18 y	0.73	0.71	0.85 (52)	0.85 (46)	
19 through 30 y	0.66	0.66	0.80 (56)	0.80 (46)	
31 through 50 y	0.66	0.66	0.80 (56)	0.80 (46)	
51 through 70 y	0.66	0.66	0.80 (56)	0.80 (46)	
> 70 y	0.66	0.66	0.80 (56)	0.80 (46)	
Pregnancy		0.88 [f]		1.1 (71)[f]	
Lactation		1.05		1.3 (71)	

[a] Dietary Reference Intakes for individual amino acids are shown in Appendix E.

[b] **EAR** = Estimated Average Requirement. An EAR is the average daily nutrient intake level estimated to meet the requirements of half of the healthy individuals in a group.

[c] **RDA** = Recommended Dietary Allowance. An RDA is the average daily dietary intake level sufficient to meet the nutrient requirements of nearly all (97–98 percent) healthy individuals in a group.

[d] **AI** = Adequate Intake. If sufficient scientific evidence is not available to establish an EAR, and thus calculate an RDA, an AI is usually developed. For healthy breast-fed infants, the AI is the mean intake. The AI for other life stage and gender groups is believed to cover the needs of all healthy individuals in the group, but a lack of data or uncertainty in the data prevents being able to specify with confidence the percentage of individuals covered by this intake.

[e] Values in parentheses ( ) are examples of the total g/day of protein calculated from g/kg/day times the reference weights in Part I, "Introduction to the Dietary Reference Intakes," Table 1.

[f] The EAR and RDA for pregnancy are only for the second half of pregnancy. For the first half of pregnancy, the protein requirements are the same as those of nonpregnant women.

PROTEIN AND AMINO ACIDS

Proteins form the major structural components of all the cells of the body. Proteins also function as enzymes, in membranes, as transport carriers, and as hormones. Amino acids are constituents of protein and act as precursors for nucleic acids, hormones, vitamins, and other important molecules. Thus, an adequate supply of dietary protein is essential to maintain cellular integrity and function, and for health and reproduction.

The requirements for protein are based on careful analyses of available nitrogen balance studies. Data were insufficient to set a Tolerable Upper Intake Level (UL). DRI values are listed by life stage group in Table 1. The Acceptable Macronutrient Distribution Range (AMDR) for protein is 5–20 percent of total calories for children 1 through 3 years of age, 10–30 percent of total calories for children 4 to 18 years of age, and 10–35 percent of total calories for adults older than 18 years of age.

For amino acids, isotopic tracer methods and linear regression analysis were used whenever possible to determine requirements. The estimated average requirements (EARs) for amino acids were used to develop amino acid scoring patterns for various age groups based on the recommended intake of dietary protein. Data were insufficient to set a Tolerable Upper Intake Level (UL) for any of the amino acids. However, the absence of a UL means that caution is warranted in using any single amino acid at levels significantly above those normally found in food.

Proteins found in animal sources such as meat, poultry, fish, eggs, milk, cheese, and yogurt provide all nine indispensable amino acids and are referred to as "complete proteins." Proteins found in plants, legumes, grains, nuts, seeds, and vegetables tend to be deficient in one or more of the indispensable amino acids and are called "incomplete proteins."

Both protein and nonprotein energy (from carbohydrates and fats) must be available to prevent protein-energy malnutrition (PEM). Similarly, if amino acids are not present in the right balance, the body's ability to use protein will be affected. Protein deficiency has been shown to affect all organs and many systems. The risk of adverse effects from excess protein intake from food appears to be very low. The data are conflicting on the potential for high-protein diets to produce gastrointestinal effects, changes in nitrogen balance, or chronic disease, such as osteoporosis or renal stones.

PROTEIN AND THE BODY

Function

Protein is the major functional and structural component of every cell in the body. All enzymes, membrane carriers, blood transport molecules, the intracellular matrices, hair, fingernails, serum albumin, keratin, and collagen are proteins, as are many hormones and a large part of membranes. Amino acids are constituents of protein and act as precursors for many coenzymes, hormones, nucleic acids, and other important molecules.

The most important aspect and defining characteristic of protein from a nutritional point of view is its amino acid composition (amino [or imino] nitrogen group). Amino nitrogen accounts for approximately 16 percent of protein weight, and so nitrogen metabolism is often considered to be synonymous with protein metabolism. Amino acids are required for the synthesis of body protein and other important nitrogen-containing compounds as mentioned above. The amino acids that are incorporated into protein are α-amino acids, with the exception of proline, which is an α-imino acid.

NUTRITIONAL AND METABOLIC CLASSIFICATION OF AMINO ACIDS

Different sources of protein widely vary in chemical composition and nutritional value. Although amino acids have been traditionally classified as indispensable (essential) and dispensable (nonessential), accumulating evidence on the metabolic and nutritional characteristics of dispensable amino acids has blurred their definition, forming a third classification called conditionally indispensable. The term conditionally indispensable recognizes that under most normal conditions, the body can synthesize these amino acids.

The nine indispensable amino acids are those that cannot be synthesized to meet the body's needs, and therefore must be obtained from the diet. The five dispensable amino acids can be synthesized in the body. Six other amino acids are conditionally indispensable because their synthesis can be limited under special pathophysiological conditions, such as prematurity in the young infant or individuals in severe catabolic stress. Table 2 lists the classification of amino acids in the human diet.

Protein Quality

The quality of a source of dietary protein depends on its ability to provide the nitrogen and amino acid requirements that are necessary for the body's growth, maintenance, and repair. This ability is determined by two factors: digestibility and amino acid composition. Digestibility affects the number and type of amino acids made available to the body. If the content of a single indispensable

TABLE 2 Indispensable, Dispensable, and Conditionally Indispensable Amino Acids in the Human Diet

Indispensable	Dispensable	Conditionally Indispensable[a]	Precursors of Conditionally Indispensable
Histidine[b]	Alanine	Arginine	Glutamine/glutamate, aspartate
Isoleucine	Aspartic acid	Cysteine	Methionine, serine
Leucine	Asparagine	Glutamine	Glutamic acid/ammonia
Lysine	Glutamic acid	Glycine	Serine, choline
Methionine	Serine	Proline	Glutamate
Phenylalanine		Tyrosine	Phenylalanine
Threonine			
Tryptophan			
Valine			

[a] Conditionally indispensable is defined as requiring a dietary source when endogenous synthesis cannot meet metabolic need.

[b] Although histidine is considered indispensable, unlike the other eight indispensable amino acids, it does not fulfill the criteria of reducing protein deposition and inducing negative nitrogen balance promptly upon removal from the diet.

amino acid in the diet is less than the individual's requirement, then this deficiency will limit the utilization of other amino acids and thus prevent normal rates of protein synthesis, even when the total nitrogen intake level is adequate. As a result, the "limiting amino acid" will determine the nutritional value of the diet's total nitrogen or protein content.

The concept of the "limiting amino acid" has led to the practice of amino acid (or chemical) scoring, whereby the indispensable amino acid composition of a given protein source is compared with that of a reference amino acid composition profile to evaluate the quality of food proteins or their capacity to efficiently meet both nitrogen and indispensable amino acid requirements.

Absorption, Metabolism, Storage, and Excretion

Amino acids are present in the body as free amino acids or as part of protein. They are available through two major pathways: dietary intake in the form of proteins or de novo synthesis by the body.

When proteins are ingested from food, they are denatured by stomach acid. In the stomach, they are also cleaved into smaller peptides by the enzyme pepsin, which is activated in response to a meal. The proteins and peptides then enter the small intestine, where a variety of enzymes hydrolyze the peptide bonds. The resulting mix of free amino acids and peptides is transported into the mucosal cells. The amino acids are then either secreted into the blood or further metabolized within the cells. Absorbed amino acids pass into the liver, where some are taken up and used and others are circulated to and used by the peripheral tissues.

About 43 percent of the total protein content of the body is present as skeletal muscle, while other structural tissues, such as skin and blood, each contain approximately 15 percent of the body's total protein. The metabolically active visceral tissues (e.g., liver and kidney tissue) contain comparatively small amounts of protein (together about 10 percent of the total). Other organs such as the brain, heart, lung, and bone contribute the remainder. Almost half of the total protein content of the body is represented by only four proteins (myosin, actin, collagen, and hemoglobin).

Amino acids are lost in the body by oxidation, excretion, or conversion to other metabolites. Metabolic products of amino acids, such as urea, creatinine, and uric acid, are excreted in the urine; fecal nitrogen losses may account for 25 percent of the obligatory loss of nitrogen. Other routes of loss of intact amino acids are through the sweat and other body secretions and through the skin, nails, and loss of hair.

PROTEIN TURNOVER

The process by which all body proteins are being continuously broken down and resynthesized is known as protein turnover. From a nutritional and metabolic point of view, it is important to recognize that protein synthesis is a continuing process that takes place within most of the body's cells. In a steady state, when neither net growth nor protein loss is occurring, protein synthesis is balanced by an equal amount of protein degradation.

The major consequence of inadequate protein intake, or of consuming diets that are low or lacking in specific indispensable amino acids, is a shift in this balance. Rates of synthesis of some body proteins decrease while protein degradation continues in order to provide an endogenous source of the amino acids most in need. The mechanism of intracellular protein degradation by which protein is hydrolyzed to free amino acids is more complex and not as well characterized at the mechanistic level as that of protein synthesis.

The daily amount of protein turned over is greater in infants and less in the elderly when compared with young adults on a body-weight basis; and some body tissues are more active than others with regard to it. Despite their rather small contribution to the total protein content of the body, the liver and the intestine together are believed to contribute as much as 50 percent of whole body protein turnover. Conversely, although skeletal muscle is the largest single component of body protein mass (43 percent), it contributes only about 25 percent to total body protein turnover.

DETERMINING DRIS

Determining Requirements

PROTEIN

The requirements for protein were based on careful analyses of available nitrogen balance studies.

AMINO ACIDS

Age-based recommendations were set for all nine of the indispensable amino acids found in dietary proteins (see Appendix E). These requirements are based on isotopic tracer methods and linear regression analysis, which were used whenever possible.

The requirements for amino acids and for total protein were used to develop a new FNB/IOM Protein Scoring Pattern for use in children aged 1 year and older and in all other age groups. The recommended amino acid scoring pattern for proteins for individuals aged 1 year and older and all other age groups is as follows (in mg/g of protein): isoleucine, 25; leucine, 55; lysine, 51; methionine + cysteine (SAA), 25; phenylalanine + tyrosine, 47; threonine, 27; tryptophan, 7; valine, 32; and histidine, 18. This pattern allows comparison of the relative nutritional quality of different protein sources by calculating a protein digestibility corrected amino acid score (PDCAAS). The calculation compares the amino acid in a test protein with the amount of that amino acid in the FNB/IOM scoring pattern multiplied by the true digestibility. Illustration of the calculation involved is detailed in *Dietary Reference Intakes for Energy, Carbohydrate, Fiber, Fat, Fatty Acids, Cholesterol, Protein, and Amino Acids* (2005).

Special Considerations

Multiparous pregnancies: Multiparous pregnancies are associated with a marked increase in low birth weight and perinatal mortality. Thus, it is logical to assume that women supporting the growth of more than one fetus have higher protein needs, and some evidence supports this assumption. Thus, it is prudent that women carrying twins should increase their protein intake by an additional 50 g/day beginning in the second trimester, as well as ensure for themselves a sufficient energy intake to utilize the protein as efficiently as possible.

Physically active individuals: It is commonly believed that athletes should consume a higher-than-normal protein intake to maintain optimum physical performance. However, since compelling evidence of additional need is lacking, no additional dietary protein is suggested for healthy adults who undertake resistance or endurance exercise.

Vegetarian diets: Individuals who restrict their diet to plant-based foods may be at risk of deficiencies in certain indispensable amino acids because the concentration of lysine, sulfur amino acids, and threonine are sometimes lower in plant proteins than in animal proteins. However, vegetarian diets that include complementary mixtures of plant proteins can provide the same quality of protein as that from animal proteins. Available evidence does not support recommending a separate protein requirement for individuals who consume complementary mixtures of plant proteins.

Criteria for Determining Protein Requirements, by Life Stage Group

Life stage group	Criterion
0 through 6 mo	Average consumption of protein from human milk
6 through 12 mo	Nitrogen equilibrium plus protein deposition
1 through 18 y	Nitrogen equilibrium plus protein deposition
> 18y	Nitrogen equilibrium
Pregnancy	Age-specific requirement plus protein deposition
Lactation	Age-specific requirement plus milk nitrogen

The AMDR

The Acceptable Macronutrient Distribution Range (AMDR) for protein is 5–20 percent of total calories for children 1 through 3 years of age, 10–30 percent of total calories for children 4 to 18 years of age, and 10–35 percent of total calories for adults older than 18 years of age (see Part II, "Macronutrients, Healthful Diets, and Physical Activity").

The UL

The Tolerable Upper Intake Level (UL) is the highest level of daily nutrient intake that is likely to pose no risk of adverse effects for almost all people. Data were insufficient to establish a UL for total protein or for any of the amino acids. However, the absence of a UL warrants caution in using any single amino acid at levels significantly above those normally found in food.

PROTEIN SOURCES

Foods

Proteins from animal sources such as meat, poultry, fish, eggs, milk, cheese, and yogurt provide all nine indispensable amino acids and are referred to as "complete proteins." Proteins from plants, legumes, grains, nuts, seeds, and vegetables tend to be deficient in one or more of the indispensable amino acids and are called "incomplete proteins."

Dietary Supplements

With the exception of discussion of amino acids from all sources, this information was not provided at the time the DRI values for protein and amino acids were set. Given limited data, caution is warranted in using any single amino acid at a level significantly above that normally found in food.

Bioavailability

(See "Protein Quality.")

Dietary Interactions

This information was not provided at the time the DRI values for protein and amino acids were set.

INADEQUATE INTAKE AND DEFICIENCY

Both protein and nonprotein energy (from carbohydrates and fats) must be available to prevent protein energy malnutrition (PEM). Similarly, if amino acids are not present in the right balance, the body's ability to use protein will be affected.

Worldwide, PEM is fairly common in both children and adults and is associated with the deaths of about 6 million children each year. In the industrialized world, PEM is predominately seen in hospitals, is associated with disease, or is often found in the elderly.

Protein deficiency has been shown to affect all of the body's organs and many of its systems, including the brain and brain function of infants and young children; the immune system, thus elevating risk of infection; gut mucosal function and permeability, which affects absorption and vulnerability to systemic disease; and kidney function.

The physical signs of protein deficiency include edema, failure to thrive in infants and children, poor musculature, dull skin, and thin and fragile hair. Biochemical changes reflecting protein deficiency include low serum albumin and low serum transferrin.

EXCESS INTAKE

Protein

The risk of adverse effects from excess protein intake from foods appears to be very low. The data are conflicting on the potential for high-protein diets to produce gastrointestinal effects, changes in nitrogen balance, or chronic disease, such as osteoporosis or renal stones. Further research is needed in these areas.

Amino Acids

There is no evidence that amino acids derived from usual or even high intakes of protein from food present any risk. Data were limited on the adverse effects of high levels of amino acid intakes from dietary supplements and therefore caution is warranted in using any single amino acid at a level significantly above that normally found in food.

Special Considerations

Maple syrup urine disease (MSUD): MSUD is the most common disorder associated with genetic anomalies in the metabolism of branched-chain amino acids (BCAAs), such as leucine, isoleucine, and valine. The condition stems from inadequate function of a multienzyme system called branched-chain ketoacid dehydrogenase and is characterized by elevated plasma levels of BCAAs, especially leucine. Although MSUD can be diagnosed in infancy, there are six other forms of the condition that begin later in life. People with MSUD must severely restrict their consumption of BCAAs. Without proper treatment and medical management, mental retardation and death may occur.

Phenylketonuria (PKU): PKU is a genetic disorder that impairs activity of the enzyme phenylalanine hydroxylase (PAH). This allows phenylalanine or by-products of its breakdown to build up in the plasma during critical periods of brain development. Chronically elevated plasma phenylalanine levels before and during infancy and childhood can cause irreversible brain damage, growth retardation, and skin abnormalities. To prevent these problems, dietary phenylalanine must be restricted within one month of birth and this restriction continued at least through childhood and adolescence. In the United States, approximately 1 of every 15,000 infants is born with PKU.

KEY POINTS FOR PROTEIN AND AMINO ACIDS

✓   Protein is the major functional and structural component of every cell in the body. All enzymes, membrane carriers, blood transport molecules, the intracellular matrices, hair, fingernails, serum albumin, keratin, and collagen are proteins, as are many hormones and a large part of membranes.

✓   The amino acids that make up proteins act as precursors for nucleic acids, hormones, vitamins, and other important molecules.

✓   The most important aspect and defining characteristic of protein from a nutritional point of view is its amino acid composition (amino [or imino] nitrogen group).

✓   Although amino acids have traditionally been classified as indispensable (essential) and dispensable (nonessential), accumulating evidence on the metabolic and nutritional characteristics of dispensable amino acids has blurred their definition, forming a third classification called conditionally indispensable.

✓   The quality of a source of dietary protein depends on its ability to provide the nitrogen and amino acid requirements that are necessary for the body's growth, maintenance, and repair.

✓   The adult requirements for protein are based primarily on nitrogen balance studies.

✓   The Acceptable Macronutrient Distribution Range (AMDR) for protein is 5–20 percent of total calories for children 1 through 3 years of age, 10–30 percent of total calories for children 4 to 18 years of age, and 10–35 percent of total calories for adults older than 18 years of age.

✓   Data were insufficient to establish a UL for total protein or amino acids.

✓   Proteins from animal sources such as meat, poultry, fish, eggs, milk, cheese, and yogurt provide all nine indispensable amino acids and are referred to as "complete proteins."

✓   Proteins from plants, legumes, grains, nuts, seeds, and vegetables tend to be deficient in one or more of the indispensable amino acids and are called "incomplete proteins."

✓   Both protein and nonprotein energy (from carbohydrates and fats) must be available to prevent protein-energy malnutrition (PEM).

✓   Protein deficiency has been shown to affect all of the body's organs and many systems.

✓   The data are conflicting on the potential for high-protein diets to produce gastrointestinal effects, changes in nitrogen balance, or chronic disease, such as osteoporosis or renal stones.

✓   There is no evidence that amino acids derived from usual or even high intakes of protein from food present any risk. Data were limited on the adverse effects of high levels of amino acid intakes from dietary supplements and therefore caution is warranted in using any single amino acid at a level significantly above that normally found in food.

TABLE 1 Dietary Reference Intakes for Water by Life Stage Group

	DRI values (L/day)[a]
	AI[b]

Life stage group[c]	
0 through 6 mo	0.7, assumed to be from human milk
7 through 12 mo	0.8 of *total*[d] water, assumed to be from human milk, complementary foods and beverages. This includes approximately 0.6 L (about 3 cups) as total fluid, including formula or human milk, juices, and drinking water.
1 through 3 y	1.3 of *total* water. This includes approximately 0.9 L (about 4 cups) as total beverages, including drinking water.
4 through 8 y	1.7 of *total* water. This includes approximately 1.2 L (about 5 cups) as total beverages, including drinking water.
9 through 13 y	
males	2.4 of *total* water. This includes approximately 1.8 L (about 8 cups) as total beverages, including drinking water.
females	2.1 of *total* water. This includes approximately 1.6 L (about 7 cups) as total beverages, including drinking water.
14 through 18 y	
males	3.3 of *total* water. This includes approximately 2.6 L (about 11 cups) as total beverages, including drinking water.
females	2.3 of *total* water. This includes approximately 1.8 L (about 8 cups) as total beverages, including drinking water.
19 through > 70y	
males	3.7 of *total* water. This includes approximately 3.0 L (about 13 cups) as total beverages, including drinking water.
females	2.7 of *total* water. This includes approximately 2.2 L (about 9 cups) as total beverages, including drinking water.

TABLE 1 Continued

	DRI values (L/day)[a]
	AI[b]

Pregnancy

14 through 50 y — 3.0 of *total* water. This includes approximately 2.3 L (about 10 cups) as total beverages, including drinking water.

Lactation

14 through 50 y — 3.8 of *total* water. This includes approximately 3.1 L (about 13 cups) as total beverages, including drinking water.

[a] Conversion factors: 1 L = 33.8 fluid oz; 1 L = 1.06 qt; 1 cup = 8 fluid oz.

[b] **AI** = Adequate Intake. If sufficient scientific evidence is not available to establish an Estimated Average Requirement (EAR), and thus calculate a Recommended Dietary Allowance (RDA), an AI is usually developed. For healthy breast-fed infants, the AI is the mean intake. The AI for other life stage and gender groups is believed to cover the needs of all healthy individuals in the group, but a lack of data or uncertainty in the data prevents being able to specify with confidence the percentage of individuals covered by this intake.

[c] Life stage groups through 8 years of age represent males and females.

[d] *Total* water (as italicized) includes all water contained in food, beverages, and drinking water. For infants, 7 through 12 months, *total* water assumed to be from human milk, complementary foods and beverages.

WATER

Water, vital for life, is the largest single constituent of the human body, averaging approximately 60 percent of body weight. It is essential for cellular homeostasis and for maintaining vascular volume. It also serves as the medium for transport within the body by supplying nutrients and removing waste.

Since data were insufficient to establish an Estimated Average Requirement (EAR) and thus calculate a Recommended Dietary Allowance (RDA) for water, an Average Intake (AI) was instead developed. The AIs for water are based on the median *total* water intake from U.S. survey data. (*Total* water intake includes drinking water, water in beverages and formula, and water that is contained in food.) These reference values represent the *total* water intake that is considered likely to prevent deleterious, primarily acute, effects of dehydration, including metabolic and functional abnormalities. Although a low intake of *total* water has been associated with some chronic diseases, this evidence is insufficient to establish water intake recommendations as a means to reduce the risk of chronic diseases.

Higher intakes of *total* water will be required for those who are physically active or exposed to hot environments. Because healthy individuals have a considerable ability to excrete excess water and thereby maintain water balance, a Tolerable Upper Intake Level (UL) was not set for water. DRI values for water are listed by life stage group in Table 1.

Over the course of a few hours, body water deficits can occur due to reduced intake or increased water loss from physical activity and environmental (heat) exposure. However, on a day-to-day basis, fluid intake, usually driven by the combination of thirst and mealtime beverage consumption, helps maintain hydration status and total body water (TBW) at normal levels.

Sources of water include beverages, food, and drinking water. Inadequate water intake leads to dehydration. Excessive water intake can lead to hyponatremia, an extremely rare condition marked by a low concentration of sodium in the blood.

WATER AND THE BODY

Function

Water is the solvent for biochemical reactions and represents the largest single constituent of the human body, averaging approximately 60 percent of body weight. Water absorbs the body heat from metabolic processes, maintains vascular volume, and serves as the medium for transport within the body by supplying nutrients and removing waste. It is also essential for cellular homeostasis. Cell hydration has been suggested to be an important signal in the regulation of cell metabolism and gene expression.

Daily water intake must be balanced with water loss in order to maintain total body water (TBW). TBW is comprised of both the intracellular (ICF) and the extracellular (ECF) fluids and varies by individual due to differences in body composition.

Absorption, Metabolism, Storage, and Excretion

Water that is consumed via liquid and food is digested and absorbed within the gastrointestinal tract. Body water is distributed between the ICF and the ECF, which contain 65 and 35 percent of TBW, respectively. Body water balance depends on the net difference between water gain and water loss. Perturbations such as exercise, heat exposure, fever, diarrhea, trauma, and burns will greatly affect the net volumes and water turnover rates between these fluid compartments.

TBW gain occurs from consumption and as a by-product of the metabolization of energy-yielding nutrients from foods. Production of metabolic water is proportional to daily energy expenditure for people eating a mixed diet. TBW loss results from respiratory, skin, renal, and gastrointestinal tract water losses, which are described as follows:

Respiratory: Physical activity generally has a greater effect on water loss through evaporation within the lungs than do environmental factors, such as ambient air temperature and humidity. Daily loss averages about 200–350 mL/day for sedentary people and can increase to 500–600 mL/day for active people who live in temperate climates at sea level.

Urinary and gastrointestinal: Renal output can vary depending on specific macronutrient, salt, and water loads. Urine output inversely varies with body hydration status (usually averaging 1–2 L/day) and also generally increases in healthy older individuals because they are unable to concentrate urine as well as younger individuals. Exercise and heat reduce urine output, while cold and hypoxia increase output. Fecal water loss in healthy adults is approximately 100–200 mL/day.

Skin: Water loss through skin occurs by insensible diffusion and secreted sweat. For the average adult, loss of water by insensible diffusion is approximately 450 mL/day. In hot weather, sweat evaporation is the primary avenue of heat loss to defend the body's core temperature. Daily sweat loss considerably varies due to differences in metabolic rate and environment (e.g., clothing worn, ambient temperatures, air motion, and solar load).

DETERMINING DRIS

Determining Requirements

Since data were insufficient to establish an EAR and thus calculate an RDA for water, an AI was instead developed. The AIs for water are based on median *total* water intakes using survey data from the Third National Health and Nutrition Examination Survey (NHANES III, 1988–1994). These reference values represent *total* water intakes that are considered likely to prevent deleterious, primarily acute, effects of dehydration, including metabolic and functional abnormalities. Although a low intake of *total* water has been associated with some chronic diseases, the evidence is insufficient to establish water intake recommendations as a means to reduce the risk of chronic diseases

As with AIs for other nutrients, for a healthy person, daily consumption below the AI may not confer additional risk because a wide range of intakes is compatible with normal hydration. In this setting, the AI should not be interpreted as a specific requirement. Higher intakes of *total* water will be required for those who are physically active or exposed to hot environments.

Over the course of a few hours, body water deficits can occur due to reduced intake or increased water loss from physical activity and environmental (heat) exposure. However, on a day-to-day basis, fluid intake, usually driven by the combination of thirst and mealtime beverage consumption, helps maintain hydration status and TBW at normal levels.

Special Considerations

Generally, groups that are more active will have a greater total water intake:

- *Active adults:* Physical activity, particularly when performed in hot weather, increases daily fluid needs. Daily water requirements for adults can double in hot weather (86°F or 30°C) and triple in very hot weather (104°F or 40°C) to make up for water lost via sweating.

- *Active children*: Children who are active produce considerably less sweat than active adults, even when exercising in hot environments. This difference in sweat production prevails until midpuberty and should be considered when determining the water requirements of active children and adolescents.
- *Elderly*: Hydration status continues to be normal in elderly individuals over a wide range of intakes. However, a deficit in thirst and fluid intake regulation, age-related impairments in renal-concentrating and sodium-conserving ability, prior history of stroke, or evidence of hypothalamic or pituitary dysfunction may contribute to increased incidence of dehydration and hypernatremia.

Factors Affecting Water Requirements

Physical activity and heat strain: Physical activity and heat strain can substantially increase water loss through sweating. The daily water requirement increases that arise from activity and ambient temperature are the result of increased sweating to meet evaporative cooling requirements. A person's sweating rate depends on climatic conditions, the clothing worn, and exercise intensity and duration. Physical fitness level has a modest effect on sweat loss, unless accompanied by heat acclimation. Studies have shown broad ranges in fluid requirements based on these influences. Examples include:

- People in very hot (e.g., desert) climates, who often have sweating rates of 0.3–1.2 L/hour while performing occupational activities
- People wearing protective clothing, who often have sweating rates of 1–2 L/hour while performing light-intensity exercise in hot weather
- Male competitive runners, who can have sweating rates of 1 to > 2 L/hour while training or racing in the heat
- Female competitive runners may increase their sweat losses from approximately 0.7 L/hour in temperate weather to approximately 1.1 L/hour in warm weather when performing the same event

Altitude and cold temperature: Altitude exposure increases respiratory water loss and hypoxia-induced diuresis. There may also be reduced fluid consumption and, for persons traversing rugged mountain terrains, elevated sweating due to high metabolic rates. The net effect can lead to dehydration. Body fluid loss in cold climates can be as high as loss in hot climates due to high rates of energy expenditure and the use of highly insulated heavy clothing. Fluid loss during cold exposure is thought to result from cold-induced diuresis and increased respiratory loss.

Diabetes mellitus: Dehydration is clearly associated with the worsening control of diabetes. In addition, uncontrolled diabetes dramatically contributes to development of severe dehydration and volume depletion due to osmotic diuresis. In people with poorly controlled diabetes, reduced water intake can also lead to dehydration owing to infection or hypotension, which can lead to delirium and an impaired ability to seek water.

Cystic fibrosis: People with cystic fibrosis have high concentrations of sodium chloride in their sweat. They may lose excessive amounts of sodium and chloride when their sweating rates are high and, unlike healthy people, their body fluid osmolality does not increase due to the high concentrations of sodium chloride in their sweat. Without elevated serum osmolality, a major trigger for thirst, cystic fibrosis patients can quickly become dehydrated during physical activity, particularly in the heat.

Diuretics and other medications: There are no medications that directly stimulate water intake. When decreased fluid intake has occurred due to illness, medications that improve metabolic and cognitive function should indirectly help people increase their fluid intake. Examples include antibiotics for infections, insulin for unstable diabetics, and analgesics for delirium-inducing pain. However, some drugs, such as diuretics, cause excess water loss. Diuretics are commonly used medications that are prescribed for the treatment of conditions such as hypertension, heart failure, and chronic kidney disease. Dehydration may occur in people who do not modify their use of diuretics in hot weather or in other situations where excess water loss occurs. Other medications, such as lithium, may interfere with the kidneys' regulatory systems, leading to excessive water loss.

Criteria for Determining *Total* Water Requirements, by Life Stage Group

Life stage group	Criterion
0 through 6 months	Average consumption from human milk content
7 through 12 months	Average consumption from human milk + complementary foods and other beverages
1 through > 70 y	Median *total* water intake using data from NHANES III
Pregnancy	Same as age-specific values for nonpregnant women
Lactation	Same as age-specific values for nonpregnant women

The UL

The Tolerable Upper Intake Level (UL) is the highest level of daily nutrient intake that is likely to pose no risk of adverse effects for almost all people. Because healthy individuals have considerable ability to excrete excess water and thereby maintain water balance, a UL was not set for water. However, acute water toxicity has been reported from the rapid consumption of large quantities of fluids that greatly exceeded the kidneys' maximal excretion rate of approximately 0.7–1.0 L/hour.

According to NHANES III (1988–1994), the highest total water intake (99th percentile) reported was 8.1 L/day. No adverse intakes have been reported with chronic high intakes of water in health people consuming a normal diet, as long as fluid intake is approximately proportional to losses.

DIETARY SOURCES

Sources of water include beverages, food, and drinking water. Fruits and vegetables contain a high percentage of water. According to data from NHANES III, adults in the United States obtained *total* water from the following sources:

- 35–54 percent from drinking water
- 49–63 percent from other beverages (with juice, carbonated drinks, coffee, and milk being the major sources)
- 19–25 percent from foods (such as fruits, vegetables, soups, ice cream, and meats)

Dietary Interactions

There is evidence that water may interact with certain nutrients and dietary substances (see Table 2).

INADEQUATE INTAKE

Inadequate water intake leads to dehydration, the effects of which include the following:

- Impaired mental function and motor control
- Diminished aerobic and endurance exercise performance
- Enhanced fever response (fever is a regulated rise in body temperature)
- Increased core temperature during exercise
- Reduced tolerance to the stress of exercise and heat
- Increased resting heart rate when standing or lying down

TABLE 2 Potential Substances That Affect Water Requirements

Substance	Potential Interaction	Notes
SUBSTANCES THAT AFFECT WATER REQUIREMENTS		
Caffeine	Due to its diuretic effect, caffeine in high amounts may lead to a total body water (TBW) deficit.	Available data were inconsistent. Unless future research proves otherwise, caffeinated beverages appear to contribute to total water intake to the same degree as noncaffeinated fluids do.
Alcohol	Alcohol intake appears to increase water excretion.	Based on limited data, ethanol ingestion did not appear to result in appreciable fluid loss over a 24-hour period. An increased excretion of water due to ethanol ingestion was transient.
Sodium	Increased sodium intake may increase urine volume.	Based on limited data, it was not possible to determine the extent to which sodium intake influences water intake.
Protein	Increased protein consumption may increase water needs. Urea, a major end product of the metabolism of dietary proteins and amino acids, requires water for excretion by the kidneys.	Studies showed that increased protein intake did not affect water intake or urine volume in the setting of *ad libitum* water consumption.
Fiber	Fecal water loss is increased with increased dietary fiber.	Limited studies showed significant increases in fecal water loss with high-fiber diets.
Carbohydrate	The presence of dietary carbohydrates may affect	On average, 100 g/day of carbohydrates (the amount needed to prevent ketosis) has been shown to decrease body water deficit by decreasing the quantity of body solutes (ketone bodies) that need to be excreted. This response is similar when ketosis occurs with the consumption of very low carbohydrate diets.

- Impaired ability to maintain blood pressure when presented with vascular challenges
- Fainting (in susceptible people)
- Reduced cardiac output during exercise and heat stress
- Apparent increased risk of life-threatening heat stroke

EXCESS INTAKE

No adverse effects have been reported with chronic high intakes of water by healthy people who consume a normal diet, as long as fluid intake is approximately proportional to fluid loss. Excessive water intake can lead to hyponatremia, which is a low concentration of sodium in the blood (defined as serum sodium concentration of less than 135 mmol/L). The lowering of the extracellular fluid sodium concentration causes fluid to move into the intracellular fluid space, resulting in central nervous system edema, lung congestion, and muscle weakness. Hyponatremia can also occur from excessive fluid intake, the under-replacement of sodium, or both, during or after prolonged endurance athletic events. In severe cases, hyponatremia can be life-threatening.

Hyponatremia is rare in healthy persons who consume an average North American diet. The condition is most often seen in infants, psychiatric patients with psychogenic polydipsia (chronic excessive thirst and fluid intake), patients on psychotropic drugs, women who have undergone surgery using a uterine distension medium, and participants in prolonged endurance events, such as military recruits.

A series of case studies has suggested that gross overconsumption of fluids (for example, more than 20 L/day) is associated with irreversible bladder lesions and possibly thinner bladder muscles, delayed bladder sensation, and flow rate impairment.

KEY POINTS FOR WATER

✓   Water, vital for life, is essential for cellular homeostasis and for maintaining vascular volume. It also serves as the medium for transport within the body by supplying nutrients and removing waste.

✓   Since data were insufficient to establish an EAR and thus calculate an RDA for water, an AI was instead developed.

✓   The AIs for water are based on the median *total* water intake from U.S. survey data. These reference values represent *total* water intakes that are considered likely to prevent deleterious, primarily acute, effects of dehydration, including metabolic and functional abnormalities.

✓   Although a low intake of *total* water has been associated with some chronic diseases, this evidence is insufficient to establish water intake recommendations as a means to reduce the risk of chronic diseases.

✓   Over the course of a few hours, body water deficits can occur due to reduced intake or increased water loss from physical activity and environmental (heat) exposure. However, on a day-to-day basis, fluid intake, driven by the combination of thirst and mealtime beverage consumption, helps maintain hydration status and total body water at normal levels.

✓   Because healthy individuals have a considerable ability to excrete excess water and thereby maintain water balance, a UL was not set for water.

✓   Acute water toxicity has been reported from the rapid consumption of large quantities of fluids that greatly exceeded the kidneys' maximal excretion rate of approximately 0.7–1.0 L/hour.

✓   Sources of water include drinking water, beverages, and food.

✓   Inadequate water intake leads to dehydration, which can impair mental function, exercise performance, exercise and heat stress tolerance, and blood pressure regulation.

✓   Excessive water intake can lead to hyponatremia, which is a low concentration of sodium in the blood. This condition leads to central nervous system edema, lung congestion, and muscle weakness.

PART III
VITAMINS AND MINERALS

Part Three of this publication summarizes information from the DRI reports titled *Dietary Reference Intakes for Vitamin C, Vitamin E, Selenium, and Carotenoids* (2000); *Dietary Reference Intakes for Water, Potassium, Sodium, Chloride, and Sulfate* (2005); *Dietary Reference Intakes for Calcium, Phosphorus, Magnesium, Vitamin D, and Fluoride* (1997); *Dietary Reference Intakes for Thiamin, Riboflavin, Niacin, Vitamin B$_6$, Folate, Vitamin B$_{12}$, Pantothenic Acid, Biotin, and Choline* (1998); and *Dietary Reference Intakes for Vitamin A, Vitamin K, Arsenic, Boron, Chromium, Copper, Iodine, Iron, Manganese, Molybdenum, Nickel, Silicon, Vanadium, and Zinc* (2001). This section is divided into chapters that are organized by nutrient for 35 individual vitamins and minerals. Each chapter provides a table of known nutrient reference values; reviews the function of a given nutrient in the human body; summarizes the known effects of deficiencies and excessive intakes; describes how a nutrient may be related to chronic disease or developmental abnormalities, where data were available; and provides the indicator of adequacy for determining the nutrient requirements.

Vitamins covered in Part Three include vitamin A, vitamin B$_6$, vitamin B$_{12}$, biotin, vitamin C, carotenoids, choline, vitamin D, vitamin E, folate, vitamin K, niacin, pantothenic acid, riboflavin, and thiamin. Minerals covered in Part Three include calcium, chromium, copper, fluoride, iodine, iron, magnesium, manganese, molybdenum, phosphorus, potassium, selenium, sodium chloride, sulfate, and zinc; there is also a chapter on other substances including arsenic, boron, nickel, silicon, and vanadium.

DEFINITIONS USED IN TABLES IN PART III

EAR = Estimated Average Requirement. An EAR is the average daily nutrient intake level estimated to meet the requirements of half of the healthy individuals in a group.

RDA = Recommended Dietary Allowance. An RDA is the average daily dietary intake level sufficient to meet the nutrient requirements of nearly all (97–98 percent) healthy individuals in a group.

AI = Adequate Intake. If sufficient scientific evidence is not available to establish an EAR, and thus calculate an RDA, an AI is usually developed. For healthy breast-fed infants, the AI is the mean intake. The AI for other life stage and gender groups is believed to cover the needs of all healthy individuals in the group, but a lack of data or uncertainty in the data prevents being able to specify with confidence the percentage of individuals covered by this intake.

UL = Tolerable Upper Intake Level. The UL is the highest level of daily nutrient intake that is likely to pose no risk of adverse health effects to almost all individuals in the general population. Unless otherwise specified, the UL represents total intake from food, water, and supplements. In the absence of a UL, extra caution may be warranted in consuming levels above the recommended intake. Members of the general population should be advised not to routinely exceed the UL. The UL is not meant to apply to individuals who are treated with the nutrient under medical supervision or to individuals with predisposing conditions that modify their sensitivity to the nutrient.

TABLE 1 Dietary Reference Intakes for Vitamin A by Life Stage Group

	DRI values (µg RAE[a]/day)					
	EAR[b]		RDA[c]		AI[d]	UL[e,f]
	males	females	males	females		
Life stage group						
0 through 6 mo					400	600
7 through 12 mo					500	600
1 through 3 y	210	210	300	300		600
4 through 8 y	275	275	400	400		900
9 through 13 y	445	420	600	600		1,700
14 through 18 y	630	485	900	700		2,800
19 through 30 y	625	500	900	700		3,000
31 through 50 y	625	500	900	700		3,000
51 through 70 y	625	500	900	700		3,000
> 70 y	625	500	900	700		3,000
Pregnancy						
≤ 18 y		530		750		2,800
19 through 50 y		550		770		3,000
Lactation						
≤ 18 y		885		1,200		2,800
19 through 50 y		900		1,300		3,000

[a] **RAE** = Retinol activity equivalent. 1 µg RAE = 1 µg retinol, 12 µg β-carotene, and 24 µg α-carotene or β-cryptoxanthin. The RAE for dietary provitamin A carotenoids in foods is twofold greater than retinol equivalents (RE), whereas the RAE for preformed vitamin A in foods is the same as RE.

[b] **EAR** = Estimated Average Requirement.

[c] **RDA** = Recommended Dietary Allowance.

[d] **AI** = Adequate Intake.

[e] **UL** = Tolerable Upper Intake Level.

[f] The UL for vitamin A applies only to preformed vitamin A (e.g., retinol, the form of vitamin A found in animal foods, most fortified foods, and supplements). It does not apply to vitamin A derived from carotenoids.

VITAMIN A

Vitamin A is a fat-soluble nutrient that is important for vision, gene expression, reproduction, embryonic development, growth, and immune function. Forms of vitamin A include retinol (preformed vitamin A), retinal, retinoic acid, and retinyl esters. The term vitamin A also includes provitamin A carotenoids that are dietary precursors of retinol. The term retinoids refers to retinol and its metabolites, and any synthetic analogues that have a similar structure.

The requirements for vitamin A are now denoted in retinol activity equivalents (RAEs), such that 1 µg RAE = 1µg all-*trans*-retinol, 12 µg β-carotene, and 24 µg α-carotene or β-cryptoxanthin. This recognizes that 50 percent less bioconversion of carotenoids to vitamin A occurs than was previously thought when vitamin A was expressed in retinol equivalents (REs). The change means that twice the amount of provitamin A–rich carotenoids contained in leafy green vegetables and certain fruits is required to provide a given amount of vitamin A activity.

The requirements for vitamin A are based on the assurance of adequate liver stores of vitamin A. The Tolerable Upper Intake Level (UL) is based on liver abnormalities as the critical endpoint. For women of childbearing age, the UL is based on teratogenicity as the critical adverse effect. DRI values are listed by life stage group in Table 1.

Preformed vitamin A (retinol) is naturally found in animal-based foods, whereas dietary carotenoids (provitamin A carotenoids), which are converted to vitamin A in the body, are present in oils, fruits, and vegetables. Common dietary sources of preformed vitamin A in the United States and Canada include liver, dairy products, and fish. Foods fortified with vitamin A are margarine and low-fat and nonfat (skim and partly skimmed) milk. Provitamin A carotenoids are found in carrots, broccoli, squash, peas, spinach, and cantaloupe.

The most specific clinical effect of vitamin A deficiency is xerophthalmia and its various stages, including night blindness, conjunctival xerosis, Bitot's spots, corneal xerosis, corneal ulceration, and scarring. Preformed vitamin A toxicity (hypervitaminosis A) due to high vitamin A intakes may be acute or chronic.

VITAMIN A AND THE BODY

Function

Vitamin A is a fat-soluble vitamin that is important for normal vision, gene expression, reproduction, embryonic development, growth, and immune function. Forms of vitamin A include retinol (preformed vitamin A), retinal, retinoic acid, and retinyl esters. Some examples of vitamin A functions include retinal, which is required by the eye to transduce light into the neural signals necessary for vision; retinoic acid, which is required to maintain normal differentiation of the cornea and conjunctival membranes, thus preventing xerophthalmia; and retinioic acid, which is required to regulate the expression of various genes that encode for structural proteins (e.g., skin keratins), enzymes (e.g., alcohol dehydrogenase), extracellular matrix proteins (e.g., laminin), and retinol binding proteins and receptors.

The term vitamin A also includes provitamin A carotenoids that are the dietary precursors of retinol. The term retinoids refers to retinol and its metabolites, and any synthetic analogues that have a similar structure to retinol. Of the more than 600 forms of carotenoids found in nature, several have provitamin A nutritional activity, but food composition data are available for only three (α-carotene, β-carotene, and β-cryptoxanthin). The proposed functions of provitamin A carotenoids are described in Part III, "Carotenoids."

Absorption, Metabolism, Storage, and Excretion

Preformed vitamin A (retinol) is absorbed in the small intestine. The efficiency of absorption of preformed vitamin A is generally high, ranging from 70 to 90 percent. Absorption is carrier-mediated and saturable, but becomes nonsaturable at high pharmacological doses. As the amount of ingested preformed vitamin A increases, its absorbability remains high.

Carotenoids are absorbed into the small intestine by passive diffusion. Efficiency of absorption has been estimated at 9–22 percent, although this decreases as the amount ingested increases. Some carotenoids (β-carotene, α-carotene, and β-cryptoxanthin) are converted to vitamin A in the body.

Along with exogenous lipids, retinal esters (newly formed in the intestine) and nonhydrolyzed carotenoids are transported from the intestine to the liver in chylomicrons and chylomicron remnants. Retinoic acid, another form of vitamin A, is absorbed via the portal system bound to albumin. Liver, lung, adipose, and other tissues possess carotene enzyme activity, and so it is presumed that carotenes may be converted to vitamin A as they are delivered to tissues.

When vitamin A intake is adequate, more than 90 percent of total body vitamin A is located in the liver, which releases the nutrient into the circulation in a process that depends on the availability of retinol binding protein (RBP). That which is not released remains stored in the liver. The majority of vitamin A metabolites are excreted in the urine; some vitamin A is also excreted in the bile. Amounts excreted via the bile increase as the liver vitamin A exceeds a critical concentration. This serves as a protective mechanism for reducing the risk of excess storage.

DETERMINING DRIS

Determining Requirements

The requirements for vitamin A are based on the assurance of adequate liver stores of vitamin A. Although a large body of observational epidemiological evidence suggests that higher blood concentrations of β-carotenes and other carotenoids obtained from foods are associated with a lower risk of several chronic diseases, there is currently insufficient evidence to support a recommendation that requires a certain percentage of dietary vitamin A to come from provitamin A carotenoids in meeting the vitamin A requirement. However, existing recommendations for the increased consumption of carotenoid-rich fruits and vegetables for their health-promoting benefits are strongly supported (see Part III, "Carotenoids"). For example, consuming the recommended 5 servings of fruits and vegetables per day could provide 5.2–6 mg/day of provitamin A carotenoids, which would constitute approximately 50–65 percent of the adult male RDA for vitamin A.

Special Considerations

Vegetarian diets: Preformed vitamin A (retinol) is found only in animal-based foods. People who do not consume such foods must meet their requirements with foods that contain sufficient provitamin A carotenoids, such as deeply colored fruits and vegetables, or with fortified foods, such as margarine, some plant-based beverages, and cereals.

Parasites and infection: Malabsorption of vitamin A can occur with diarrhea and intestinal infections, such as those observed in developing countries. With infection and fever, the requirement for vitamin A may be greater than the requirements listed in this chapter, which are based on generally healthy individuals.

Retinol Activity Equivalents (RAEs)

Based on data demonstrating that the efficiency of absorption of β-carotene is less than what has been traditionally thought, retinol activity equivalents (RAEs) were developed to address the new findings about reduced absorption of β-carotene. The requirements for vitamin A are now denoted in RAEs rather than retinol equivalents (REs). Using μg RAEs, the vitamin A activity of provitamin A carotenoids is half of the vitamin A activity that is assumed when using μg REs. This change in equivalency values is based on data demonstrating that the vitamin A activity of purified β-carotene in oil is half of the activity of vitamin A. It is also based on recent data demonstrating that the vitamin A activity of dietary β-carotene is one-sixth, rather than one-third, of the vitamin activity of purified β-carotene in oil. This change in bioconversion means that a larger amount of provitamin A carotenoids, and therefore darkly colored, carotene-rich fruits and vegetables, is needed to meet the vitamin A requirement. It also means that, in the past, vitamin A intake has been overestimated. The RAEs for dietary β-carotene, α-carotene, and β-cryptoxanthin are 12, 24, and 24 μg, respectively, compared to the corresponding REs of 6, 12, and 12 μg reported by the National Research Council in 1989 (see Figure 1).

Nutrient databases will need to be revised to provide total vitamin A activity in μg RAE. In the meantime, it is possible to estimate total vitamin A activity in μg RAE from existing tables that list μg RE. For foods, such as liver, that

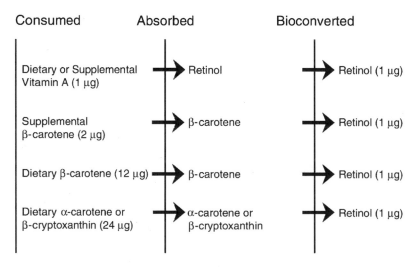

FIGURE 1 Absorption and bioconversion of ingested provitamin A carotenoids to retinol based on new equivalency factors (retinol equivalency ratio).

contain only vitamin A activity from preformed vitamin A (retinol), no adjustment is necessary. Vitamin A values for foods that contain only plant sources (provitamin A carotenoids) of vitamin A can be adjusted by dividing the μg RE by two. For foods that contain both plant and animal sources of vitamin A (e.g., a casserole containing meat and vegetables), the adjustment process is more complex. (See Appendix F for more information on determining the vitamin A content of foods.)

Supplemental β-carotene has a higher bioconversion to vitamin A than does dietary β-carotene. With low doses, the conversion is as high as 2:1; developers of composition information for dietary supplements should use this higher conversion factor. Little is known about the bioconversion of the forms of β-carotene that are added to foods, so fortification of forms of β-carotene should be assumed to have the same bioconversion as food forms, 12:1.

Food and supplement labels usually state vitamin A levels in International Units (IUs). One IU of retinol is equivalent to 0.3 μg of retinol, or 0.3 μg RAE. One IU of β-carotene in supplements is equivalent to 0.5 IU of retinol, or 0.15 μg RAE (0.3 × 0.5). One IU of dietary β-carotene is equivalent to 0.165 IU retinol, or 0.05 μg RAE (0.3 × 0.165). One IU of other dietary provitamin A carotenoids is equivalent to 0.025 μg RAE.

Equivalency examples:
- Example 1. A diet contains 500 μg retinol, 1,800 μg β-carotene and 2,400 μg β-carotene: 500 + (1,800 ÷ 12) + (2,400 ÷ 24) = 750 μg RAE
- Example 2. A diet contains 1,666 IU of retinol and 3,000 IU of β-carotene: (1,666 × 0.3) + (3,000 × 0.05) = 650 μg RAE
- Example 3. A supplement contains 5,000 IU of vitamin A: 5,000 × 0.3 = 1,500 μg RAE

For more information on vitamin A conversions, please see Appendix F.

Criteria for Determining Vitamin A Requirements, by Life Stage Group

Life stage group	Criterion
0 through 6 mo	Average vitamin A intake from human milk
7 through 12 mo	Extrapolation from 0 through 6 mo AI
1 through 18 y	Extrapolation from adult EAR
19 through > 70 y	Adequate liver vitamin A stores

Pregnancy

≤18 y	Age-specific requirement + estimated daily accumulation by fetus
19 through 50 y	Age-specific requirement + estimated daily accumulation by fetus

Lactation

≤18 y	Age-specific requirement + average amount of vitamin A secreted in human milk
19 through 50 y	Age-specific requirement + average amount of vitamin A secreted in human milk

The UL

The Tolerable Upper Intake Level (UL) is the highest level of daily nutrient intake that is likely to pose no risk of adverse effects for almost all people. Members of the general population should not routinely exceed the UL, which for vitamin A applies to the chronic intake of preformed vitamin A from foods, fortified foods, and some supplements. The UL for adults is based on liver abnormalities as the critical adverse effect; for women of childbearing age, the UL is based on teratogenicity as the critical adverse effect. High β-carotene intakes have not been shown to cause hypervitaminosis A.

Based on data from the Third National Health and Nutrition Examination Survey (NHANES III, 1994–1996), the highest median intake of preformed vitamin A for any gender and life stage group was 895 µg/day for lactating women. The highest reported intake at the 95th percentile was 1,503 µg/day for lactating women. For U.S. adults who took supplements containing vitamin A, intakes at the 95th percentile ranged from approximately 1,500 to 3,000 µg/day. Fewer than 5 percent of pregnant women had dietary and supplemental intake levels that exceeded the UL. The risk of exceeding the UL for vitamin A appears to be small based on the intakes cited above.

Special Considerations

Individuals susceptible to adverse effects: People with high alcohol intake, pre-existing liver disease, hyperlipidemia, or severe protein malnutrition may be distinctly susceptible to the adverse effects of excess preformed vitamin A intake. These individuals may not be protected by the UL for vitamin A for the general population. The UL is not meant to apply to communities of malnourished individuals prophylactically receiving vitamin A, either periodically or through fortification, as a means to prevent vitamin A deficiency, or for individuals being treated with vitamin A for diseases such as retinitis pigmentosa.

DIETARY SOURCES

Foods

Preformed vitamin A (retinol) is found naturally in animal-based foods, whereas dietary carotenoids, which are converted to vitamin A in the body, are present in oils, fruits, and vegetables. Common dietary sources of preformed vitamin A in the United States and Canada include liver, dairy products, and fish. However, according to data from the Continuing Survey of Food Intakes by Individuals (CSFII, 1994–1996), in the United States the major contributors of vitamin A from foods were grains (fortified with vitamin A) and vegetables (which contain provitamin A carotenoids) at approximately 55 percent, followed by dairy and meat products at approximately 30 percent.

Foods fortified with vitamin A are margarine and low-fat and non-fat (skim and partly skimmed) milk. Major contributors as provitamin A carotenoids to dietary intake include: β-carotene found in carrots, broccoli, squash, peas, spinach, and cantaloupe; carrots as α-carotene; and fruits as the sole contributors of β-cryptoxanthin.

Dietary Supplements

According to NHANES III data, the median intake of vitamin A from supplements was approximately 1,430 μg RAE/day for men and women. According to U.S. data from the 1986 National Health Interview Survey (NHIS), approximately 26 percent of adults in the United States took supplements that contained vitamin A.

Bioavailability

Factors such as dietary fat intake, intestinal infections, the food matrix, and food processing can affect the absorption of vitamin A by the body. Dietary fat appears to enhance absorption, whereas absorption is diminished in individuals with diarrhea, intestinal infections, and infestations. The matrix of foods affects the ability of carotenoids to be released from food. For example, serum β-carotene concentration was significantly lower when individuals consumed β-carotene from carrots than from β-carotene supplements. Food processing affects the absorption of carotenoids. For example, absorption is greater from cooked compared to raw carrots and spinach.

Dietary Interactions

There is evidence that vitamin A may interact with certain nutrients and dietary substances (see Table 2).

TABLE 2 Potential Interactions with Other Dietary Substances

Substance	Potential Interaction	Notes
SUBSTANCES THAT AFFECT VITAMIN A		
Dietary fat	Dietary fat may enhance the absorption of vitamin A and provitamin A carotenoids.	Research results in this area are mixed.
Iron	Iron deficiency may negatively affect vitamin A status.	It was reported that iron deficiency alters the distribution of vitamin A concentration between the plasma and liver.
Zinc	Zinc deficiency may negatively affect vitamin A status.	Zinc deficiency influences the mobilization of vitamin A from the liver and its transport into the circulation. However, human studies have not established a consistent relationship between zinc and vitamin A status. It has been suggested that zinc intake may positively affect vitamin A status only in individuals with moderate to severe protein-energy malnutrition.
Alcohol	Alcohol consumption may negatively affect vitamin A status.	Because both retinol and ethanol are alcohols, there is potential for overlap in the metabolic pathways of these two compounds. Ethanol consumption results in a depletion of liver vitamin A stores in humans. Although the effect on vitamin A is due, in part, to liver damage associated with chronic alcohol intake and to malnutrition, the reduction in liver stores of vitamin A is also a direct effect of alcohol consumption.
VITAMIN A AFFECTING OTHER SUBSTANCES		
Iron	Vitamin A deficiency may negatively affect iron status.	Studies suggest that vitamin A deficiency impairs iron mobilization from stores and that, therefore, vitamin A supplementation improves hemoglobin concentrations.

INADEQUATE INTAKE AND DEFICIENCY

The most specific clinical effect of inadequate vitamin A intake is xerophthalmia, which is estimated to affect 3 million to 10 million children (mostly in developing countries) annually. Of those affected, 250,000 to 300,000 go blind every year. Xerophthalmia is an irreversible drying of the conjunctiva and cornea. Various stages of the disease include night blindness (impaired dark adaptation due to the slowed regeneration of rhodopsin), conjunctival xerosis, Bitot's spots, corneal xerosis, corneal ulceration, and scarring, all related to vitamin A deficiency. Night blindness is the first ocular symptom to be observed with vitamin A deficiency; however, it does respond rapidly to treatment with vitamin A.

Other adverse effects associated with vitamin A deficiency include decreased immune function and an increased risk of infectious morbidity and mortality, such as respiratory infection and diarrhea. Although vitamin A supplementation has been shown to reduce the severity of diarrhea, it has had little effect on the risk or severity of respiratory infections, except when associated with measles. The World Health Organization (WHO) recommends treating children who suffer from xerophthalmia, measles, prolonged diarrhea, wasting malnutrition, and other acute infections with vitamin A. Furthermore, the American Academy of Pediatrics recommends vitamin A supplementation for children in the United States who are hospitalized with measles.

EXCESS INTAKE

Preformed vitamin A toxicity (hypervitaminosis A) due to high vitamin A intakes may be acute or chronic. (High β-carotene intake has not been shown to produce vitamin A toxicity.) Acute toxicity usually produces transient effects resulting from single or short-term large doses of retinol $\geq$ 150,000 μg in adults and proportionately less in children and is characterized by the following:

- Nausea
- Vomiting
- Headache
- Increased cerebrospinal fluid pressure
- Vertigo
- Blurred vision
- Muscular incoordination
- Bulging fontanel (in infants)

Chronic toxicity is usually associated with the ingestion of large doses of retinol $\geq$ 30,000 μg/day for months or years. Chronic toxicity generally produces less specific and more varied symptoms, such as birth defects, liver abnormalities, reduced bone mineral density, and disorders of the central nervous system. More research is needed to clarify whether chronic vitamin A intake may lead to loss in bone mineral density and a consequent increased risk of hip fracture in certain population groups, particularly among premenopausal and postmenopausal women.

Human and animal data show a strong causal association between excess vitamin A intake and liver abnormalities because the liver is the main storage site and target organ for vitamin A toxicity. These abnormalities range from reversibly elevated liver enzymes to widespread fibrosis, cirrhosis, and sometimes death.

Special Considerations

Teratogenicity: Concern for the possible teratogenicity of high vitamin A intake in humans is based on the unequivocal demonstration of human teratogenicity following high-dose supplementation of vitamin A. The critical period for susceptibility appears to be during the first trimester of pregnancy. The primary birth defects associated with excess vitamin A intake are those derived from cranial neural crest cells, such as craniofacial malformations and abnormalities of the central nervous system (except neural tube defects), thymus, and heart. Most of the human data on teratogenicity of vitamin A involve doses ≥ 7,800 μg/day.

Adverse effects in infants and children: There are several case reports of toxic effects of vitamin A in infants, toddlers, and children who have ingested excess vitamin A for a period of months to years. Of particular concern are intracranial (bulging fontanel) and skeletal abnormalities that can result in infants who are given vitamin A doses of 5,500–6,750 μg/day. Other effects of toxicity in infants and children include bone tenderness and pain, increased intracranial pressure, desquamation, brittle nails, mouth fissures, alopecia, fever, headache, lethargy, irritability, weight loss, vomiting, and hepatomegaly.

KEY POINTS FOR VITAMIN A

✓   Vitamin A is a fat-soluble vitamin that is important for normal vision, gene expression, reproduction, embryonic development, growth, and immune function.

✓   The requirements for vitamin A are now denoted in retinol activity equivalents (RAEs), such that 1 RAE = 1 µg all-*trans*-retinol, 12 µg β-carotene, and 24 µg α-carotene or β-cryptoxanthin.

✓   The requirements for vitamin A are based on the assurance of adequate liver stores of vitamin A. The UL is based on liver abnormalities as the critical endpoint; for women of childbearing age, the UL is based on teratogenicity as the critical adverse effect.

✓   People with high alcohol intake, preexisting liver disease, hyperlipidemia, or severe protein malnutrition may not be protected by the UL set for the general population.

✓   Food and supplement labels usually state vitamin A levels in International Units, or IUs. One IU of retinol is equivalent to 0.3 µg of retinol, or 0.3 µg RAE.

✓   There is currently insufficient evidence to support a recommendation that requires a certain percentage of dietary vitamin A to come from provitamin A carotenoids in meeting the vitamin A requirement. However, existing recommendations for the increased consumption of carotenoid-rich fruits and vegetables for their health-promoting benefits are strongly supported.

✓   Preformed Vitamin A (retinol) is found naturally only in animal-based foods.

✓   Good sources of provitamin A carotenoids are fruits and vegetables, including carrots, broccoli, squash, peas, spinach, and cantaloupe.

✓   The most specific clinical effect of inadequate vitamin A intake and deficiency is xerophthalmia, an irreversible drying of the conjunctiva and cornea.

✓   Vitamin A toxicity (hypervitaminosis A) may be acute or chronic. (High β-carotene intake has not been shown to produce vitamin A toxicity.) The adverse effects of excess vitamin A are from excessive intake of preformed vitamin A, or retinol.

TABLE 1 Dietary Reference Intakes for Vitamin B$_6$ by Life Stage Group

	DRI values (mg/day)					
	EAR[a]		RDA[b]		AI[c]	UL[d]
	males	females	males	females		
Life stage group						
0 through 6 mo					0.1	ND[e]
7 through 12 mo					0.3	ND
1 through 3 y	0.4	0.4	0.5	0.5		30
4 through 8 y	0.5	0.5	0.6	0.6		40
9 through 13 y	0.8	0.8	1.0	1.0		60
14 through 18 y	1.1	1.0	1.3	1.2		80
19 through 30 y	1.1	1.1	1.3	1.3		100
31 through 50 y	1.1	1.1	1.3	1.3		100
51 through 70 y	1.4	1.3	1.7	1.5		100
> 70 y	1.4	1.3	1.7	1.5		100
Pregnancy						
≤ 18 y		1.6		1.9		80
19 through 50 y		1.6		1.9		100
Lactation						
≤ 18 y		1.7		2.0		80
19 through 50 y		1.7		2.0		100

[a] **EAR** = Estimated Average Requirement.

[b] **RDA** = Recommended Dietary Allowance.

[c] **AI** = Adequate Intake.

[d] **UL** = Tolerable Upper Intake Level. Unless otherwise specified, the UL represents total intake from food, water, and supplements.

[e] **ND** = Not determinable. This value is not determinable due to the lack of data of adverse effects in this age group and concern regarding the lack of ability to handle excess amounts. Source of intake should only be from food to prevent high levels of intake.

VITAMIN B$_6$

V itamin B$_6$ (pyridoxine and related compounds) functions as a coenzyme in the metabolism of amino acids, glycogen, and sphingoid bases. Vitamin B$_6$ comprises a group of six related compounds: pyridoxal (PL), pyridoxine (PN), pyridoxamine (PM), and their respective 5'-phosphates (PLP, PNP, and PMP). The major forms found in animal tissue are PLP and PMP; plant-derived foods primarily contain PN and PNP, sometimes in the form of a glucoside.

The primary criterion used to estimate the requirements for vitamin B$_6$ is a plasma pyridoxal 5'-phosphate value of at least 20 nmol/L. The Tolerable Upper Intake Level (UL) is based on sensory neuropathy as the critical adverse effect. DRI values are listed by life stage group in Table 1.

Rich food sources of vitamin B$_6$ include highly fortified cereals, beef liver and other organ meats, and highly fortified, soy-based meat substitutes. The clinical signs and symptoms of vitamin B$_6$ deficiency have only been observed during depletion with very low levels of the vitamin and have never been seen at intakes of 0.5 mg/day or more. No adverse effects have been associated with high intakes of the vitamin from food sources. Very large oral doses (2,000 mg/day or more on a chronic basis) of supplemental pyridoxine have been associated with the development of sensory neuropathy and dermatological lesions.

VITAMIN B$_6$ AND THE BODY

Function

Vitamin B$_6$ functions as a coenzyme in the metabolism of amino acids, glycogen, and sphingoid bases. Vitamin B$_6$ comprises a group of six related compounds: pyridoxal (PL), pyridoxine (PN), pyridoxamine (PM), and their respective 5'-phosphates (PLP, PNP, and PMP). The major forms found in animal tissue are PLP and PMP; plant-derived foods primarily contain PN and PNP, sometimes in the form of a glucoside.

Absorption, Metabolism, Storage, and Excretion

Absorption of vitamin B$_6$ in the gut occurs via phosphatase-mediated hydrolysis followed by the transport of the nonphosphorylated form into the mucosal cell. Transport occurs by nonsaturable passive diffusion. Even large doses of the nutrient are well absorbed.

Most of the absorbed nonphosphorylated vitamin B_6 goes to the liver, and certain forms of the vitamin (pyridoxal, pyridoxine, and pyridoxamine) are converted to their respective 5'-phosphates by pyridoxal kinase. Vitamin B_6 can be bound to proteins in tissues, which limits accumulation at very high intakes. When this capacity is exceeded, nonphosphorylated forms of vitamin B_6 are released by the liver and other tissues into the circulation. At pharmacological doses of vitamin B_6, high amounts accumulate in the muscle, plasma, and erythrocytes when other tissues are saturated.

Most of the body's vitamin B_6 is found in the muscle; the muscle pool of the vitamin appears to very slowly turn over. Vitamin B_6 is oxidized in the liver and then released and primarily excreted in the urine.

DETERMINING DRIS

Determining Requirements

The primary criterion used to estimate the requirements for vitamin B_6 is a plasma 5'-pyridoxal phosphate value of at least 20 nmol/L.

Criteria for Determining Vitamin B_6 Requirements, by Life Stage Group

Life stage group	Criterion
0 through 6 mo	Human milk content
7 through 12 mo	Mean of extrapolation from younger infants and from adults
1 through 18 y	Extrapolation from adults
19 through > 70 y	Plasma pyridoxal 5'-phosphate level
Pregnancy	
≤ 18 y through 50 y	Plasma pyridoxal 5'-phosphate level
Lactation	
≤ 18 y through 50 y	Amount of vitamin B_6 secreted in milk

The UL

The Tolerable Upper Intake Level (UL) is the highest level of daily nutrient intake that is likely to pose no risk of adverse effects for almost all people. Members of the general population should not routinely consume more than the UL. For adults, the UL for Vitamin B_6 represents total intake from food, water, and supplements and is based on sensory neuropathy as the critical adverse effect. The UL is not meant to apply to individuals who are receiving vitamin B$_6$ under medical supervision.

Based on data from the Third National Health and Nutrition Examination Survey (NHANES III, 1988–1994), 9 mg/day was the highest mean intake of vitamin B$_6$ from food and supplements reported for any life stage and gender group. The highest reported intake at the 95th percentile was 21 mg/day in pregnant females aged 14 through 55 years, most of which was pyridoxine from supplements. The risk of adverse effects resulting from excess intake of vitamin B$_6$ from food and supplements appears to be very low at these intake levels.

DIETARY SOURCES

Foods

Data from the Continuing Survey of Food Intakes by Individuals (CSFII, 1994–1996) indicated that the greatest contribution to the vitamin B$_6$ intake of the U.S. adult population came from fortified, ready-to-eat cereals; mixed foods (including sandwiches) with meat, fish, or poultry as the main ingredient; white potatoes and other starchy vegetables; and noncitrus fruits. Especially rich sources of vitamin B$_6$ include highly fortified cereals; beef liver and other organ meats; and highly fortified, soy-based meat substitutes.

Dietary Supplements

Approximately 26 percent of all adults reported taking a supplement containing vitamin B$_6$, according to the 1986 National Health Interview Survey (NHIS) in the United States. For adults over age 60 years who took supplements and participated in the Boston Nutritional Status Survey (1981–1984), the median supplemental vitamin B$_6$ intake was 2.2 mg/day for both men and women.

Bioavailability

The bioavailability of vitamin B$_6$ from a mixed diet is approximately 75 percent.

Dietary Interactions

This information was not provided at the time the DRI values for this nutrient were set.

INADEQUATE INTAKE AND DEFICIENCY

In controlled studies, clinical signs and symptoms of vitamin B_6 deficiency have only been observed during depletion with very low levels of the vitamin and have never been seen at intakes of 0.5 mg/day or more. The signs and symptoms of vitamin B_6 deficiency include the following:

- Seborrheic dermatitis
- Microcytic anemia (from decreased hemoglobin synthesis)
- Epileptiform convulsions
- Depression and confusion

Special Considerations

Medications: Drugs that can react with carbonyl groups have the potential to interact with a form of vitamin B_6. For example, isoniazid, which is used in the treatment of tuberculosis, and L-DOPA, which is metabolized to dopamine, have been reported to reduce plasma concentrations of vitamin B_6.

Oral contraceptives: Studies have shown decreased vitamin B_6 status in women who receive high-dose oral contraceptives. Plasma concentrations of the nutrient are lowered, but the decrease is quite small. (It should be noted that these studies were conducted when the level of estrogen in oral contraceptives was three to five times higher than current levels.)

Alcohol: Chronic alcoholics tend to have low vitamin B_6 status, which is distinct from deficiency caused by liver disease or by poor diet. The extent to which this causes an increased vitamin B_6 requirement is not known.

Preeclampsia: Lowered vitamin B_6 status is observed in preeclampsia and eclampsia, suggesting a potentially increased requirement for the vitamin in preeclampsia.

EXCESS INTAKE

No adverse effects have been associated with high intakes of vitamin B_6 from food sources. Very large oral doses (2,000 mg/day or more) of supplemental pyridoxine, which are used to treat many conditions, including carpal tunnel syndrome, painful neuropathies, seizures, premenstrual syndrome, asthma, and sickle cell disease, have been associated with the development of sensory neuropathy and dermatological lesions.

KEY POINTS FOR VITAMIN B$_6$

✓   Vitamin B$_6$ (pyridoxine and related compounds) functions as a coenzyme in the metabolism of amino acids, glycogen, and sphingoid bases.

✓   The requirements for vitamin B$_6$ are based on a plasma pyridoxal 5′-phosphate value of at least 20 nmol/L. The UL is based on sensory neuropathy as the critical adverse effect.

✓   Rich food sources of vitamin B$_6$ include highly fortified cereals, beef liver and other organ meats, and highly fortified, soy-based meat substitutes. Other contributors to vitamin B$_6$ intake include mixed foods with meat, fish, or poultry as the main ingredient; white potatoes and other starchy vegetables; and noncitrus fruits.

✓   Clinical signs and symptoms of vitamin B$_6$ deficiency have only been observed during depletion with very low levels of the vitamin and have never been seen at intakes of 0.5 mg/day or more.

✓   The signs and symptoms of vitamin B$_6$ deficiency are seborrheic dermatitis, microcytic anemia, epileptiform convulsions, and depression and confusion.

✓   No adverse effects have been associated with high intakes of vitamin B$_6$ from food sources.

✓   Very large oral doses (2,000 mg/day or more) of supplemental pyridoxine have been associated with the development of sensory neuropathy and dermatological legions.

TABLE 1 Dietary Reference Intakes for Vitamin B_{12} by Life Stage Group

	DRI values (µg/day)					
	EAR[a]		RDA[b]		AI[c]	UL[d]
	males	females	males	females		
Life stage group						
0 through 6 mo					0.4	
7 through 12 mo					0.5	
1 through 3 y	0.7	0.7	0.9	0.9		
4 through 8 y	1.0	1.0	1.2	1.2		
9 through 13 y	1.5	1.5	1.8	1.8		
14 through 18 y	2.0	2.0	2.4	2.4		
19 through 30 y	2.0	2.0	2.4	2.4		
31 through 50 y	2.0	2.0	2.4	2.4		
51 through 70 y	2.0	2.0	2.4[e]	2.4[e]		
> 70 y	2.0	2.0	2.4[e]	2.4[e]		
Pregnancy						
≤ 18 y		2.2		2.6		
19 through 50 y		2.2		2.6		
Lactation						
≤ 18 y		2.4		2.8		
19 through 50 y		2.4		2.8		

[a] **EAR** = Estimated Average Requirement.

[b] **RDA** = Recommended Dietary Allowance.

[c] **AI** = Adequate Intake.

[d] **UL** = Tolerable Upper Intake Level. Data were insufficient to set a UL. In the absence of a UL, extra caution may be warranted in consuming levels above the recommended intake.

[e] Because 10 to 30 percent of older people may malabsorb food-bound vitamin B_{12}, for adults over 50 years old it is advisable for most of this amount to be obtained by consuming foods fortified with vitamin B_{12} or a vitamin B_{12}-containng supplement.

VITAMIN B₁₂

Vitamin B$_{12}$ (cobalamin) functions as a coenzyme for a critical reaction that converts homocysteine to methionine and in the metabolism of fatty acids of odd chain length. An adequate supply of vitamin B$_{12}$ is essential for normal blood formation and neurological function.

The requirements for vitamin B$_{12}$ are based on the amount needed to maintain hematological status and normal serum vitamin B$_{12}$ values. An assumed absorption of 50 percent is included in determining the Estimated Average Requirement (EAR). Data were insufficient to set a Tolerable Upper Intake Level (UL). DRI values are listed by life stage group in Table 1.

Because 10–30 percent of older people may be unable to absorb naturally occurring vitamin B$_{12}$, most likely due to atrophic gastritis, it is advisable for those older than 50 years to meet their needs mainly by consuming foods fortified with vitamin B$_{12}$ or by taking a supplement that contains it. Individuals with vitamin B$_{12}$ deficiency caused by a lack of intrinsic factor require medical treatment.

Naturally occurring vitamin B$_{12}$ is found primarily in foods of animal origin. Many plant-based foods are fortified with the vitamin. The major cause of vitamin B$_{12}$ deficiency is pernicious anemia, a condition in which the stomach does not produce intrinsic factor. The hematological effects that occur with this deficiency are identical to those that accompany folate deficiency. No adverse effects have been associated with excess vitamin B$_{12}$ intake from food or supplements in healthy individuals. The apparent low toxicity of the vitamin may be because, when high doses are given orally, only a small percentage of it can be absorbed from the gastrointestinal tract.

VITAMIN B₁₂ AND THE BODY

Function

Vitamin B$_{12}$ (cobalamin) functions as a coenzyme for a critical reaction that converts homocysteine to methionine and for a separate reaction in the metabolism of fatty acids and amino acids. An adequate supply of vitamin B$_{12}$ is essential for normal blood formation and neurological function. Although the preferred scientific use of the term vitamin B$_{12}$ is usually restricted to cyanocobalamin, in this publication vitamin B$_{12}$ refers to all potentially biologically active cobalamins.

Absorption, Metabolism, Storage, and Excretion

Small amounts of vitamin B_{12} are absorbed by an active process that requires an intact stomach, intrinsic factor (a glycoprotein that the parietal cells of the stomach secrete after being stimulated by food), pancreatic sufficiency, and a normally functioning terminal ileum. Vitamin B_{12} is processed in the stomach and the small intestine before being released into the circulation. The liver takes up approximately 50 percent of circulating nutrient; the remainder is transported to other tissues.

There is a lack of data on the absorption of vitamin B_{12} from many foods. Therefore, for this publication, a conservative adjustment for the bioavailability of naturally occurring vitamin B_{12} was used. In particular, it is assumed that 50 percent of dietary vitamin B_{12} is absorbed by healthy adults with normal gastric function.

If there is a lack of intrinsic factor (as in the case of pernicious anemia), malabsorption of the vitamin results. If untreated, this may lead to potentially irreversible neurological damage and possibly life-threatening anemia. Malabsorption also results from atrophic gastritis with low stomach acid secretion, a condition estimated to occur in 10–30 percent of people older than 50 years.

Vitamin B_{12} is continually secreted in the bile. In healthy individuals, most of it is reabsorbed and available for metabolic functions. However, in the absence of intrinsic factor, essentially all the vitamin B_{12} from the bile is excreted in the stool rather than recirculated. Thus, deficiency develops more rapidly in individuals who have no intrinsic factor or who malabsorb vitamin B_{12} for other reasons than it does in those who do not ingest it (such as those with complete vegetarian diets). The excretion of vitamin B_{12} is proportional to body stores; it is excreted mainly in the stool but also in the urine and through the skin.

DETERMINING DRIS

Determining Requirements

The requirements for vitamin B_{12} are based on the amount needed to maintain hematological status and normal serum vitamin B_{12} values. An assumed absorption of 50 percent is included in determining the EAR.

Special Considerations

Aging and atrophic gastritis: Vitamin B_{12} status tends to decline with age, perhaps due to a decrease in gastric acidity and the presence of atrophic gastritis and of bacterial overgrowth accompanied by malabsorption of food-bound vitamin B_{12}. It is estimated that approximately 10–30 percent of elderly people have atrophic gastritis, although the condition may often go undiagnosed. Thus, it is advisable for those older than 50 years to meet their needs mainly by consuming foods fortified with vitamin B$_{12}$ or by taking a supplement that contains it.

Infants of vegan mothers: Infants of vegan mothers should be supplemented with vitamin B$_{12}$ at the level of the AI from birth because their stores at that time are low and their mothers' milk may supply very small amounts of the vitamin.

Individuals with increased needs: A person with any malabsorption syndrome will likely require increased amounts of vitamin B$_{12}$. Patients with pernicious anemia or Crohn's disease involving the terminal ileum and patients who have had a gastrectomy, gastric bypass surgery, or ileal resection will require the nutrient under a physician's direction. People who are HIV-positive with chronic diarrhea may also require either increased oral or parenteral vitamin B$_{12}$. Patients with atrophic gastritis, pancreatic insufficiency, or prolonged omeprazole treatment will have decreased bioavailability of food-bound vitamin B$_{12}$ and will require normal amounts of crystalline vitamin B$_{12}$ (either in fortified foods or in a supplement).

Criteria for Determining Vitamin B$_{12}$ Requirements, by Life Stage Group

Life stage group	Criterion
0 through 6 mo	Human milk content
7 through 12 mo	Extrapolation from younger infants
1 through 18 y	Extrapolation from adults
19 through > 70 y	Amount needed to maintain hematological status and normal serum vitamin B$_{12}$ values
Pregnancy	
≤ 18 y through 50 y	Age-specific requirement + fetal deposition of the vitamin B$_{12}$
Lactation	
≤ 18 y through 50 y	Age-specific requirement + amount of vitamin B$_{12}$ secreted in human milk

The UL

The Tolerable Upper Intake Level (UL) is the highest level of daily nutrient intake that is likely to pose no risk of adverse effects for almost all people. Due to inadequate data on adverse effects of excess vitamin B$_{12}$ consumption, a UL for the vitamin could not be determined.

Based on data from the Third National Health and Nutrition Examination Survey (NHANES III, 1988–1994), the highest median intake of B_{12} from diet and supplements for any life stage and gender group was 17 µg/day; the highest reported intake at the 95th percentile was 37 µg/day. Furthermore, there appear to be no risks associated with intakes from supplemental B_{12} that are more than two orders of magnitude higher than the 95th percentile intake. However, this does not mean that there is no potential for adverse effects to occur with high intakes.

DIETARY SOURCES

Foods

Vitamin B_{12} is naturally found in foods of animal origin. It is also found in plant-based foods that have been fortified, such as ready-to-eat cereals and meal replacement formulas. Particularly rich sources of natural vitamin B_{12} such as shellfish, organ meats such as liver, some game meats (such as venison and rabbit), and some fish (such as herring, sardines, and trout) are not a regular part of many people's diets. According to the Continuing Survey of Food Intakes by Individuals (CSFII, 1994–1996), the greatest contributors to vitamin B_{12} intake in U.S. adults were mixed foods (including sandwiches) with meat, fish, or poultry as the main ingredient. For women, the second highest contributor to intake was milk and milk beverages; for men it was beef. Fortified ready-to-eat cereals contributed a greater proportion of dietary vitamin B_{12} for women than for men.

Although milk is a good source of vitamin B_{12}, cooking it may greatly reduce its vitamin content. For example, boiling milk for 10 minutes reduces vitamin B_{12} content by about 50 percent.

Dietary Supplements

In the United States, cyanocobalamin is the only commercially available vitamin B_{12} preparation used in supplements and pharmaceuticals. It is also the principal form used in Canada. Approximately 26 percent of all adults reported taking a supplement that contained vitamin B_{12}, according to the 1986 National Health Interview Survey (NHIS). For adults over age 60 years who took supplements and participated in the Boston Nutritional Status Survey, median supplemental vitamin B_{12} intakes were 5.0 µg/day for men and 6.0 µg/day for women.

Bioavailability

Data on the bioavailability of vitamin B_{12} are few. Studies have found the absorption of the nutrient in healthy adults to be 65 percent from mutton, 11 percent from liver, 24–36 percent from eggs, 60 percent from chicken, and 25–47 percent from trout. Because of a lack of data on dairy foods and most forms of red meat and fish, a conservative adjustment for the bioavailability of naturally occurring vitamin B_{12} was used for this publication. In particular, it is assumed that 50 percent of dietary vitamin B_{12} is absorbed by healthy adults with normal gastric function.

Dietary Interactions

There is evidence that vitamin B_{12} may interact with certain nutrients (see Table 2).

TABLE 2 Potential Interactions with Other Nutrients

Substance	Potential Interaction	Notes
NUTRIENTS THAT AFFECT VITAMIN B₁₂		
Folate	Adequate or high folate intake may mitigate the effects of a vitamin B_{12} deficiency on normal blood formation.	There is no evidence that folate intake or status changes the requirement for vitamin B_{12}.

INADEQUATE INTAKE AND DEFICIENCY

The clinical effects of vitamin B_{12} deficiency are hematological, neurological, and gastrointestinal:

- *Hematological effects:* The major cause of vitamin B_{12} deficiency is pernicious anemia, a condition in which the gastric mucosa of the stomach does not produce intrinsic factor. The hematological effects of vitamin B_{12} deficiency include weakness, fatigue, shortness of breath, and palpitations. These effects are identical to those observed in folate deficiency. As in folate deficiency, the underlying mechanism of anemia is an interference with normal deoxyribonucleic acid (DNA) synthesis. This results in megaloblastic change, which causes the production of larger-than-normal erythrocytes (macrocytosis). By the time anemia is established, there is usually also some degree of neutropenia and thrombocytopenia because the megaloblastic process affects all rapidly dividing bone-marrow elements. The hematological complications are completely reversed by treatment with vitamin B_{12}.

- *Neurological effects:* Neurological complications are present in 75–90 percent of individuals with clinically observable vitamin B_{12} deficiency and may, in about 25 percent of cases, be the only clinical manifestation of deficiency. Evidence is mounting that the occurrence of neurological complications is inversely correlated with the degree of anemia; that is, patients who are less anemic show more prominent neurological complications, and vice versa. Neurological manifestations include tingling and numbness in the extremities (worse in the lower limbs), gait disturbances, and cognitive changes such as loss of concentration, memory loss, disorientation, and dementia, with or without mood changes. Visual disturbances, insomnia, impotency, and impaired bowel and bladder control.
- *Gastrointestinal effects:* Vitamin B_{12} deficiency is also frequently associated with various gastrointestinal complaints, including sore tongue, loss of appetite, flatulence, and constipation. Some of these gastrointestinal effects may be related to the underlying gastric disorder in pernicious anemia.

EXCESS INTAKE

No adverse effects have been associated with excess vitamin B_{12} intake from food or supplements in healthy individuals. The apparent low toxicity of the vitamin may be because, when high doses are orally given, only a small percentage of it can be absorbed from the gastrointestinal tract. Although there are extensive data showing no adverse effects associated with high intakes of supplemental vitamin B_{12}, the studies in which such intakes were reported were not designed to assess adverse effects.

KEY POINTS FOR VITAMIN B$_{12}$

✓   Vitamin B$_{12}$ (cobalamin) functions as a coenzyme for a reaction that converts homocysteine to methionine and for a separate reaction in the metabolism of certain fatty acids and amino acids.

✓   Although the preferred scientific use of the term vitamin B$_{12}$ is usually restricted to cyanocobalamin, in this publication vitamin B$_{12}$ refers to all potentially biologically active cobalamins.

✓   The requirements for vitamin B$_{12}$ are based on the amount needed to maintain hematological status and normal serum vitamin B$_{12}$ values.

✓   Data were insufficient to set a UL.

✓   Because 10–30 percent of older people may be unable to absorb naturally occurring vitamin B$_{12}$, it is advisable for those older than 50 years to meet their needs mainly by consuming foods fortified with vitamin B$_{12}$ or by taking a supplement that contains vitamin B$_{12}$.

✓   A person with any malabsorption syndrome will likely require increased amounts of vitamin B$_{12}$.

✓   Individuals with vitamin B$_{12}$ deficiency caused by a lack of intrinsic factor require medical treatment.

✓   Vitamin B$_{12}$ is naturally found in foods of animal origin. It is also found in plant-based foods that have been fortified, such as ready-to-eat cereals and meal replacement formulas. Although milk is a good source, cooking it may greatly reduce its vitamin B$_{12}$ content.

✓   The major cause of vitamin B$_{12}$ deficiency is pernicious anemia, a condition in which the gastric mucosa of the stomach does not produce intrinsic factor. The hematological effects that occur with this deficiency are identical to those observed in folate deficiency.

✓   No adverse effects have been associated with excess vitamin B$_{12}$ intake from food or supplements in healthy individuals. The apparent low toxicity of the vitamin may be because, when high doses are orally given, only a small percentage of it can be absorbed from the gastrointestinal tract.

TABLE 1 Dietary Reference Intakes for Biotin by Life Stage Group

	DRI values (μg/day)	
	AI[a]	UL[b]
Life stage group[c]		
0 through 6 mo	5	
7 through 12 mo	6	
1 through 3 y	8	
4 through 8 y	12	
9 through 13 y	20	
14 through 18 y	25	
19 through 30 y	30	
31 through 50 y	30	
51 through 70 y	30	
> 70 y	30	
Pregnancy		
≤ 18 y	30	
19 through 50 y	30	
Lactation		
≤ 18 y	35	
19 through 50 y	35	

[a] **AI** = Adequate Intake.

[b] **UL** = Tolerable Upper Intake Level. Data were insufficent to set a UL. In the absence of a UL, extra caution may be warranted in consuming levels above the recommended intake.

[c] All groups except Pregnancy and Lactation represent males and females.

BIOTIN

Biotin functions as a coenzyme in bicarbonate-dependent carboxylation reactions. It exists both as free biotin and in protein-bound forms in foods. Little is known about how protein-bound biotin is digested.

Since data were insufficient to set an Estimated Average Requirement (EAR) and thus calculate a Recommended Dietary Allowance (RDA) for biotin, an Adequate Intake (AI) was instead developed. The AIs for biotin are based on data extrapolation from the amount of biotin in human milk. Data were insufficient to set a Tolerable Upper Intake Level (UL). DRI values are listed by life stage group in Table 1.

The biotin content of foods is generally not documented. It is widely distributed in natural foods, but its concentration varies. Signs of biotin deficiency have been conclusively demonstrated in individuals consuming raw egg whites over long periods and in patients receiving total parenteral nutrition (TPN) solutions that do not contain biotin. No adverse effects have been documented for biotin at any intake tested.

BIOTIN AND THE BODY

Function

Biotin functions as a coenzyme in bicarbonate-dependent carboxylation reactions.

Absorption, Metabolism, Storage, and Excretion

Biotin exists both as free biotin and in protein-bound forms in foods. Little is known about how protein-bound biotin is digested. It appears to be absorbed in both the small intestine and the colon. The mechanism of biotin transport to the liver and other tissues after absorption has not been well established. Avidin, a protein found in raw egg white, has been shown to bind to biotin in the small intestine and prevent its absorption. The mechanism of biotin transport to the liver and other tissues after absorption has not been well established. Biotin is excreted in the urine.

DETERMINING DRIS

Determining Requirements

Since data were insufficient to establish an EAR and thus calculate an RDA, an AI was instead developed. The AIs for biotin are based on extrapolation from the amount of biotin in human milk. Most major nutrition surveys do not report biotin intake.

Special Considerations

Individuals with increased needs: People who receive hemodialysis or peritoneal dialysis may have an increased requirement for biotin, as do those with genetic biotinidase deficiency.

Criteria for Determining Biotin Requirements, by Life Stage Group

Life stage group	Criterion
0 through 6 mo	Human milk content
7 through 12 mo	Extrapolation from infants
1 through > 70 y	Extrapolation from infants
Pregnancy	
≤ 18 through 50 y	Extrapolation from infants
Lactation	
≤ 18 through 50 y	To cover the amount of biotin secreted in milk, the AI is increased by 5 µg/day

The UL

The Tolerable Upper Intake Level (UL) is the highest level of daily nutrient intake that is likely to pose no risk of adverse effects for almost all people. Due to insufficient data on the adverse effects of excess biotin consumption, a UL for biotin could not be determined.

DIETARY SOURCES

Foods

Biotin content has been documented for relatively few foods, and so it is generally not included in food composition tables. Thus, intake tends to be underestimated in diets. Although biotin is widely distributed in natural foods, its concentration significantly varies. For example, liver contains biotin at about 100 µg/100 g, whereas fruits and most meats contain only about 1 µg/100 g.

Dietary Supplements

According to the 1986 National Health Interview Survey (NHIS), approximately 17 percent of U.S. adults reported taking a supplement that contained biotin. Specific data on intake from supplements were not available.

Bioavailability

This information was not provided at the time the DRI values for this nutrient were set.

Dietary Interactions

This information was not provided at the time the DRI values for this nutrient were set.

INADEQUATE INTAKE AND DEFICIENCY

Signs of biotin deficiency have been conclusively demonstrated in individuals consuming raw egg whites over long periods and in patients receiving total parenteral nutrition (TPN) solutions that do not contain biotin. The effects of biotin deficiency include the following:

- Dermatitis (often appearing as a red scaly rash around the eyes, nose, and mouth)
- Conjunctivitis
- Alopecia
- Central nervous system abnormalities, such as depression, lethargy, hallucinations, and paresthesia of the extremities

Symptoms of deficiency in infants on biotin-free TPN appear much earlier after the initiation of the TPN regimen than in adults. In biotin-deficient infants, hypotonia, lethargy, and developmental delays, along with a peculiar withdrawn behavior, are all characteristic of a neurological disorder resulting from a lack of biotin.

EXCESS INTAKE

There have been no reported adverse effects of biotin in humans or animals. Toxicity has not been reported in patients given daily doses of biotin up to 200 mg orally and up to 20 mg intravenously to treat biotin-responsive inborn errors of metabolism and acquired biotin deficiency.

KEY POINTS FOR BIOTIN

✓ Biotin functions as a coenzyme in bicarbonate-dependent carboxylation reactions.

✓ Since data were insufficient to establish an EAR and thus calculate an RDA, an AI was instead developed.

✓ The AIs for biotin are based on extrapolation from the amount of biotin in human milk.

✓ People who receive hemodialysis or peritoneal dialysis may have an increased requirement for biotin, as may those with genetic biotinidase deficiency.

✓ Data were insufficient to set a UL.

✓ The biotin content of foods is generally not documented. It is widely distributed in natural foods, but its concentration varies.

✓ Signs of biotin deficiency have been conclusively demonstrated in individuals consuming raw egg whites over long periods and in patients receiving total parenteral nutrition (TPN) solutions that do not contain biotin.

✓ The effects of biotin deficiency include dermatitis, alopecia, conjunctivitis, and abnormalities of the central nervous system.

✓ No adverse effects have been associated with high intakes of biotin.

TABLE 1 Dietary Reference Intakes for Vitamin C by Life Stage Group

	DRI values (mg/day)					
	EAR[a]		RDA[b]		AI[c]	UL[d]
	males	females	males	females		
Life stage group						
0 through 6 mo					40	ND[e]
7 through 12 mo					50	ND
1 through 3 y	13	13	15	15		400
4 through 8 y	22	22	25	25		650
9 through 13 y	39	39	45	45		1,200
14 through 18 y	63	56	75	65		1,800
19 through 30 y	75	60	90	75		2,000
31 through 50 y	75	60	90	75		2,000
51 through 70 y	75	60	90	75		2,000
≥ 70 y	75	60	90	75		2,000
Pregnancy						
≤ 18 y		66		80		1,800
19 through 50 y		70		85		2,000
Lactation						
≤ 18 y		96		115		1,800
19 through 50 y		100		120		2,000

[a] **EAR** = Estimated Average Requirement.

[b] **RDA** = Recommended Dietary Allowance.

[c] **AI** = Adequate Intake.

[d] **UL** = Tolerable Upper Intake Level. Unless otherwise specified, the UL represents total intake from food, water, and supplements.

[e] **ND** = Not determinable. This value is not determinable due to the lack of data of adverse effects in this age group and concern regarding the lack of ability to handle excess amounts. Source of intake should only be from food to prevent high levels of intake.

VITAMIN C

Vitamin C (ascorbic acid) is a water-soluble nutrient that acts as an anti-oxidant and a cofactor in enzymatic and hormonal processes. It also plays a role in the biosynthesis of carnitine, neurotransmitters, collagen, and other components of connective tissue, and modulates the absorption, transport, and storage of iron.

The adult requirements for vitamin C are based on estimates of body pool or tissue vitamin C levels that are deemed adequate to provide antioxidant protection. Smokers have an increased requirement. The adverse effects upon which the Tolerable Upper Intake Level (UL) is based are osmotic diarrhea and gastrointestinal disturbances. DRI values are listed by life stage group in Table 1. Foods rich in vitamin C include fruits and vegetables, including citrus fruits, tomatoes, potatoes, strawberries, spinach, and cruciferous vegetables. Vitamin C deficiency is by and large not a problem in the United States and Canada, and the risk of adverse effects of excess intake appears to be very low at the highest usual Vitamin C intakes.

VITAMIN C AND THE BODY

Function

Vitamin C (ascorbic acid) is a water-soluble nutrient that acts as an antioxidant by virtue of its high reducing power. It has a number of functions: as a scavenger of free radicals; as a cofactor for several enzymes involved in the biosynthesis of carnitine, collagen, neurotransmitters, and in vitro processes; and as a reducing agent. Evidence for in vivo antioxidant functions of ascorbate include the scavenging of reactive oxidants in activated leukocytes, lung, and gastric mucosa, and diminished lipid peroxidation as measured by urinary isoprostane excretion.

Absorption, Metabolism, Storage, and Excretion

Vitamin C is absorbed in the intestine via a sodium-dependent active transport process that is saturable and dose-dependent. As intake increases, absorption decreases. At low intestinal concentrations of vitamin C, active transport is the primary mode of absorption. When intestinal concentrations of vitamin C are high, passive diffusion becomes the main form of absorption.

Besides dose-dependent absorption, body vitamin C content is also regulated by the kidneys, which conserve or excrete unmetabolized vitamin C. Renal excretion of vitamin C increases proportionately with higher intakes of the vitamin. These processes allow the body to conserve vitamin C during periods of low intake and to limit plasma levels of vitamin C at high intakes.

The amount of vitamin C stored in different body tissues widely varies. High levels are found in the pituitary and adrenal glands, leukocytes, eye tissues and humors, and the brain, while low levels are found in plasma and saliva. A total body pool of less than 300 mg is associated with symptoms of scurvy, a disease of severe vitamin C deficiency; maximum body pools (in adults) are limited to about 2,000 mg.

With high intakes, unabsorbed vitamin C degrades in the intestine, which may account for the diarrhea and gastrointestinal upset sometimes reported by people taking large doses. At very low ascorbate intakes, essentially no ascorbate is excreted unchanged and a minimal loss occurs.

DETERMINING DRIS

Determining Requirements

The requirements for vitamin C are based on estimates of body pool or tissue vitamin C levels that are deemed adequate to provide antioxidant protection with minimal urinary loss. Although some studies have reported a possible protective effect of vitamin C against diseases such as cardiovascular disease, cancer, lung disease, cataracts, and even the common cold, others have failed to do so. Additionally, the majority of evidence accumulated thus far has been largely observational and epidemiological and thus does not prove cause and effect.

Special Considerations

Gender: Women tend to have higher blood levels of vitamin C than men of the same age, even when intake levels are the same, making the requirements for women lower than for men. The difference in vitamin C requirements of men and women is assumed based on mean differences in body size, total body water, and lean body mass.

Age: No consistent differences in the absorption or metabolism of vitamin C due to aging have been demonstrated at median vitamin C intakes. This suggests that reports of low blood concentrations of vitamin C in elderly populations may be due to poor dietary intakes, chronic disease or debilitation, or other factors, rather than solely an effect of aging. Therefore, the requirements of older adults do not differ from those of younger adults.

Smoking: Studies have shown that smokers have decreased plasma and leukocyte levels of vitamin C compared to nonsmokers, even after adjusting for vitamin C intake from foods. Metabolic turnover of the vitamins has been shown to be about 35 mg/day greater in smokers. This means that smokers need 35 mg/day more to maintain the same body pool as nonsmokers. The mechanism by which smoking compromises vitamin C status has not been well established.

Exposure to environmental tobacco smoke: Increased oxidative stress and vitamin C turnover have been observed in nonsmokers who are regularly exposed to tobacco smoke. Although the available data were insufficient to estimate a special requirement, these nonsmokers are urged to ensure that they meet the RDA for vitamin C.

Certain pregnant subpopulations: Pregnant women who smoke, abuse drugs or alcohol, or regularly take aspirin may have increased requirements for vitamin C.

Individuals susceptible to adverse effects: People with hemochromatosis, glucose-6-phosphate dehydrogenase deficiency, and renal disorders may be particularly susceptible to the adverse effects of excess vitamin C intake and therefore should be cautious about ingesting vitamin C at levels greater than the RDA. Vitamin C may enhance iron absorption and exacerbate iron-induced tissue damage in individuals with hemochromatosis, while those with renal disorders may have increased risk of oxalate kidney stone formation from excess vitamin C intake.

Criteria for Determining Vitamin C Requirements, by Life Stage Group

Life stage group	Criterion
0 through 6 mo	Human milk content
7 through 12 mo	Human milk + solid food
1 through 18 y	Extrapolation from adult
19 through 30 y	Near-maximal neutrophil concentration
31 through > 70 y	Extrapolation of near-maximal neutrophil concentration from 19 through 30 y

Pregnancy	
≤ 18 y through 50 y	Age-specific requirement + tansfer to the fetus

Lactation	
≤ 18 y through 50 y	Age-specific requirement + vitamin C secreted in human milk

The UL

The Tolerable Upper Intake Level (UL) is the highest level of daily nutrient intake that is likely to pose no risk of adverse effects for almost all people. Members of the general population should not routinely exceed the UL, which for vitamin C applies to intake from both food and supplements. Osmotic diarrhea and gastrointestinal disturbances are the critical endpoints upon which the UL for vitamin C is based.

Based on data from the Third National Health and Nutrition Examination Survey (NHANES III, 1988–1994), the highest mean intake of vitamin C from diet and supplements for any gender and lifestage group was estimated to be about 200 mg/day (for males aged 51 through 70 years and females aged 51 years and older). The highest reported intake at the 99th percentile was greater than 1,200 mg/day in males aged 31 through 70 years and in females aged 51 through 70 years. The risk of adverse effects resulting from excess intake of vitamin C from food and supplements appears to be very low.

DIETARY SOURCES

Foods

Almost 90 percent of vitamin C found in the typical diet comes from fruits and vegetables, with citrus fruits and juices, tomatoes and tomato juice, and potatoes being major contributors. Other sources include brussels sprouts, cauliflower, broccoli, strawberries, cabbage, and spinach. Some foods are also fortified with vitamin C. The vitamin C content of foods can vary depending on growing conditions and location, the season of the year, the stage of maturity, cooking practices, and the storage time prior to consumption.

Dietary Supplements

Data from the Boston Nutritional Status Survey (1981–1984) estimated that 35 percent of men and 44 percent of women took some form of vitamin C supplements; of them, 19 percent of men and 15 percent of women had intakes greater than 1,000 mg/day.

Bioavailability

There does not appear to be much variability in the bioavailability of vitamin C between different foods and dietary supplements. Approximately 70–90 percent of usual dietary intakes of vitamin C (30–180 mg/day) is absorbed by the body. However, absorption falls to 50 percent or less as intake increases to doses of 1,000 mg/day or more.

TABLE 2 Potential Interactions with Other Dietary Substances

Substance	Potential Interaction	Notes
VITAMIN C AFFECTING OTHER SUBSTANCES		
Iron	Vitamin C may enhance the absorption of nonheme iron.	Vitamin C added to meals facilitates the intestinal absorption of nonheme iron, possibly due to lowering of gastrointestinal iron to the more absorbable ferrous state or to countering the effect of substances that inhibit iron absorption. However, studies in which the vitamin was added to meals over long periods have not shown significant improvement of body iron status, indicating that ascorbic acid has a lesser effect on iron bioavailability than has been predicted from tests involving single meals.
Copper	Vitamin C may reduce copper absorption.	Excess vitamin C may reduce copper absorption, but the significance of this potential effect in humans is questionable because the data have been mixed.
Vitamin B_{12}	Large doses of vitamin C may reduce vitamin B_{12} levels.	Low serum B_{12} values reported in people receiving megadoses of vitamin C are likely to be artifacts of the effect of vitamin C on the radiotope assay for B_{12}, and thus not a true nutrient–nutrient interaction.

Dietary Interactions

There is evidence that vitamin C may interact with certain nutrients and dietary substances (see Table 2).

INADEQUATE INTAKE AND DEFICIENCY

Severe vitamin C deficiency is rare in industrialized countries, but it is occasionally seen in people whose diets lack fruits and vegetables or in those who abuse alcohol or drugs. In the United States, low blood levels of vitamin C are more common in men, particularly elderly men, than in women, and in populations of lower socioeconomic status.

The classic disease of severe vitamin C deficiency is scurvy, which is characterized by the symptoms related to connective tissue defects. Scurvy usually occurs at a plasma concentration of less than 11 μmol/L (0.2 mg/dL). The signs and symptoms of scurvy include the following:

- Follicular hyperkeratosis
- Petechiae

- Ecchymoses
- Coiled hairs
- Inflamed and bleeding gums
- Perifollicular hemorrhages
- Joint effusions
- Arthralgia
- Impaired wound healing

Other signs and symptoms include dyspnea, edema, Sjögren's syndrome (dry eyes and mouth), weakness, fatigue, and depression. In experimental subjects who were made vitamin C deficient but not frankly scorbutic, gingival inflammation and fatigue were among the most sensitive markers of deficiency.

Vitamin C deficiency in infants, known as infantile scurvy, may result in bone abnormalities, hemorrhagic symptoms, and anemia. Infantile scurvy is rarely seen because human milk provides an adequate supply of vitamin C and infant formulas are fortified with the vitamin.

EXCESS INTAKE

Adverse effects from vitamin C intake have been associated primarily with large doses (> 3,000 mg/day) and may include diarrhea and other gastrointestinal disturbances. There is no evidence suggesting that vitamin C is carcinogenic or teratogenic or that it causes adverse reproductive effects.

Special Considerations

Blood and urine tests: Vitamin C intakes of 250 mg/day or higher have been associated with false-negative results for detecting stool and gastric occult blood. Therefore, high-dose vitamin C supplements should be discontinued at least 2 weeks before physical exams to avoid interference with blood and urine tests.

KEY POINTS FOR VITAMIN C

✓   Vitamin C (ascorbic acid) is a water-soluble nutrient that acts as an antioxidant and a cofactor in enzymatic and hormonal processes. It also plays a role in the biosynthesis of carnitine, neurotransmitters, collagen, and other components of connective tissue, and modulates the absorption, transport, and storage of iron.

✓   Vitamin C requirements for adults are based on estimates of body pool or tissue vitamin C levels that are deemed adequate to provide antioxidant protection. The adverse effects upon which the UL is based are osmotic diarrhea and gastrointestinal disturbances.

✓   Although some studies have reported a possible protective effect of vitamin C against diseases such as cardiovascular disease, cancer, lung disease, cataracts, and even the common cold, others have failed to do so.

✓   Because smokers suffer increased oxidative stress and metabolic turnover of vitamin C, the requirements are raised by 35 mg/day.

✓   Increased oxidative stress and vitamin C turnover have been observed in nonsmokers who are regularly exposed to tobacco smoke, and thus nonsmokers are urged to ensure that they meet the RDA for vitamin C.

✓   The risk of adverse effects resulting from excess vitamin C intake appears to be very low.

✓   Almost 90 percent of vitamin C found in the typical diet comes from fruits and vegetables, with citrus fruits and juices, tomatoes and tomato juice, and potatoes being major contributors. Other sources include brussels sprouts, cauliflower, broccoli, strawberries, cabbage, and spinach.

✓   Low blood concentrations of vitamin C in elderly populations may be due to poor dietary intakes, chronic disease or debilitation, or other factors, rather than solely an effect of aging.

✓   The classic disease of severe vitamin C deficiency is scurvy, the signs and symptoms of which include follicular hyperkeratosis, petechiae, ecchymoses, coiled hairs, inflamed and bleeding gums, perifollicular hemorrhages, joint effusions, arthralgia, and impaired wound healing.

✓   Severe vitamin C deficiency is rare in industrialized countries, but it is occasionally seen in people whose diets lack fruits and vegetables or in those who abuse alcohol or drugs.

✓   Adverse effects have been associated primarily with large doses (> 3,000 mg/day) and may include diarrhea and other gastrointestinal disturbances.

CAROTENOIDS

C arotenoids are natural pigments found in plants, and are abundant in deeply colored fruits and vegetables. The most prevalent carotenoids in North American diets are α-carotene, β-carotene, lycopene, lutein, zeaxanthin, and β-cryptoxanthin. Of these, α-carotene, β-carotene, and β-cryptoxanthin can be converted into retinol (vitamin A) in the body and are called provitamin A carotenoids. Lycopene, lutein, and zeaxanthin have no vitamin A activity and are called nonprovitamin A carotenoids. The only known function of carotenoids in humans is to act as a source of vitamin A in the diet (provitamin A carotenoids only).

There are no DRIs specifically for carotenoids (see Part III, "Vitamin A" for vitamin A DRIs and the contribution of carotenoids to vitamin A intake). Although epidemiological evidence suggests that higher blood concentrations of β-carotene and other carotenoids obtained from foods are associated with a lower risk of several chronic diseases, other evidence suggests possible harm arising from very large doses in population subgroups, such as smokers and asbestos workers. Currently, there is insufficient evidence to recommend that a certain percentage of dietary vitamin A should come from provitamin A carotenoids. However, existing recommendations calling for the increased consumption of carotenoid-rich fruits and vegetables for their health-promoting benefits are strongly supported.

Based on evidence that β-carotene supplements have not been shown to aid in the prevention or cure of major chronic diseases, and may cause harm in certain population subgroups, β-carotene supplements are not advisable other than as a provitamin A source and for the prevention and control of vitamin A deficiency in at-risk populations.

Foods rich in carotenoids include deep yellow-, red-, and orange-colored fruits and vegetables and green leafy vegetables. Carotenoids found in ripe fruits and cooked yellow tubers are more efficiently converted into vitamin A than are carotenoids from equal amounts of dark green, leafy vegetables. If adequate retinol (vitamin A) is provided in the diet, there are no known clinical effects of consuming diets low in carotenes over the short term; carotenodermia or lycopenodermia (skin discoloration) are the only proven adverse effects associated with excess consumption of carotenoids.

CAROTENOIDS AND THE BODY

Function

In plants, carotenoids function as pigments. In humans, the only known function of carotenoids is their provitamin A activity. Carotenoids may have additional functions, such as enhancing immune function and decreasing the risk of macular degeneration, cataracts, some cardiovascular events, and some types of cancer (particularly lung, oral cavity, pharyngeal, and cervical cancers), but the evidence is inconclusive. The risks for some diseases appear to be increased in certain population subgroups when large doses of β-carotene are taken.

Absorption, Metabolism, Storage, and Excretion

Dietary carotenoids are fat-soluble and are absorbed in the intestine via bile acid micelles. The uptake of β-carotene by intestinal mucosal cells is believed to occur by passive diffusion. Once inside the mucosal cells, carotenoids or their metabolic products (e.g., vitamin A) are incorporated into chylomicrons and released into the lymphatic system. Carotenoids are either absorbed intact or, in the case of provitamin A carotenoids, cleaved to form vitamin A prior to secretion into the lymph.

Carotenoids are transported in the blood by lipoproteins and stored in various body tissues, including the adipose tissue, liver, kidneys, and adrenal glands. (The adipose tissue and liver appear to be the main storage sites.) Excretion occurs via the bile and urine.

DETERMINING DRIS

Determining Requirements

Data were inadequate to estimate the requirements for β-carotene and other carotenoids. Although epidemiological evidence suggests that higher blood concentrations of β-carotene and other carotenoids obtained from foods are associated with a lower risk of several chronic diseases, this evidence could not be used to establish a requirement for β-carotene or other carotenoid intake because the observed effects may be due to other substances found in carotenoid-rich food, or other behavioral correlates of increased fruit and vegetable consumption. Other evidence suggests possible harm arising from very large doses in population subgroups, such as smokers and asbestos workers.

Currently, there is insufficient evidence to recommend that a certain percentage of dietary vitamin A should come from provitamin A carotenoids. Although no DRI values are proposed for carotenoids, existing recommendations calling for the increased consumption of carotenoid-rich fruits and vegetables for their health-promoting benefits are strongly supported. The existing recommendation to consume 5 or more servings of fruits and vegetables per day would provide 3–6 mg/day of β-carotene.

(For vitamin A DRIs, the contribution of carotenoids to vitamin A intake, and conversion factors of the various carotenoids to retinol activity equivalents [RAEs], see Part III, "Vitamin A," and Appendix F.)

The UL

There were insufficient data available on the potential adverse effects of excess carotenoid intake to derive a Tolerable Upper Intake Level (UL). However, in light of research indicating an association between high-dose β-carotene supplements and lung cancer in smokers (see "Excess Intake"), β-carotene supplements are not advisable for the general population. No adverse effects other than carotenodermia (skin discoloration) have been reported from the consumption of carotenoids in food.

DIETARY SOURCES

Foods

Foods rich in carotenoids include deep yellow-, red-, and orange-colored fruits and vegetables and green leafy vegetables. Major contributors of β-carotene to the diets of U.S. women of childbearing age include carrots (the major contributor), cantaloupe, broccoli, vegetable-beef or chicken soup, spinach, and collard greens. Major contributors of α-carotene, β-cryptoxanthin, lycopene, and lutein and zeaxanthin, respectively, are carrots, orange juice and orange juice blends, tomatoes and tomato products, and spinach and collard greens.

Carotenoids are not added to most infant formulas (milk- or soy-based), and the carotenoid content of human milk highly varies depending on the carotenoid content of the mother's diet.

Dietary Supplements

β-Carotene, α-carotene, β-cryptoxanthin, lutein and zeaxanthin, and lycopene are available as dietary supplements. However, there are no reliable estimates of the amount being consumed by people in the United States or Canada.

Bioavailability

The extent of conversion of a highly bioavailable source of dietary β-carotene to vitamin A in humans has been shown to be between 60 and 75 percent, with an additional 15 percent of the β-carotene absorbed intact. However, absorption of most carotenoids from foods is considerably lower and can be as low as 2 percent. Several other factors affect the bioavailability and absorption of carotenoids, including:

Food matrix: The food matrix in which ingested carotenoids are found affects bioavailability the most. For example, the absorption of β-carotene supplements that are solubilized with emulsifiers and protected by antioxidants can be 70 percent or more; absorption from fruits exceeds tubers, and the absorption from raw carrots can be as low as 5 percent.

Cooking techniques: Cooking appears to improve the bioavailability of some carotenoids. For example, the bioavailability of lycopene from tomatoes is vastly improved when tomatoes are cooked with oil. Steaming also improves carotenoid bioavailability in carrots and spinach. However, prolonged exposure to high temperatures, through boiling, for example, may reduce the bioavailability of carotenoids from vegetables.

Dietary fat: Studies have shown that to optimize carotenoid absorption, dietary fat must be consumed during the same meal as the carotenoid.

Other factors: Lipid-lowering drugs, olestra, plant sterol–enriched margarines, and dietary pectin supplements have all been shown to reduce carotenoid absorption.

Dietary Interactions

Different carotenoids may compete with each other for absorption. This is more likely to occur in people who take supplements of a particular carotenoid than in people who consume a variety of carotenoid rich fruits and vegetables. For example, β-carotene supplements reduce lutein absorption from food; and when carotene and lutein are given as supplements, β-carotene absorption increases.

INADEQUATE INTAKE AND DEFICIENCY

If adequate retinol (vitamin A) is provided in the diet, there are no known clinical effects of consuming diets low in carotenes over the short term.

Special Considerations

Smoking: Smokers tend to have lower plasma concentrations of carotenoids compared to nonsmokers. It is unknown whether this is attributable solely to poor intake or if tobacco smoke somehow reduces the circulating levels of carotenoids. The greater the intensity of smoking (the number of cigarettes per day), the greater the decrease in serum carotenoid concentrations. Although smoking may result in a need for higher intakes of dietary carotenoids to achieve optimal plasma concentrations, caution is warranted because studies have shown an increased risk of lung cancer in smokers who took β-carotene supplements (see "Excess Intake"). Recommendations made to smokers to increase carotenoid intake should emphasize foods, not supplements, as the source.

Alcohol consumption: As with tobacco, alcohol intake is inversely associated with serum carotenoid concentrations. Those who chronically consume large quantities of alcohol are often deficient in many nutrients, but it is unknown whether the deficiency is the result of poor diet or of the metabolic consequences of chronic alcoholism or the synergistic effect of both.

EXCESS INTAKE

Harmless skin discoloration in the form of carotenodermia (yellow discoloration) or lycopenodermia (orange discoloration) is the only proven adverse effect associated with the excess consumption of carotenoids from food and supplements. This condition has been reported in adults who took supplements containing 30 mg/day or more of β-carotene for long periods of time or who consumed high levels of carotenoid-rich foods, such as carrots. Skin discoloration is also the primary effect of excess carotenoid intake noted in infants, toddlers, and young children. The condition is reversible when carotene ingestion is discontinued.

Special Considerations

Increased risk of lung cancer in smokers: In the Alpha-Tocopherol, Beta-Carotene Cancer Prevention (ATBC) Trial, an increase in lung cancer was associated with supplemental β-carotene in doses of 20 mg/day or greater (for 5 to 8 years) in current smokers. Another multicenter lung cancer prevention trial, the Carotene and Retinol Efficacy Trial (CARET), which involved smokers and asbestos-exposed workers, reported more lung cancer cases in a group supplemented with a nutrient combination that contained both β-carotene and retinol than in a group that received placebos. In contrast, the Physicians' Health Study, conducted in the United States, reported no significant effect of 12 years of supplementation with β-carotene (50 mg every other day) on cancer or total mortality, even among smokers who took the supplements for up to 12 years.

Supplemental forms of β-carotene have markedly greater bioavailability than β-carotene from foods, and the concentrations associated with possible adverse effects are well beyond the concentrations achieved through foods. So, although 20 mg/day of supplemental β-carotene is enough to raise blood concentrations to a range associated with increased lung cancer risk, the same amount of β-carotene in foods is not.

Individuals with increased needs: Supplemental β-carotene can be used as a provitamin A source or for the prevention of vitamin A deficiency in populations with inadequate vitamin A nutriture. Long-term supplementation with β-carotene in people with adequate vitamin A status does not increase the concentration of serum retinol. For vitamin A-deficient individuals and for people suffering from erythropoietic protoporphyria (a photosensitivity disorder), treatment using higher doses may be called for, but only under a physician's direction.

KEY POINTS FOR CAROTENOIDS

✓   Carotenoids are natural pigments found in plants, and are abundant in deeply colored fruits and vegetables. Certain carotenoids function as a source of vitamin A in humans.

✓   There are no DRIs specifically for carotenoids.

✓   Currently, there is insufficient evidence to recommend that a certain percentage of dietary vitamin A should come from provitamin A carotenoids.

✓   Carotenoids may enhance immune function and decrease the risk of macular degeneration, cataracts, some vascular events, and some types of cancer. But carotenoids have also been linked to an increased incidence of cancer in certain population subgroups, such as smokers and asbestos workers.

✓   Foods rich in carotenoids include deep yellow-, red-, and orange-colored fruits and vegetables and green leafy vegetables. Carotenoids found in ripe fruits and cooked yellow tubers are more efficiently converted into vitamin A than are carotenoids from equal amounts of dark green, leafy vegetables.

✓   Several factors influence the bioavailability and absorption of carotenoids, including the food matrix, cooking techniques, the presence of dietary fat, and lipid-lowering drugs and dietary constituents.

✓   If adequate retinol (vitamin A) is provided in the diet, there are no known clinical effects of consuming diets low in carotenes over the short term.

✓   Harmless skin discoloration can result from excess consumption of carotenoids from food or supplements.

✓   Based on evidence that β-carotene supplements have not been shown to aid in the prevention of major chronic diseases, and may cause harm in certain population subgroups, β-carotene supplements are not advisable other than as a provitamin A source and for the prevention and control of vitamin A deficiency in at-risk populations.

TABLE 1 Dietary Reference Intakes for Choline by Life Stage Group

| | DRI values (mg/day) | | |
| | AI[a,b] | | UL[c] |
	males	females	
Life stage group			
0 through 6 mo	125	125	ND[d]
7 through 12 mo	150	150	ND
1 through 3 y	200	200	1,000
4 through 8 y	250	250	1,000
9 through 13 y	375	375	2,000
14 through 18 y	550	400	3,000
19 through 30 y	550	425	3,500
31 through 50 y	550	425	3,500
51 through 70 y	550	425	3,500
> 70 y	550	425	3,500
Pregnancy			
≤ 18 y		450	3,000
19 through 50 y		450	3,500
Lactation			
≤ 18 y		550	3,000
19 through 50 y		550	3,500

[a] **AI** = Adequate Intake.

[b] Although AIs have been set for choline, there are few data to assess whether a dietary supply of choline is needed at all stages of the life cycle. It may be that the choline requirement can be met by endogenous synthesis at some of these stages.

[c] **UL** = Tolerable Upper Intake Level. Unless otherwise specified, the UL represents total intake from food, water, and supplements.

[d] **ND** = Not determinable. This value is not determinable due to the lack of data of adverse effects in this age group and concern regarding the lack of ability to handle excess amounts. Source of intake should only be from food to prevent high levels of intake.

CHOLINE

Choline is required for the structural integrity of cell membranes. It is also involved in methyl metabolism, cholinergic neurotransmission, transmembrane signaling, and lipid and cholesterol transport and metabolism. Choline in the diet is available as free choline or is bound as esters such as phosphocholine, glycerophosphocholine, sphingomyelin, or phosphatidylcholine.

Since data were insufficient to set an Estimated Average Requirement (EAR) and thus calculate a Recommended Dietary Allowance (RDA) for choline, an Adequate Intake (AI) was instead developed. The AIs for choline are based on the intake required to maintain liver function, as assessed by measuring serum alanine aminotransferase levels. The Tolerable Upper Intake Level (UL) is based on hypotension as the critical effect, with fishy body odor as the secondary consideration.

Although AIs have been set for choline, there are few data to assess whether a dietary supply of choline is needed at all stages of the life cycle. It may be that the choline requirement can be met by endogenous synthesis at some of these stages. DRI values are listed by life stage group in Table 1.

Foods rich in choline include milk, liver, eggs, and peanuts. Lecithin, a food additive used as an emulsifying agent, also adds choline to the diet. Although choline is clearly essential to life, few data exist on the effects of inadequate dietary intake in healthy people. The signs and symptoms associated with excess choline intake are fishy body odor, sweating, vomiting, salivation, hypotension, gastrointestinal effects, and liver toxicity.

CHOLINE AND THE BODY

Function

Choline is required for the structural integrity of cell membranes. It is also involved in methyl metabolism, cholinergic neurotransmission, transmembrane signaling, and lipid and cholesterol transport and metabolism. For example, choline accelerates the synthesis and release of acetylcholine, an important neurotransmitter involved in memory and muscle control. It is also a precursor for the synthesis of phospholipids, including phosphatidylcholine (a membrane constituent important for the structure and function of membranes), for intracellular signaling and hepatic export of very low density lipoproteins. Lecithin, a substance commonly added to foods as an emulsifying agent, is rich in phosphatidylcholine. The term lecithin is often interchangeably used with phosphatidylcholine.

Absorption, Metabolism, Storage, and Excretion

Dietary choline is absorbed in the small intestine. Before it can be absorbed from the gut, some is metabolized by bacteria to form betaine, which may be absorbed and used as a methyl donor, and methylamines, which are not methyl donors.

Choline is found in foods as free choline and as esterified forms such as phosphocholine, glycerophosphocholine, sphingomyelin, and phosphatidylcholine. Pancreatic enzymes can liberate choline from some of the latter to form free choline. Free choline enters the portal circulation of the liver, whereas phosphatidylcholine may enter the lymph in chylomicrons. All tissues, including the brain, liver, and kidneys, accumulate choline by diffusion and mediated transport. Some choline is excreted in the urine unchanged but most is oxidized in the kidneys to form betaine.

DETERMINING DRIS

Determining Requirements

Since data were not sufficient for deriving an EAR, and thus calculating an RDA, an Adequate Intake (AI) was instead developed. The AIs for choline are based on the prevention of liver damage, as assessed by measuring serum alanine aminotransferase levels. The estimate is uncertain because it is based on a single published study and may need revision when data are available. This amount is influenced by the availability of methionine and folate in the diet (see "Dietary Interactions"). It may also be influenced by gender, pregnancy, lactation, and stage of development. Although AIs are set for choline, it may be that the requirement can be met by endogenous synthesis at some of these life stages.

Most major nutrition surveys in the United States and Canada do not report choline intake. The choline content of foods is also not included in major nutrient databases.

Criteria for Determining Choline Requirements, by Life Stage Group

Life stage group	Criterion
0 through 6 mo	Human milk content
7 through 12 mo	Extrapolation from infants or from adults
1 through 3 y	Extrapolation from adults
4 through >70 y	Serum alanine aminotransferase levels

Pregnancy

≤ 18 y through 50 y   Age-specific + fetal and placental accumulation of choline

Lactation

≤ 18 y through 50 y   Age-specific + choline secreted in human milk

The UL

The Tolerable Upper Intake Level (UL) is the highest level of daily nutrient intake that is likely to pose no risk of adverse effects for almost all people. Members of the general population should not routinely consume more than the UL. The UL for choline represents total intake from food, water, and supplements. Hypotension was selected as the critical effect in deriving a UL for choline, with fishy body odor selected as the secondary consideration.

Because there is no information from national surveys on choline intakes or on supplement usage, the risk of adverse effects within the United States or Canada cannot be characterized.

Special Considerations

Individuals susceptible to adverse effects: People with fish odor syndrome (trimethylaminuria), renal disease, liver disease, depression, and Parkinson's disease may have an increased susceptibility to the adverse effects of choline intakes at the UL.

DIETARY SOURCES

Foods

Most choline in foods is in the form of phophatidylcholine in membranes. Foods that are especially rich in choline include milk, liver, eggs, and peanuts. It is possible for usual dietary intakes to provide as much as 1,000 mg/day of choline. Lecithin added during food processing may increase the average daily per-capita consumption of phosphatidylcholine by 1.5 mg/kg of body weight for adults.

Dietary Supplements

Choline is available as a dietary supplement as choline chloride or choline bitartrate and as lecithin, which usually contains approximately 25 percent phosphatidylcholine or 3–4 percent choline by weight. There are no reliable estimates of the frequency of use or the amount of these supplements consumed by individuals in the United States and Canada.

Bioavailability

This information was not provided at the time the DRI values for this nutrient were set.

Dietary Interactions

Choline, methionine, and folate metabolism interact at the point that homocysteine is converted into methionine. Disturbing the metabolism of one of these methyl donors can affect the metabolism of the others.

INADEQUATE INTAKE AND DEFICIENCY

Although choline is clearly essential to life, few data exist on the effects of inadequate dietary intake in healthy people. Based on one study examining the effects of artificially induced choline deficiency in healthy men who consumed an otherwise adequate diet, liver damage occurred, resulting in elevated levels of alanine aminotransferase in the blood. Fatty infiltration of the liver has also been shown to occur in individuals fed with total parenteral nutrition (TPN) solutions devoid of choline.

EXCESS INTAKE

Choline doses that are in orders of magnitude greater than estimated intake from food have been associated with fishy body odor (trimethylaminuria), sweating, salivation, hypotension, and hepatotoxicity in humans. There are no indications in the literature that excess choline intake produces any additional adverse effects in humans. Fishy body odor results from the excretion of excessive amounts of trimethylamine, a choline metabolite, as the result of bacterial action. Lecithin does not present a risk of fishy body odor.

KEY POINTS FOR CHOLINE

✓   Choline is required for the structural integrity of cell membranes. It is also involved in methyl metabolism, cholinergic neurotransmission, transmembrane signaling, and lipid and cholesterol transport and metabolism.

✓   Since data were insufficient to set an EAR and thus calculate an RDA for choline, an AI was instead developed.

✓   The AIs for choline are based on the prevention of liver damage, as assessed by measuring serum alanine aminotransferase levels.

✓   Although AIs have been set for choline, there are few data to assess whether a dietary supply of choline is needed at all stages of the life cycle. It may be that the requirement can be met by endogenous synthesis at some of these stages.

✓   The UL is based on hypotension as the critical effect, with fishy body odor as the secondary consideration.

✓   People with fish odor syndrome (trimethylaminuria), renal disease, liver disease, depression, and Parkinson's disease may have an increased susceptibility to the adverse effects of choline intakes at the UL.

✓   Foods rich in choline include milk, liver, eggs, and peanuts. Lecithin, a food additive used as an emulsifying agent, also adds choline to the diet.

✓   Although choline is clearly essential to life, few data exist on the effects of inadequate dietary intake in healthy people. Based on one study examining the effects of induced inadequate dietary intake in healthy men who consumed an otherwise adequate diet, liver damage occurred.

✓   Choline doses that are in orders of magnitude greater than estimated intake from food have been associated with fishy body odor (trimethylaminuria), sweating, salivation, hypotension, and hepatotoxicity in humans. There are no indications in the literature that excess choline intake produces any additional adverse effects in humans.

TABLE 1 Dietary Reference Intakes for Vitamin D by Life Stage Group

	DRI values (μg/day)	
	AI[a,b,c]	UL[d]
Life stage group[e]		
0 through 6 mo	5	25
7 through 12 mo	5	25
1 through 3 y	5	50
4 through 8 y	5	50
9 through 13 y	5	50
14 through 18 y	5	50
19 through 30 y	5	50
31 through 50 y	5	50
51 through 70 y	10	50
> 70 y	15	50
Pregnancy		
≤ 18 y	5	50
19 through 50 y	5	50
Lactation		
≤ 18 y	5	50
19 through 50 y	5	50

[a] **AI** = Adequate Intake.
[b] As cholecalciferol. 1μg cholecalciferol = 40 IU vitamin D.
[c] In the absence of adequate exposure to sunlight.
[d] **UL** = Tolerable Upper Intake Level. Unless otherwise specified, the UL represents total intake from food, water, and supplements.
[e] All groups except Pregnancy and Lactation represent males and females.

VITAMIN D

Vitamin D (calciferol) is involved in bone health and is naturally found in very few foods. Synthesized in the skin through exposure to ultraviolet B rays in sunlight, its major biological function is to aid in the absorption of calcium and phosphorus, thereby helping maintain normal serum levels of these minerals. Vitamin D also functions as an antiproliferation and prodifferentiation hormone, but the exact role it plays is not yet known.

The AIs for vitamin D are based on serum 25-hydroxyvitamin D [25(OH)D], which is the form that represents vitamin D storage. The Tolerable Upper Intake Level (UL) was derived using studies of the effect of vitamin D intake on serum calcium concentrations (to prevent hypercalcemia) in humans. Since data were inadequate to determine an Estimated Average Requirement (EAR) and thus calculate a Recommended Dietary Allowance (RDA) for vitamin D, an Average Intake (AI) was instead developed. DRI values are listed by life stage group in Table 1.

Foods naturally rich in vitamin D include the flesh of fatty fish, some fish-liver oils, and eggs from hens fed vitamin D. Fortified milk products and breakfast cereals are also good sources of vitamin D. Vitamin D deficiency can impair normal bone metabolism, which may lead to rickets in children or osteomalacia (undermineralized bone) or osteoporosis (porous bones) in adults. In contrast, excess vitamin D intake can cause high blood calcium, high urinary calcium, and the calcification of soft tissues, such as blood vessels and certain organs.

VITAMIN D AND THE BODY

Function

The primary function of vitamin D in the body is to aid in the intestinal absorption of calcium and phosphorus, thereby helping maintain normal serum levels of these minerals in the body. Other roles in cellular metabolism involve antiproliferation and prodifferentiation actions.

Vitamin D is fat-soluble and occurs in many forms, but the two dietary forms are vitamin D_2 (ergocalciferol) and vitamin D_3 (cholecalciferol). Vitamin D_2 originates from the yeast and plant sterol, ergosterol; vitamin D_3 originates from 7-dehydrocholesterol, a precursor of cholesterol, when synthesized in the skin. Vitamin D_2 and vitamin D_3 are similarly metabolized. Vitamin D without a subscript represents either vitamins D_2 or D_3, or both, and is biologically inert. The biologically active hormone form of vitamin D is 1,25-dihydroxyvitamin D [1,25(OH)$_2$D].

Absorption, Metabolism, Storage, and Excretion

Vitamin D is either synthesized in the skin through exposure to ultraviolet B rays in sunlight or ingested as dietary vitamin D. After absorption of dietary fat-soluble vitamin D in the small intestine, it is incorporated into the chylomicron fraction and absorbed through the lymphatic system.

Whether from the skin or from the lymphatic system, vitamin D accumulates in the liver, where it is hydroxylated to 25-hydroxyvitamin D [25(OH)D] and then enters the circulation. The circulating 25(OH)D concentration is a good indicator of vitamin D status. In order to have biological activity at physiological concentrations, 25(OH)D must be hydroxylated to 1,25(OH)$_2$D. This conversion occurs in the kidneys and is tightly regulated by parathyroid hormone in response to serum calcium and phosphorus levels. Vitamin D is absorbed in the small intestine and is principally excreted in the bile after metabolites are inactivated. A variety of vitamin D metabolites are excreted by the kidney into the urine.

DETERMINING DRIS

Determining Requirements

Because sufficient data were not available to establish an EAR and thus calculate an RDA, an AI was instead developed. The AIs for vitamin D are based on serum 25(OH)D concentrations; they assume that no vitamin D is available from sun-mediated cutaneous synthesis. The AI is the intake value that appears to be needed to maintain (in a defined group of healthy individuals with limited but uncertain sun exposure and stores) serum 25-hydroxyvitamin D concentrations above a defined amount. The latter is that concentration below which vitamin D deficiency rickets or osteomalacia occurs. When consumed by an individual, the AI is sufficient to minimize the risk of low serum 25(OH)D.

Because human milk contains very little vitamin D, breast-fed infants who are not exposed to sunlight are unlikely to obtain adequate amounts of vitamin D from mother's milk to satisfy their needs beyond early infancy. Therefore, the AI for infants aged 0 through 12 months does not assume vitamin D synthesis from sunlight exposure and is based on the lowest dietary intake associated with adequate serum 25(OH)D concentrations.

Accurate estimates of vitamin D intakes in the United States are lacking, in part because the vitamin D composition of fortified foods highly varies and also because many surveys do not include estimates of vitamin D intake.

Special Considerations

Older adults: Older adults, especially those who live in northern industrialized cities of the world, are more prone to developing vitamin D deficiency.

Infants: Whether fed human milk or formula, infants have the same requirements for dietary vitamin D if they have not been exposed to sunlight. Most standard infant formulas contain enough vitamin D to meet needs, but because human milk has very little vitamin D, breast-fed infants who are not exposed to sunlight are unlikely to obtain adequate amounts of vitamin D from mother's milk to satisfy their needs beyond early infancy.

For infants who live in far-northern latitudes or whose sunlight exposure is restricted, a minimal intake of 2.5 μg (100 IU)/day of vitamin D will likely prevent rickets. However, at this intake and in the absence of sunlight, many infants will have serum 25(OH)D concentrations within the range that is often observed in cases of rickets. For this reason, and assuming that infants are not obtaining any vitamin D from sunlight, an AI of at least 5 μg (200 IU)/day is recommended.

Criteria for Determining Vitamin D Requirements, by Life Stage Group

Life stage group	Criterion
For all life stage groups	Serum 25(OH)D

The UL

The Tolerable Upper Intake Level (UL) is the highest level of daily nutrient intake that is likely to pose no risk of adverse effects for almost all people. Members of the general population should not routinely exceed the UL. The DRI for vitamin D was derived using studies of the effect of vitamin D intake on serum calcium concentrations (to prevent hypercalcemia) in humans and represents total intake from food, water, and supplements.

Because milk is fortified to contain 10 μg (400 IU)/quart of vitamin D in the United States and 8.8 μg (352 IU)/liter of vitamin D in Canada, people with high milk intakes also may have relatively high vitamin D intakes. The 1986 National Health Interview Survey (NHIS) estimated that the 95th percentile of intake by users of vitamin D supplements was 20 μg (800 IU)/day for men and 17.2 μg(686) IU/day for women. For most people, vitamin D intake from food and supplements is unlikely to exceed the UL. However, people who are at the upper end of the ranges for both sources of intake, particularly those who use many supplements and those with high intakes of fish or fortified milk, may be at risk for vitamin D toxicity.

Special Considerations

Granulomatous diseases: People with granulomatous diseases (such as sarcoidosis, tuberculosis, and histoplasmosis), who are receiving glucocorticoids may require supplemental vitamin D. Granulomatous diseases are characterized by hypercalcemia or hypercalciuria, or both, in individuals with normal or less-than-normal vitamin D intakes or with exposure to sunlight (see "Inadequate Intake and Deficiency").

SOURCES OF VITAMIN D

Sunlight

Exposure to ultraviolet B rays through sunlight is a primary way by which humans obtain vitamin D. However, several factors can limit the skin's synthesis of vitamin D, including the use of sunscreen, increased levels of skin melanin, the distance one is from the Equator, the time of day, and the season of the year. Above and below latitudes of approximately 40 degrees N and 40 degrees S, vitamin D_3 in the skin is absent during most of the 3–4 winter months. The far-northern and southern latitudes extend this period for up to 6 months.

Foods

Vitamin D naturally occurs in very few foods, mainly in the flesh of fatty fish, some fish-liver oils, and eggs from hens fed vitamin D. Most people's dietary intake of vitamin D comes from foods fortified with vitamin D. In Canada, all milks and margarines must be fortified. In the United States, milk products, breakfast cereals, and some fruit juices are fortified.

Dietary Supplements

In the 1986 NHIS, the use of vitamin D supplements was reported in more than one-third of children 2 to 6 years of age, more than one-fourth of women, and almost one-fifth of men. The median supplement dose was the same for all users: 10 μg (400 IU).

Bioavailability

This information was not provided at the time the DRI values for this nutrient were set.

Dietary interactions

There is evidence that vitamin D may interact with certain other nutrients and dietary substances (see Table 2).

TABLE 2 Potential Interactions with Other Dietary Substances

Substance	Potential Interaction	Notes
SUBSTANCES THAT AFFECT VITAMIN D		
Magnesium	Magnesium deficiency may affect the body's response to pharmacological vitamin D.	Individuals with hypocalcemia and magnesium deficiency are resistant to pharmacological doses of vitamin D, 1,α-hydroxyvitamin D, and 1,25-dihydroxyvitamin D.

INADEQUATE INTAKE AND DEFICIENCY

Vitamin D deficiency results in the inadequate bone mineralization or demineralization of the skeleton. The potential effects of vitamin D deficiency include the following:

- Rickets (in children)
- Osteomalacia (in adults)
- Elevated serum parathyroid hormone
- Decreased serum phosphorus
- Elevated serum alkaline phosphatase
- Osteoporosis (porous bones)

Epidemiological studies have found an association between vitamin D deficiency and an increased risk of colon, breast, and prostate cancer in people who live at higher latitudes. However, additional studies are needed to further explore this association.

Special Considerations

Older adults: As adults age, their ability to synthesize vitamin D in the skin significantly decreases. Adults over the age of 65 years produce four times less vitamin D in the skin compared with adults aged 20 to 30 years.

Sunlight and skin pigmentation: The major source of vitamin D for humans is the exposure of the skin to sunlight, which initiates the conversion of 7-dehydrocholesterol to previtamin D_3 in the skin. An increase in skin melanin pigmentation or the topical use of sunscreen reduces the production of vitamin D_3 in the skin.

Malabsorption disorders: Conditions that cause fat malabsorption, such as severe liver failure, Crohn's disease, Whipple's disease, and celiac sprue, are associated with vitamin D deficiency because people with these conditions are unable to absorb vitamin D.

Medications: Glucocorticoids inhibit vitamin D–dependent intestinal calcium absorption and therefore can cause osteopenia. Individuals on glucocorticoid therapy may require supplemental vitamin D to maintain normal serum levels of 25(OH)D. Medications used to control seizures, such as phenobarbital and dilantin, can alter the metabolism and circulating half-life of vitamin D. People taking these medications (particularly those without exposure to sunlight) may require supplemental vitamin D.

EXCESS INTAKE

Excess intake of vitamin D can cause hypervitaminosis D, which is characterized by a considerable increase in the serum levels of 25(OH)D (to 400–1,250 nmol/L). The adverse effects of hypervitaminosis D are probably largely mediated via hypercalcemia. The potential effects of the hypercalcemia associated with hypervitaminosis D include the following:

- Polyuria
- Polydipsia
- Hypercalciuria
- Calcification of soft tissues (including the kidneys, blood vessels, heart, and lungs)
- Anorexia
- Nausea
- Vomiting
- Reduced renal function

There is no evidence that vitamin D obtained through sun exposure can contribute to vitamin D toxicity because there is a limit to the amount of vitamin D_3 formed. Once this amount is reached, the previtamin and vitamin D_3 remaining in the skin are destroyed with continued sunlight exposure.

KEY POINTS FOR VITAMIN D

✓   Vitamin D (calciferol) is involved in bone health. It aids in the absorption of calcium and phosphorus, thereby helping maintain normal serum levels of these minerals.

✓   Vitamin D is either synthesized in the skin through exposure to ultraviolet B rays in sunlight or ingested as dietary vitamin D. As adults age, their ability to synthesize vitamin D in the skin significantly decreases.

✓   Since data were inadequate to determine an EAR and thus calculate an RDA for vitamin D, an AI was instead developed.

✓   The AIs for vitamin D are based on serum 25(OH)D, which is the form that represents vitamin D storage.

✓   The UL was derived using studies of the effect of vitamin D intake on serum calcium concentrations (to prevent hypercalcemia) in humans.

✓   For most people, dietary vitamin D intake is unlikely to exceed the UL.

✓   Most standard infant formulas contain enough vitamin D to meet needs, but because human milk has very little vitamin D, breast-fed infants who are not exposed to sunlight are unlikely to obtain adequate amounts of vitamin D from mother's milk to satisfy their needs beyond early infancy.

✓   Exposure to ultraviolet B rays through sunlight is a primary way by which humans obtain vitamin D. However, several factors can limit the skin's synthesis of vitamin D, including the use of sunscreen, increased levels of skin melanin, the distance one is from the Equator, the time of day, and the season of the year.

✓   Vitamin D naturally occurs in very few foods, mainly in the flesh of fatty fish, some fish-liver oils, and eggs from hens fed vitamin D. In Canada, all milks and margarines must be fortified. In the United States, milk products, breakfast cereals, and some fruit juices are fortified.

✓   Vitamin D deficiency can impair normal bone metabolism, which may lead to rickets in children and osteomalacia in adults. It is also implicated in osteoporosis in adults.

✓ Older adults, especially those who live in northern industrialized cities of the world, are more prone to developing vitamin D deficiency.

✓ There is no evidence that vitamin D obtained through sun exposure can contribute to vitamin D toxicity.

✓ Excess intake of vitamin D can cause hypervitaminosis D, the effects of which include hypercalcemia, hypercalciuria, and calcification of soft tissues, such as blood vessels and certain organs.

TABLE 1 Dietary Reference Intakes for Vitamin E (α-Tocopherol^a) by Life Stage Group

| | DRI values (mg^a/day) | | | |
	EAR^b	RDA^c	AI^d	UL^{e,f}
Life stage group^g				
0 through 6 mo			4	ND^h
7 through 12 mo			5	ND
1 through 3 y	5	6		200
4 through 8 y	6	7		300
9 through 13 y	9	11		600
14 through 18 y	12	15		800
19 through 30 y	12	15		1,000
31 through 50 y	12	15		1,000
51 through 70 y	12	15		1,000
> 70 y	12	15		1,000
Pregnancy				
≤ 18 y	12	15		800
19 through 50 y	12	15		1,000
Lactation				
≤ 18 y	16	19		800
19 through 50 y	16	19		1,000

^{a} For the EAR, RDA, and AI: α-Tocopherol includes *RRR*-α-tocopherol, the only form of α-tocopherol that occurs naturally in foods, and the 2*R*-stereoisomeric forms of α-tocopherol (*RRR*-, *RSR*-, *RRS*-, and *RSS*-α-tocopherol) that occur in fortified foods and supplements. This does not include the 2*S*-stereoisomeric forms of α-tocopherol (*SRR*-, *SSR*-, *SRS*-, and *SSS*-α-tocopherol), also found in fortified foods and supplements. The 2*S*-stereoisomers are not stored in the body.
^{b} **EAR** = Estimated Average Requirement.
^{c} **RDA** = Recommended Dietary Allowance.
^{d} **AI** = Adequate Intake.
^{e} **UL** = Tolerable Upper Intake Level. Unless otherwise specified, the UL represents total intake from food, water, and supplements.
^{f} As α-tocopherol; applies to any form of supplemental α-tocopherol since all are absorbed and can potentially contribute to vitamin E toxicity. The UL applies to synthetic forms obtained from supplements, fortified foods, or a combination of the two. Little information exists on the adverse effects that might result from ingestion of other forms.
^{g} All groups except Pregnancy and Lactation represent males and females.
^{h} **ND** = Not determinable. This value is not determinable due to the lack of data of adverse effects in this age group and concern regarding the lack of ability to handle excess amounts. Source of intake should only be from food to prevent high levels of intake.

VITAMIN E

Vitamin E is a fat-soluble nutrient that functions as a chain-breaking antioxidant in the body by preventing the spread of free-radical reactions. Of the eight naturally occurring forms of vitamin E only the α-tocopherol form of the vitamin is maintained in the plasma.

The requirements for vitamin E are based on the prevention of hydrogen peroxide–induced hemolysis. The Estimated Average Requirement (EAR), Recommended Dietary Allowance (RDA), and Adequate Intake (AI) values for vitamin E only apply to intake of the 2R-stereoisomeric forms of α-tocopherol from food, fortified foods, and supplements. Other naturally occurring forms of vitamin E do not meet the vitamin E requirement because they are not converted to α-tocopherol in humans and are poorly recognized by the α-tocopherol transfer protein in the liver.

The Tolerable Upper Intake Level (UL) is based on the adverse effect of increased tendency to hemorrhage. The UL for vitamin E applies to any forms of supplemental α-tocopherol because all are absorbed; these forms of synthetic vitamin E are almost exclusively used in supplements, food fortification, and pharmacological agents. Little information exists on the adverse effects that might result from the ingestion of other forms of vitamin E. DRI values are listed by life stage group in Table 1.

Food sources of vitamin E include vegetable oils and spreads, unprocessed cereal grains, nuts, fruits, vegetables, and meats (especially the fatty portion). Overt deficiency of vitamin E in the United States and Canada is rare and is generally only seen in people who are unable to absorb the vitamin or who have inherited conditions that prevent the maintenance of normal blood concentrations. There is no evidence of adverse effects from the consumption of vitamin E naturally occurring from foods. The possible chronic effects of lifetime exposures to high supplemental levels of α-tocopherol remain uncertain.

VITAMIN E AND THE BODY

Function

Unlike most nutrients, vitamin E does not appear to play a specific role in certain metabolic pathways. Its major function seems to be as a nonspecific chain-breaking antioxidant that prevents the spread of free-radical reactions. It scavenges peroxyl radicals and protects polyunsaturated fatty acids within membrane phospholipids and in plasma lipoproteins.

On the molecular level, vitamin E (α-tocopherol form) inhibits protein kinase C activity (involved in cell proliferation and differentiation) in smooth muscle cells, platelets, and monocytes. It may also improve vasodilation and inhibit platelet aggregation by enhancing the release of prostacyclin.

Absorption, Metabolism, Storage, and Excretion

Vitamin E is absorbed in the intestine, although the precise rate of absorption is not known. All of the forms of vitamin E appear to have similar low absorption efficiency. Absorbed vitamin E in the form of chylomicron remnants is taken up by the liver, and then only one form of vitamin E, α-tocopherol, is preferentially secreted in very low density lipoproteins. Thus, it is the liver, not the intestine, that discriminates between tocopherols. Tissues take up vitamin E from the plasma. Vitamin E rapidly transfers between various lipoproteins and also between lipoproteins and membranes, which may enrich membranes with vitamin E. Vitamin E is excreted in both the urine and feces, with fecal elimination being the major mode of excretion.

DETERMINING DRIS

There are eight naturally occurring forms, or isomers, of vitamin E: four tocopherols (α-, β-, γ-, and δ-tocopherols) and four tocotrienols (α-, β-, γ-, and δ-tocotrienols). These various forms of vitamin E are not interconvertible in humans, and thus do not behave the same metabolically. Of the eight, only α-tocopherol is maintained in the plasma.

The isomer α-tocopherol has eight possible stereoisomers: four in the 2R-stereoisomeric form (RRR-, RSR-, RRS-, and RSS-α-tocopherol) and four in the 2S-stereoisomeric form (SRR-, SSR-, SRS-, and SSS-α-tocopherol). Of these, only one—the RRR form—naturally occurs in foods. All eight stereoisomers are represented by synthetic forms (together called all-rac-α-tocopherol) and are present in fortified foods and in vitamin supplements.

Of the eight stereoisomers of α-tocopherol, the only forms that are maintained in the plasma are naturally occurring RRR-α-tocopherol and the 2R-stereoisomeric forms present in synthetic forms. Since the 2S-stereoisomers are not maintained in the plasma or tissues, they are not included in the definition of active components for vitamin E activity in humans.

For the purpose of establishing the requirements, vitamin E activity is defined here as being limited to the 2R-stereoisomeric forms of α-tocopherol. However, all eight stereoisomeric forms of supplemental α-tocopherol are used as the basis for establishing the UL for vitamin E. This is because all eight forms are absorbed. These recommended intakes and ULs vary from past definitions and recommendations for vitamin E.

Determining Requirements

The adult requirements for vitamin E are based largely on induced vitamin E deficiency in humans and the intake that correlated with in vitro hydrogen peroxide–induced red blood cell hemolysis and plasma α-tocopherol concentrations. Although some studies have reported a possible protective effect of vitamin E on conditions such as cardiovascular and neurological diseases, cancer, cataracts, and diseases of the immune system, the data are inadequate to support population-wide dietary recommendations that are specifically based on preventing these diseases.

The EAR, RDA, and AI values for vitamin E apply only to intake of the 2R-stereoisomeric forms of α-tocopherol from food, fortified foods, and supplements. The other naturally occurring isomers of vitamin E (β-, γ-, and δ-tocopherols and α-, β-, γ-, and δ-tocotrienols) do not contribute to meeting the vitamin E requirement because they are not converted to α-tocopherol in humans; these forms of synthetic vitamin E are almost exclusively used in supplements, food fortification, and pharmacological agents. Little information exists on the adverse effects that might result from ingestion of excess amounts of other isomeric forms (such as γ- and β-tocopherol).

Currently, most nutrient databases, as well as nutrition labels, do not distinguish among all the different forms of vitamin E found in food. These databases often present the data as α-tocopherol equivalents (α-TE), and thus include the contributions of all eight naturally occurring forms of vitamin E, after adjustment for bioavailability using previously determined equivalencies. It is recommended that the use of α-TE be abandoned due to the lack of evidence of bioavailability via transport in the plasma or tissues. Because these other forms of vitamin E occur in foods, the intake of α-TE is greater than the intake of α-tocopherol alone. The values above were converted from α-TE to α-tocopherol using a factor of 0.8 as described later in this chapter (see "Dietary Sources").

Criteria for Determining Vitamin E Requirements, by Life Stage Group

Life stage group	Criterion
0 through 6 mo	Human milk content
7 through 12 mo	Extropolation from 0 to 5.9 mo
1 through 18 y	Extrapolation from adult
19 through 30 y	Prevention of hydrogen peroxide–induced hemolysis
31 through > 70 y	Extrapolation of hydrogen peroxide–induced hemolysis from 19 through 30 y

Pregnancy

≤ 18 y through 50 y   Age-specific requirement + plasma concentration

Lactation

≤ 18 y through 50 y   Age-specific requirement + vitamin E secreted in milk

The UL

The Tolerable Upper Intake Level (UL) is the highest level of daily nutrient intake that is likely to pose no risk of adverse effects for almost all people. Members of the general population should not routinely consume more than the UL. The UL for vitamin E is based on the adverse effect of increased tendency to hemorrhage. The UL applies to all supplemental α-tocopherol forms of vitamin E (*RRR*-α-tocopherol and *all-rac*-α-tocopherol), since all are absorbed and can thus potentially contribute to vitamin E toxicity.

Sources of vitamin E available as supplements are usually labeled as international units (IUs) of natural vitamin E and its esters or as synthetic vitamin E and its esters. Table 2 shows the IUs of various sources of supplemental vitamin E that are equivalent to the UL for adults of 1,000 mg/day of any form of supplemental α-tocopherol.

Based on the Third National Health and Nutrition Examination Survey (NHANES III, 1988–1994) data, the highest mean reported intake of vitamin E from food and supplements for all life stage and gender groups was approximately 45 mg/day of α-tocopherol equivalents (reported by women aged 51 to 70 years). This group also had the highest reported intake at the 99th percentile, at 508 mg/day of α-tocopherol equivalents, which is well below the UL of 1,000 mg/day for any form of α-tocopherol. Vitamin E supplement use is high in the U.S. population. In the 1986 National Health Interview Survey (NHIS), supplements containing vitamin E were used by 23 percent of men, 29 percent of women, and 37 percent of young children in the United States. The risk of adverse effects resulting from excess intake of α-tocopherol from food and supplements appears to be very low based on this information.

Special Considerations

Vitamin K deficiency or anticoagulant therapy: The UL for vitamin E pertains to individuals in the general population with adequate vitamin K intake. Individuals who are deficient in vitamin K or who are on anticoagulant therapy are at increased risk of coagulation defects and should be monitored when taking vitamin E supplements.

**TABLE 2 Amounts in International Units (IU) of Any Forms of
α-Tocopherol*ᵃ* Contained in Vitamin E*ᵇ* Supplements Equivalent to
the UL for Adults*ᶜ***

Sources of Vitamin E Available as Supplements	UL for Adults Total α-Tocopherol (mg/day)	IU from Source Providing Adult UL
Synthetic Vitamin E and Esters		
dl-α-Tocopheryl acetate	1,000	1,100
dl-α-Tocopheryl succinate	1,000	1,100
dl-α-Tocopherol	1.000	1,100
Natural Vitamin E and Esters		
d-α-Tocopheryl acetate	1,000	1,500
d-α-Tocopheryl succinate	1,000	1,500
d-α-Tocopherol	1,000	1,500

ᵃ All forms of supplemental α-tocopherol include all eight stereoisomers of α-tocopherol. The UL is based on animal studies feeding either *all racemic-* or *RRR-*α-tocopherol, both of which resulted in equivalent adverse effects.

ᵇ Vitamin E supplements have been historically, although incorrectly, labeled *d-* or *dl-*α-tocopherol. Sources of vitamin E include the *all racemic-* (*dl-*α-tocopherol [*RRR-, RRS-, RSR-, RSS-, SSS-, SRS-, SSR-,* and *SRR-*] or synthetic) form and its esters. All of these forms of vitamin E may be present in supplements.

ᶜ The conversion factors used in this table are based on 2S-forms contributing to the adverse effects

DIETARY SOURCES

Foods

The main dietary sources of vitamin E are vegetable oils, such as wheat-germ oil, sunflower oil, cottonseed oil, safflower oil, canola oil, olive oil, palm oil, and rice-bran oil. Fats and oils in the form of spreads often contribute to vitamin E intake. Other sources of vitamin E include unprocessed cereal grains, nuts, fruits, vegetables, and meats (especially the fatty portion). As previously stated, only the natural form of α-tocopherol (*RRR-*α-tocopherol) found in these unfortified foods counts toward meeting the RDA. Other non-α-tocopherol forms of vitamin E present in food do not.

It is important to note that because vitamin E is generally found in fat-containing foods and is more easily absorbed from fat-containing meals, intakes of vitamin E by people who consume low-fat diets may be less than optimal unless food choices are carefully made to enhance vitamin E intake.

Estimating α-tocopherol content of foods and diets: As discussed, many databases of nutrient content and many food-intake surveys list vitamin E in the form of α-tocopherol equivalents (α-TE) rather than α-tocopherol. To estimate α-tocopherol content, multiply the number of α-tocopherol equivalents by a factor of 0.8:

$$\text{mg of } \alpha\text{-tocopherol in a meal} = \text{mg of } \alpha\text{-TEs in a meal} \times 0.8$$

Dietary Supplements

Vitamin E supplement use appears to be high in the U.S. population. Data from the Boston Nutritional Status Survey (1981–1984) on adults aged 60 years and older found that 38 percent of men took dietary supplements and, of them, 68 percent took a vitamin E supplement. Of the women surveyed, 49 percent used supplements, and 73 percent of them took a vitamin E supplement. In the 1986 NHIS, 26 percent of all adults reported using supplements that contained vitamin E.

Converting IUs to mg of α-tocopherol: To determine the milligrams of α-tocopherol in a dietary supplement labeled in international units (IUs), one of two conversion factors may be used:

- If the form of the supplemental vitamin E is naturally occurring or *RRR*-α-tocopherol (which has been historically and incorrectly labeled as *d*-α-tocopherol), the correct factor is 0.67 mg/IU. Thus, 30 IUs of *RRR*-α-tocopherol (labeled as *d*-α-tocopherol) in a multivitamin supplement would equate to 20 mg of α-tocopherol (30 × 0.67). The same factor is used for 30 IUs of either *RRR*-α-tocopherol acetate or *RRR*-α-tocopherol succinate because the amount in grams of these forms in a capsule has been adjusted based on their molecular weight.

  Mg of α-tocopherol in food, fortified food, or multivitamin = IU of the *RRR*-α-tocopherol compound × 0.67

- If the form of the supplement is *all-rac*-α-tocopherol (historically and incorrectly labeled as *dl*-α-tocopherol), the appropriate factor is 0.45 mg/IU. (This reflects the inactivity of the 2S-stereoisomers.) Thus, 30 IU of *all-rac*-α-tocopherol (labeled as *dl*-α-tocopherol) in a multivitamin supplement would equate to 13.5 mg of α-tocopherol (30 × 0.45). The same factor is used for the *all-rac*-α-tocopherol acetate and succinate forms.

  Mg of α-tocopherol in food, fortified food, or multivitamin = IU of the *all-rac*-α-tocopherol compound × 0.45

See Appendix F on conversion factors on converting IUs of vitamin E to α tocopherol.

Bioavailability

Because vitamin E is a fat-soluble nutrient, its absorption is enhanced when it is consumed in a meal that contains fat; however, the optimal amount of fat to enhance absorption has not been reported. This is probably more of a consideration for people who take vitamin E in supplement form, rather than for those who consume it from foods, since most dietary vitamin E is found in foods that contain fat.

Dietary Interactions

There is evidence that vitamin E may interact with certain dietary substances (see Table 3).

TABLE 3 Potential Interactions with Other Dietary Substances

Substance	Potential Interaction	Notes
SUBSTANCES THAT AFFECT VITAMIN E		
Polyunsaturated fatty acids (PUFAs)	Vitamin E requirements may increase when intakes of PUFAs are increased.	High PUFA intakes should be accompanied by increased vitamin E intakes.

INADEQUATE INTAKE AND DEFICIENCY

Vitamin E deficiency is very rare; overt symptoms of deficiency in healthy individuals consuming diets low in vitamin E have never been described. Vitamin E deficiency occurs only as a result of genetic abnormalities of vitamin E metabolism, fat malabsorption syndromes, or protein-energy malnutrition. The signs and symptoms of deficiency include the following:

- Peripheral neuropathy (primary symptom)
- Spinocerebellar ataxia
- Skeletal myopathy
- Pigmented retinopathy
- Increased erythrocyte fragility
- Increased ethane and pentane production

EXCESS INTAKE

There is no evidence of adverse effects from the excess consumption of vitamin E naturally occurring in foods. With regard to supplemental vitamin E intake in the form of synthetic α-tocopherol (as a supplement, food fortificant, or pharmacological agent), most studies in humans showing the safety of vitamin E were conducted in small groups of individuals who received supplemental amounts of 3,200 g/day or less (usually less than 2,000 mg/day) of α-tocopherol for periods of a few weeks to a few months Thus, the possible chronic effects of longer exposure to high supplemental levels of α-tocopherol remain uncertain and some caution must be exercised in judgments regarding the safety of supplemental doses of α-tocopherol over multiyear periods. The potential adverse effects of excess vitamin E intake include hemorrhagic toxicity and diminished blood coagulation in individuals who are deficient in vitamin K or on anticoagulant therapy.

Special Considerations

Premature infants: Hemolytic anemia due to vitamin E deficiency is of frequent concern in premature infants. However, its management via vitamin E supplementation must be carefully controlled because small premature infants are particularly vulnerable to the toxic effects of α-tocopherol.

KEY POINTS FOR VITAMIN E

✓   Vitamin E (α-tocopherol) is a fat-soluble nutrient that functions as a chain-breaking antioxidant in the body by preventing the spread of free-radical reactions.

✓   The adult requirements for vitamin E are based on prevention of hydrogen peroxide–induced hemolysis. The UL is based on the adverse effect of increased tendency to hemorrhage.

✓   The EAR, RDA, and AI values for vitamin E apply only to intake of the 2*R*-stereoisomeric forms of α-tocopherol from food, fortified foods, and supplements. The UL applies to any form of supplemental α-tocopherol because all are absorbed; these forms of synthetic vitamin E are almost exclusively used in supplements, food fortification, and pharmacological agents.

✓   Food sources of vitamin E include vegetable oils and spreads, unprocessed cereal grains, nuts, fruits, vegetables, and meats (especially the fatty portion).

✓   Vitamin E deficiency is very rare in the United States and Canada, generally occurring only as the result of genetic abnormalities of vitamin E metabolism, fat malabsorption syndromes, or protein-energy malnutrition. The primary effect of vitamin E deficiency is peripheral neuropathy.

✓   There is no evidence of adverse effects from the consumption of vitamin E naturally occurring in foods.

✓   The primary known adverse effect resulting from excessive supplemental vitamin E intake is hemorrhagic toxicity.

TABLE 1 Dietary Reference Intakes for Folate by Life Stage Group

	DRI values (µg /day[a])					
	EAR[b]		RDA[c]		AI[d]	UL[e,f]
	males	females	males	females		
Life stage group						
0 through 6 mo					65	ND[g]
7 through 12 mo					80	ND
1 through 3 y	120	120	150	150		300
4 through 8 y	160	160	200	200		400
9 through 13 y	250	250	300	300		600
14 through 18 y	330	330	400	400[h]		800
19 through 30 y	320	320	400	400[h]		1,000
31 through 50 y	320	320	400	400[h]		1,000
51 through 70 y	320	320	400	400		1,000
> 70 y	320	320	400	400		1,000
Pregnancy						
≤ 18 y		520		600[i]		800
19 through 50 y		520		600[i]		1,000
Lactation						
≤ 18 y		450		500		800
19 through 50 y		450		500		1,000

[a] As dietary folate equivalents (DFEs). 1 DFE = 1 µg food folate = 0.6 µg of folic acid from fortified food or as a supplement consumed with food = 0.5 µg of folic acid from a supplement taken on an empty stomach.

[b] **EAR** = Estimated Average Requirement.

[c] **RDA** = Recommended Dietary Allowance.

[d] **AI** = Adequate Intake.

[e] **UL** = Tolerable Upper Intake Level. Unless otherwise specified, the UL represents total intake from food, water, and supplements.

[f] The UL for folate applies to synthetic forms obtained from supplements, fortified foods, or a combination of the two.

[g] **ND** = Not determinable. This value is not determinable due to the lack of data of adverse effects in this age group and concern regarding the lack of ability to handle excess amounts. Source of intake should only be from food to prevent high levels of intake.

[h] To reduce risk of neural tube defects, women capable of becoming pregnant should take 400 µg of folic acid daily from fortified foods, supplements, or both, in addition to consuming food folate from a varied diet.

[i] It is assumed that women will continue consuming 400 µg from supplements or fortified food until their pregnancy is confirmed and they enter prenatal care, which ordinarily occurs after the end of the periconceptional period—the critical time for formation of the neural tube.

FOLATE

Folate is a B vitamin that functions as a coenzyme in the metabolism of nucleic and amino acids. Folate is a generic term that includes both the naturally occurring form of the vitamin (food folate or pteroyl-polyglutamates) and the monoglutamate form (folic acid or pteroylmonoglutamic acid), which is used in fortified foods and dietary supplements.

The requirements for folate are based on the amount of dietary folate equivalents (DFEs, with values adjusted for differences in the absorption of food folate and folic acid) needed to maintain erythrocyte folate. DFEs adjust for the nearly 50 percent lower bioavailability of food folate compared to that of folic acid. The Tolerable Upper Intake Level (UL) is based on the precipitation or exacerbation of neuropathy in vitamin B_{12}–deficient individuals as the critical endpoint and represents total intake from fortified food or dietary supplements. The UL does not include naturally occurring food folate. Although epidemiological evidence suggests that folate may protect against vascular disease, cancer, and mental disorders, the evidence was not sufficient to use risk reduction of these conditions as a basis for setting folate requirements. DRI values are listed by life stage group in Table 1.

Rich food sources of folate include fortified grain products, dark green vegetables, and beans and legumes. Chronic inadequate folate intake results in macrocytic anemia. The adverse effect of consuming excess supplemental folate is the onset or progression of neurological complications in people with vitamin B_{12} deficiency. Excess folate can obscure or mask and thus potentially delay the diagnosis of vitamin B_{12} deficiency, which can result in an increased risk of progressive, unrecognized neurological damage.

To reduce the risk of neural tube defects, women able to become pregnant should take 400 µg of folic acid daily from fortified foods, supplements, or both, in addition to consuming food folate from a varied diet. It is important to note that this recommendation specifically calls for folic acid, which is more bioavailable than food folate. Since foods fortified to a level of 400 µg are not available in Canada, the recommendation is to consume a multivitamin containing 400 µg of folic acid every day in addition to the amount of folate in a healthful diet.

FOLATE AND THE BODY

Function

Folate is a water-soluble B-complex vitamin that functions as a coenzyme in the metabolism of nucleic and amino acids. The term folate refers to two forms: naturally occurring folates in food, referred to here as food folates (pteroylpolyglutamates), and folic acid (pteroylmonoglutamic acid), which is rarely naturally found in foods but is the form used in dietary supplements and fortified foods. Folic acid is the most stable form of folate.

Absorption, Metabolism, Storage, and Excretion

Folate is absorbed from the gut across the intestinal mucosa via a saturable, pH-dependent active transport process. When pharmacological doses of folic acid are consumed, it is also absorbed by nonsaturable passive diffusion. Folate is taken up from the portal circulation by the liver, where it is metabolized and retained or released into the blood or bile. Approximately two-thirds of folate in plasma is bound to protein. Some folate is excreted in the urine, bile, and feces.

DETERMINING DRIS

Determining Requirements

The requirements for folate are based on the amount of dietary folate equivalents (DFEs) needed to maintain erythrocyte folate; ancillary data on plasma homocysteine and plasma folate concentrations were also considered. DFEs adjust for the nearly 50 percent lower bioavailability of food folate compared with that of folic acid (see "Bioavailability"), such that:

> 1 DFE = 1 μg food folate = 0.6 μg of folic acid from fortified food or as a supplement consumed with food = 0.5 μg of folic acid from a supplement taken on an empty stomach

Currently, nutrition labels do not distinguish between sources of folate (food folate and folic acid) or express the folate content in DFEs. Although epidemiological evidence suggests that folate may protect against vascular disease, cancer, and mental disorders, the evidence was not sufficient to use risk reduction of these conditions as a basis for setting folate requirements.

Special Considerations

Individuals with increased needs: Intakes of folate higher than the RDA may be needed by women who are carrying more than one fetus, mothers nursing more than one infant, individuals with chronic heavy intake of alcohol, and individuals on chronic anticonvulsant or methotrexate therapy.

To reduce the risk of neural tube defects, women able to become pregnant should take 400 μg of folic acid daily from fortified foods, supplements, or both, in addition to consuming food folate from a varied diet. It is important to note that this recommendation specifically calls for folic acid, which is more bioavailable than food folate. Since foods fortified to a level of 400 μg are not available in Canada, the recommendation is to consume a multivitamin containing 400 μg of folic acid every day in addition to the amount of folate in a healthful diet.

Intake of Folate

Currently nutrient databases and nutrition labels do not express the folate content of food in DFEs, which take into account the different bioavailabilities of folate sources. (See Box 1 for information on how DFEs and types of folate are

---

BOX 1 The Relationship Between DFEs and Types of Folate

DFEs and types of folate are related as follows:

1 μg of DFEs	= 1.0 μg of food folate
	= 0.6 μg of folate added to foods (as a fortificant or folate supplement with food)
	= 0.5 μg of folate taken as a supplement (on an empty stomach)

1 μg food folate	= 1.0 μg of DFEs
1 μg of folate added as a fortificant or as a supplement consumed with meals	= 1.7 μg of DFEs
1 μg of folate supplement taken on an empty stomach	= 2.0 μg of DFEs

When intakes of folate in an individual's diet are assessed, it is possible to approximate the DFE intake by estimating the amount present that has been added in fortification and the amount present that naturally occurs as food folate by using the relationship of 1 μg of folate added as a fortificant = 1.7 μg of DFEs (the reciprocal of 1 μg of DFEs = 0.6 μg folate added to food).

related.) Thus, nutrient intake data substantially underestimates the actual current intake. This is due to problems associated with analyzing the folate content of food, underreported intake, and the change in U.S. fortification laws instituted in 1998 (see "Dietary Sources" for information on fortification).

Criteria for Determining Folate Requirements, by Life Stage Group

Life stage group	Criterion
0 through 6 mo	Human milk content
7 through 12 mo	Extrapolation from younger infants and from adults
1 through 18 y	Extrapolation from adults
19 through > 70 y	Maintenance of normal erythrocyte folate, plasma homocysteine, plasma or serum folate

Pregnancy	
≤ 18 y through 50 y	Maintenance of normal erythrocyte and serum folate levels

Lactation	
≤ 18 y through 50 y	Folate intake necessary to replace folate secreted in human milk + folate needed to maintain folate status

The UL

The Tolerable Upper Intake Level (UL) is the highest level of daily nutrient intake that is likely to pose no risk of adverse effects for almost all people. Members of the general population should not routinely consume more than the UL. The UL for folate is from fortified foods or dietary supplements, or both. The UL does not include naturally occurring food folate and is based on the precipitation or exacerbation of neuropathy in vitamin B_{12}–deficient individuals as the critical endpoint. It has been recognized that excessive intake of folate supplements may obscure or mask and potentially delay the diagnosis of vitamin B_{12} deficiency.

The intake of folate in the United States is currently higher than indicated by the National Health and Nutrition Examination Survey (NHANES III, 1988–1994) because enriched cereal grains in the U.S. food supply, to which no folate was added previously, are now fortified with folate at 140 μg/100 g of cereal grain. The Food and Drug Administration (FDA) estimated that those who follow the guidance of the U.S. Food Guide Pyramid (1992) and consume cereal grains at the upper end of the recommended range might obtain an additional 440 μg/day of folate under the U.S. fortification regulations. Using this estimate and with the assumption of regular use of an over-the-counter supplement (400 μg per dose), it is unlikely that the intake of folate would regularly exceed 1,000 μg/day for members of any life stage or gender group.

Special Considerations

Individuals at increased risk: People who are at risk of vitamin B_{12} deficiency include those who follow a vegan diet, older adults with atrophic gastritis, and those with pernicious anemia and bacterial overgrowth of the gut. These individuals may place themselves at an increased risk of neurological disorders if they consume excess folate because folate may mask vitamin B_{12} deficiency.

Females of childbearing age: In general, the prevalence of vitamin B_{12} deficiency in women of the childbearing years is very low and the consumption of supplemental folate at or above the UL in this subgroup is unlikely to produce adverse effects.

DIETARY SOURCES

Foods

Rich food sources of folate include fortified grain products, dark green vegetables, and beans and legumes. According to data from the Continuing Survey of Food Intakes by Individuals (CSFII, 1994–1996), the greatest contribution to folate intake in U.S. adults came from fortified ready-to-eat cereals and a category called "other vegetables." This category includes vegetables such as green beans, green peas, lettuces, cabbages, and vegetable soups. Many of the vegetables in the "other vegetables" category have lower folate content than dark green vegetables, but are so commonly eaten that their contribution to total folate intake is relatively high compared to other sources such as citrus juices and legumes.

During the period when data were collected for CSFII (1994–1996), the only grain products fortified with folate were mainly hot and cold breakfast cereals. However, as of January 1, 1998, in the United States, all enriched cereal grains, such as bread, pasta, flour, breakfast cereal, and rice, are required to be fortified with folic acid at 1.4 mg/kg of grain. In Canada, the fortification of all white flour and cornmeal with folate is at a level of 1.5 mg/kg and fortification of alimentary paste is at a level of at least 2.0 mg/kg. Because enriched grains are widely consumed in Canada and the United States, these foods are now an important contributor to folate intake.

It is estimated that folate fortification will increase the folate intake of most U.S. women by 80 μg/day (136 μg DFE/day) or more. This amount could be provided by 1 cup of pasta plus 1 slice of bread. Depending on the cereal grains chosen and the amount consumed, 5 servings daily might add 220 µg/day or more of folate from fortified foods (nearly 400 µg DFE/day) to the diet.

Dietary Supplements

Folic acid supplements in doses of 400 µg are widely available over the counter. Supplements containing 1,000 µg or more are available by prescription in the United States and Canada.

In a nationwide telephone survey conducted by the Centers for Disease Control and Prevention (CDC) during January and February 1997, 43 percent of women of childbearing age reported taking some form of vitamin supplement containing folic acid; 32 percent reported taking a folic acid supplement daily and 12 percent reported taking a supplement less frequently.

Bioavailability

The bioavailability of folate varies, depending on the form of the vitamin ingested and whether it is consumed with or without food. Folic acid supplements taken on an empty stomach are nearly 100 percent bioavailable. No published information was found regarding the effect of food on the bioavailability of folate supplements. Folate in the form of folic acid added to foods is about 85 percent bioavailable. Naturally occurring food folates are about 50 percent bioavailable.

Dietary Interactions

There is evidence that folate may interact with certain nutrients, dietary substances, and drugs (see Table 2).

INADEQUATE INTAKE AND DEFICIENCY

Inadequate folate intake first leads to a decrease in serum folate concentration, then to a decrease in erythrocyte folate concentration, a rise in homocysteine concentration, and megaloblastic changes in the bone marrow and other tissues with rapidly dividing cells. These changes ultimately lead to macrocytic anemia, at first evidenced by a low erythrocyte count and eventually by a low hematocrit and hemoglobin, as well. The effects of moderate to severe macrocytic anemia may include the following:

- Weakness
- Fatigue
- Difficulty in concentrating
- Irritability

TABLE 2 Potential Interactions with Other Dietary Substances

Substance	Potential Interaction	Notes
SUBSTANCES THAT AFFECT FOLATE		
Alcohol	Inadequate folate intake in people with chronic alcoholism leads to folate deficiency.	Ethanol intake may aggravate folate deficiency by impairing intestinal folate absorption and hepatobiliary metabolism and by increasing renal folate excretion.
Cigarettes	Chronic smoking may lead to folate deficiency.	Low intake, rather than an increased requirement, in smokers may account for the poorer folate status of smokers.
Nonsteroidal anti-inflammatory drugs (NSAIDS): aspirin, ibuprofen, and acetaminophen	Very large therapeutic doses (e.g., 3,900 mg/day) of NSAIDS may exert antifolate activity.	Routine use of low doses of these drugs has not been reported to impair folate status.
Anticonvulsant drugs	Chronic use of anti-convulsant drugs, such as diphenylhydantoin and phenobarbital, may impair folate status.	Few studies have controlled for folate intake between groups of anticonvulsant users. Therefore, definitive conclusions could not be drawn regarding the potential adverse effects of these drugs on folate status.
Methotrexate	Chronic methotrexate therapy may impair folate status.	It has been recommended that patients undergoing chronic methotrexate therapy for rheumatoid arthritis increase their folate consumption or consider folate supplements (1 mg/day).
Other drugs with antifolate activity	Pyrimethamine (for malaria), trimethoprim (for bacterial infections), triamterene (for hypertension), trimetrexate (for *Pneumocystis carinii* infection), and sulfasalazine (for chronic ulcerative colitis) have been shown to exert antifolate activity.	

- Headache
- Palpitations
- Shortness of breath
- Atrophic glossitis

Special Considerations

Coexisting deficiencies: Coexisting iron or vitamin B_{12} deficiencies may interfere with the diagnosis of folate deficiency. In contrast to folate deficiency, iron deficiency leads to a decrease in mean cell volume. When there is a deficiency of both iron and folate, the interpretation of hematological changes may be unclear. A vitamin B_{12} deficiency results in the same hematological changes that occur with folate deficiency because the vitamin B_{12} deficiency results in a secondary folate deficiency.

EXCESS INTAKE

No adverse effects have been associated with the excess consumption of the amounts of folate normally found in fortified foods. The adverse effect that may result from excess intake of supplemental folate is the onset or progression of neurological complications in people with vitamin B_{12} deficiency. Excess folate may obscure or mask and thus potentially delay the diagnosis of vitamin B_{12} deficiency, which can result in an increased risk of progressive, unrecognized neurological damage.

KEY POINTS FOR FOLATE

✓ Folate is a B vitamin that functions as a coenzyme in the metabolism of nucleic and amino acids.

✓ Folate is a generic term that includes both the naturally occurring form of the vitamin (food folate) and the monoglutamate form (folic acid), which is used in fortified foods and dietary supplements.

✓ The requirements for folate are based on the amount of DFEs needed to maintain erythrocyte folate; plasma homocysteine and plasma folate concentrations were also considered. The UL is based on precipitation or exacerbation of neuropathy in vitamin B_{12}–deficient individuals as the critical endpoint.

✓ Although epidemiological evidence suggests that folate may protect against vascular disease, cancer, and mental disorders, the evidence was not sufficient to use risk reduction of these conditions as a basis for setting folate requirements.

✓   DFEs adjust for the nearly 50 percent lower bioavailability of food folate compared with that of folic acid, such that 1 DFE = 1 µg food folate = 0.6 µg of folic acid from fortified food or as a supplement consumed with food = 0.5 µg of folic acid from a supplement taken on an empty stomach.

✓   The UL for adults is from fortified foods or supplements. The UL does not include naturally occurring food folate.

✓   To reduce the risk of neural tube defects, women able to become pregnant should take 400 µg of folic acid daily from fortified foods, supplements, or both, in addition to consuming food folate from a varied diet. It is important to note that this recommendation specifically calls for folic acid, which is more bioavailable than food folate.

✓   Rich food sources of folate include fortified grain products, dark green vegetables, and beans and legumes.

✓   Chronic inadequate folate intake results in macrocytic anemia.

✓   Coexisting iron or vitamin B_{12} deficiency may interfere with the diagnosis of folate deficiency.

✓   No adverse effects have been associated with the excess consumption of the amounts of folate normally found in fortified foods.

✓   The adverse effect that may result from excess intake of supplemental folate is the onset or progression of neurological complications in people with vitamin B_{12} deficiency. Excess folate can obscure or mask and thus potentially delay the diagnosis of vitamin B_{12} deficiency, which can result in an increased risk of progressive, unrecognized neurological damage.

TABLE 1 Dietary Reference Intakes for Vitamin K by Life Stage Group

	DRI values (µg /day)		
	AI[a]		UL[b]
	males	females	
Life stage group			
0 through 6 mo	2.0	2.0	
7 through 12 mo	2.5	2.5	
1 through 3 y	30	30	
4 through 8 y	55	55	
9 through 13 y	60	60	
14 through 18 y	75	75	
19 through 30 y	120	90	
31 through 50 y	120	90	
51 through 70 y	120	90	
> 70 y	120	90	
Pregnancy			
≤ 18 y		75	
19 through 50 y		90	
Lactation			
≤ 18 y		75	
19 through 50 y		90	

[a] **AI** = Adequate Intake.
[b] **UL** = Tolerable Upper Intake Level. Data were insufficient to set a UL. In the absence of a UL, extra caution may be warranted in consuming levels above the recommended intake.

VITAMIN K

Vitamin K functions as a coenzyme for biological reactions involved in blood coagulation and bone metabolism. Phylloquinone, the plant form of vitamin K, is the major form in the diet. Menaquinone forms are produced by bacteria in the lower bowel.

Since data were insufficient to set an Estimated Average Requirement (EAR) and thus calculate a Recommended Dietary Allowance (RDA) for vitamin K, an Average Intake (AI) was instead developed. The AIs for vitamin K are based on median intakes of the nutrient. Data were insufficient to set a Tolerable Upper Intake Level (UL). DRI values are listed by life stage group in Table 1.

Rich dietary sources of vitamin K include leafy green vegetables, soy and canola oils, and margarine. Vegetables particularly rich in vitamin K include collard greens, spinach, and salad greens. Clinically significant vitamin K deficiency is extremely rare in the general population, with cases being limited to individuals with malabsorption syndromes or to those treated with drugs known to interfere with vitamin K metabolism. No adverse effects have been reported with high intakes of vitamin K from food or supplements.

VITAMIN K AND THE BODY

Function

Vitamin K functions as a coenzyme for biological reactions involved in blood coagulation and bone metabolism. It also plays an essential role in the conversion of certain residues in proteins into biologically active forms. These proteins include plasma prothrombin (coagulation factor II) and the plasma procoagulants, factors VII, IX, and X. Two structurally related vitamin K–dependent proteins have received recent attention as being proteins with possible roles in the prevention of chronic disease. They are osteocalcin, found in bone, and matrix Gla protein, originally found in bone, but now known to be more widely distributed,

Absorption, Metabolism, Storage, and Excretion

Phylloquinone is the major form of vitamin K in the diet. It is absorbed in the small intestine in a process that is enhanced by the presence of dietary fat and dependent on the normal flow of bile and pancreatic juice. The absorbed phylloquinone is then secreted into the lymph and enters the circulation as a component of chylomicrons. The circulating vitamin K is taken up by the liver and other tissues.

The liver, which contains the highest concentration of vitamin K in the body, rapidly accumulates ingested phylloquinone. Skeletal muscle contains little phylloquinone, but significant concentrations are found in the heart and some other tissues. Turnover in the liver is rapid and hepatic reserves are rapidly depleted when dietary intake of vitamin K is restricted. Vitamin K is excreted primarily in the bile, but also, to a lesser extent, in the urine.

Menaquinone forms of vitamin K are produced by bacteria in the lower bowel, where the forms appear in large amounts. However, their contribution to the maintenance of vitamin K status has been difficult to assess. Although the content is extremely variable, the human liver contains about 10 times as much vitamin K as a mixture of menaquinones than as phylloquinone.

DETERMINING DRIS

Determining Requirements

Since data were insufficient to set an EAR and thus calculate an RDA for vitamin K, an AI was instead developed. The AIs for vitamin K are based on the median intakes of the nutrient indicated by the Third National Health and Nutrition Examination Survey (NHANES III, 1988–1994).

It has been suggested that vitamin K may have roles in osteoporosis and vascular health. However, this is difficult to establish on the basis of the studies performed thus far. Clinical intervention studies investigating the relationship between vitamin K and osteoporosis are currently being conducted in North America and Europe. Whether vitamin K status within the range of normal intake plays a significant role in the development of atherosclerosis requires further investigation and should be verified in studies that employ rigorous experimental designs.

Special Considerations

Newborns: Vitamin K is poorly transported across the placenta, which puts newborn infants at risk for vitamin K deficiency. Poor vitamin K status, added to the fact that the concentrations of most plasma clotting factors are low at the time of birth, increases the risk of bleeding during the first few weeks of life, a condition known as hemorrhagic disease of the newborn (HDNB). Because HDNB can be effectively prevented by administering vitamin K, infants born in the United States and Canada routinely receive 0.5–1 mg of phylloquinone intramuscularly or 2.0 mg orally within 6 hours of birth. This practice is supported by both U.S. and Canadian pediatric societies.

Criteria for Determining Vitamin K Requirements, by Life Stage Group

Life stage group	Criterion
0 through 6 mo	Average vitamin K intake from human milk
7 through 12 mo	Extrapolation from 0 through 6 mo AI
1 through > 70 y	Median intake of vitamin K from NHANES III

Pregnancy

≤ 18 y	Adolescent female median intake
19 through 50 y	Adult female median intake

Lactation

≤ 18 y	Adolescent female median intake
19 through 50 y	Adult female median intake

The UL

The Tolerable Upper Intake Level (UL) is the highest level of daily nutrient intake that is likely to pose no risk of adverse effects for almost all healthy people. Data were insufficient to set a UL for vitamin K.

DIETARY SOURCES

Foods

Only a relatively small number of food items substantially contribute to the dietary phylloquinone intake of most people. A few green vegetables (collards, spinach, and salad greens) contain in excess of 300 µg of phylloquinone/100 g, while broccoli, brussels sprouts, cabbage, and bib lettuce contain between 100 and 200 µg of phylloquinone/100 g. Other green vegetables contain smaller amounts.

Plant oils and margarine are the second major source of phylloquinone in the diet. The phylloquinone content of plant oils varies, with soybean and canola oils containing greater than 100 µg of phylloquinone/100 g. Cottonseed oil and olive oil contain about 50 µg/100 g, and corn oil contains less than 5 µg/100 g. According to the Food and Drug Administration's (FDA's) Total Diet Study (1991–1997), spinach, collard greens, broccoli, and iceberg lettuce are the major contributors of vitamin K in the diets of U.S. adults and children.

The hydrogenation of plant oils to form solid shortenings results in some conversion of phylloquinone to 2′,3′-dihydrophylloquinone. This form of vitamin K is more prevalent in margarines, infant formulas, and processed foods, and it can represent a substantial portion of total vitamin K in some diets. Some cheeses may also supply a substantial amount of vitamin K (40–80 μg/100 g) in the form of menaquinone. However, as earlier mentioned, the contribution of menaquinones to the maintenance of vitamin K status has been difficult to assess.

Dietary Supplements

According to data from NHANES III, median intakes of vitamin K from food and supplements were 93–119 μg/day for men and 82–90 mg/day for women (for those who reported consuming supplements).

Bioavailability

Studies on the bioavailability of vitamin K (in the form of phylloquinone) have been limited. Until more data are available, the bioavailability of phylloquinone obtained from vegetables should not be considered to be less than 20 percent as available as phylloquinone obtained from supplements. It is known, however, that the absorption of vitamin K from vegetables is enhanced by the presence of dietary fat.

Dietary Interactions

The main interaction of concern regarding vitamin K involves anticoagulant medications, such as warfarin. Chronic use of these drugs results in an acquired cellular vitamin K deficiency and a decrease in the synthesis of vitamin K–dependent clotting factors. Alterations in vitamin K intake can influence the efficacy of these drugs.

Individuals on chronic warfarin therapy may require dietary counseling on how to maintain steady vitamin K intake levels. Because habitual vitamin K intake may modulate warfarin dosage in patients using this anticoagulant, these individuals should maintain their normal dietary and supplementation patterns once an effective dose of warfarin has been established. Short-term, day-to-day variations in vitamin K intake from food sources do not appear to interfere with anticoagulant status and therefore do not need to be carefully monitored. However, changes in supplemental vitamin K intake should be avoided, since the bioavailability of synthetic (supplemental) phylloquinone is considerably greater than the bioavailability of phylloquinone from food sources.

There is evidence that vitamin K may also interact with other nutrients and dietary substances (see Table 2).

TABLE 2 Potential Interactions with Other Dietary Substances

Substance	Potential Interaction	Notes
SUBSTANCES THAT AFFECT VITAMIN K		
Vitamin E	Elevated intakes of vitamin E may antagonize the action of vitamin K.	Increased intakes of vitamin E have not been reported to antagonize vitamin K status in healthy humans. However, in one study, patients receiving anticoagulation therapy who were supplemented with approximately 400 IU/day of α-tocopherol experienced nonstatistically significant decreases in prothrombin time over a 4-week period. The metabolic basis for the potential antagonism of vitamin K by vitamin E has not been completely determined.

INADEQUATE INTAKE AND DEFICIENCY

Studies conducted over a number of years have indicated that the simple restriction of vitamin K intake to levels almost impossible to achieve in any nutritionally adequate, self-selected diet does not impair normal hemostatic control in healthy subjects. Although there is some interference in the hepatic synthesis of the vitamin K–dependent clotting factors that can be measured by sensitive assays, standard clinical measures of procoagulant potential are not changed. In general, clinically significant vitamin K deficiency is extremely rare in the general population, with cases being limited to individuals with various lipid malabsorption syndromes or to those treated with drugs known to interfere with vitamin K metabolism. However, a clinically significant vitamin K deficiency has usually been defined as a vitamin K–responsive hypoprothrombinemia and is associated with an increase in prothrombin time and, in severe cases, bleeding.

There have also been case reports of bleeding occurring in patients taking antibiotics, and the use of these drugs has often been associated with an acquired vitamin K deficiency resulting from a suppression of menaquinone-synthesizing organisms. But the reports are complicated by the possibility of general malnutrition in this given patient population and by the antiplatelet action of many of the same drugs.

EXCESS INTAKE

No adverse effects have been reported with high intakes of vitamin K from food or supplements in healthy individuals who are not intentionally blocking vitamin K activity with anticoagulation medications. A search of the literature revealed no evidence of toxicity associated with the intake of either the phylloquinone or the menaquinone forms of vitamin K. Menadione, a synthetic form of the vitamin, has been associated with liver damage and is no longer therapeutically used.

KEY POINTS FOR VITAMIN K

✓   Vitamin K functions as a coenzyme for biological reactions involved in blood coagulation and bone metabolism.

✓   Since data were insufficient to set an EAR and thus calculate an RDA for vitamin K, an AI was instead developed.

✓   The AIs for vitamin K are based on the median intakes indicated by NHANES III.

✓   Infants born in the United States and Canada routinely receive 0.5–1 mg of phylloquinone intramuscularly or 2.0 mg orally within 6 hours of birth. This practice is supported by both U.S. and Canadian pediatric societies.

✓   Data were insufficient to set a UL.

✓   Although epidemiological evidence indicates that vitamin K may play a role in osteoporosis prevention, more research in this area is needed.

✓   Only a relatively small number of food items contribute substantially to the dietary phylloquinone intake of most people. A few green vegetables (collards, spinach, and salad greens) contain in excess of 300 µg of phylloquinone/100 g, while broccoli, brussels sprouts, cabbage, and bib lettuce contain between 100 and 200 µg of phylloquinone/100 g.

✓   The main interaction of concern regarding vitamin K involves anticoagulant medications, such as warfarin. Patients on chronic warfarin therapy may require dietary counseling on how to maintain steady vitamin K intake levels.

✓   In general, clinically significant vitamin K deficiency is extremely rare in the general population, with cases being limited to individuals with malabsorption syndromes or those treated with drugs known to interfere with vitamin K metabolism. However, the classic sign of vitamin K deficiency is a vitamin K–responsive increase in prothrombin time and, in severe cases, bleeding.

✓   No adverse effects have been reported with high intakes of vitamin K from food or supplements in healthy individuals who are not intentionally blocking vitamin K activity with anticoagulation medications.

TABLE 1 Dietary Reference Intakes for Niacin by Life Stage Group

	DRI values (mg/day)					
	EAR[a,b]		RDA[a,c]		AI[a,d]	UL[e,f]
	males	females	males	females		
Life stage group						
0 through 6 mo					2	ND[g]
7 through 12 mo					4	ND
1 through 3 y	5	5	6	6		10
4 through 8 y	6	6	8	8		15
9 through 13 y	9	9	12	12		20
14 through 18 y	12	11	16	14		30
19 through 30 y	12	11	16	14		35
31 through 50 y	12	11	16	14		35
51 through 70 y	12	11	16	14		35
> 70 y	12	11	16	14		35
Pregnancy						
≤ 18 y		14		18		30
19 through 50 y		14		18		35
Lactation						
≤ 18 y		13		17		30
19 through 50 y		13		17		35

[a] As niacin equivalents (NE). 1 mg of niacin = 60 mg of tryptophan; 0–6 months = preformed niacin (not NE).

[b] **EAR** = Estimated Average Requirement.

[c] **RDA** = Recommended Dietary Allowance.

[d] **AI** = Adequate Intake.

[e] **UL** = Tolerable Upper Intake Level. Unless otherwise specified, the UL represents total intake from food, water, and supplements.

[f] The UL for niacin applies to synthetic forms obtained from supplements, fortified foods, or a combination of the two. The UL is not expressed in NEs.

[g] **ND** = Not determinable. This value is not determinable due to the lack of data of adverse effects in this age group and concern regarding the lack of ability to handle excess amounts. Source of intake should only be from food to prevent high levels of intake.

NIACIN

The term niacin refers to nicotinamide (nicotinic acid amide), nicotinic acid (pyridine-3-carboxylic acid), and derivatives that exhibit the biological activity of nicotinamide. Niacin is involved in many biological reactions, including intracellular respiration and fatty acid synthesis. The amino acid tryptophan is converted in part into nicotinamide and thus can contribute to meeting the requirement for niacin.

The primary method used to estimate the requirements for niacin intake relates intake to the urinary excretion of niacin metabolites. The requirements are expressed in niacin equivalents (NEs), allowing for some conversion of the amino acid tryptophan to niacin (1 mg niacin = 60 mg tryptophan). The Tolerable Upper Intake Level (UL) is based on flushing as the critical adverse effect. The UL applies to synthetic forms obtained from supplements, fortified foods, or a combination of the two. (The UL is in mg of preformed niacin and is not expressed in NEs.) DRI values are listed by life stage group in Table 1.

Meat, liver, poultry, and fish are rich sources of niacin. Other contributors to niacin intake include enriched and whole-grain breads and bread products and fortified ready-to-eat cereals. The classic disease of niacin deficiency is pellagra, which in industrialized nations generally only occurs in people with chronic alcoholism or conditions that inhibit the metabolism of tryptophan. There are no adverse effects associated with the excess consumption of naturally occurring niacin in foods, but they can result from excess intakes from dietary supplements, fortified foods, and pharmacological agents. The potential adverse effects of excess niacin intake include flushing, nausea, vomiting, liver toxicity, and blurred vision.

NIACIN AND THE BODY

Function

The term niacin refers to nicotinamide, nicotinic acid, and derivatives that exhibit the biological activity of nicotinamide. Niacin acts as a donor or acceptor of a hydride ion in many biological reduction–oxidation reactions, including intracellular respiration, the oxidation of fuel molecules, and fatty acid and steroid synthesis. The amino acid tryptophan is converted in part into nicotinamide and thus can contribute to meeting the requirement for niacin.

Absorption, Metabolism, Storage, and Excretion

Absorption of niacin from the stomach and intestine is rapid. At low concentrations, absorption is mediated by sodium ion–dependent facilitated diffusion. At higher concentrations, absorption is by passive diffusion. Niacin is stored in various body tissues. The niacin coenzymes NAD (nicotinamide adenine dinucleotide) and NADP (nicotinamide adenine dinucleotide phosphate) are synthesized in all body tissues from nicotinic acid or nicotinamide.

The body's niacin requirement is met not only by nicotinic acid and nicotinamide present in the diet, but also by conversion from dietary protein containing tryptophan.

DETERMINING DRIS

Determining Requirements

The requirements for niacin are based on the urinary excretion of niacin metabolites. The EAR and RDA are expressed in niacin equivalents (NEs), allowing for some conversion of the amino acid tryptophan to niacin (1 mg niacin = 60 mg tryptophan).

Special Considerations

Individuals with increased needs: The RDAs for niacin are not expected to be sufficient to meet the needs of people with Hartnup's disease, liver cirrhosis, or carcinoid syndrome, or the needs of individuals on long-term isoniazid treatment for tuberculosis. Extra niacin may also be required by those being treated with hemodialysis or peritoneal dialysis, those with malabsorption syndrome, and women who are carrying more than one fetus or breastfeeding more than one infant.

Criteria for Determining Niacin Requirements, by Life Stage Group

Life stage group	Criterion
0 through 6 mo	Human milk content
7 through 12 mo	Extrapolation from adults
1 through 18 y	Extrapolation from adults
19 through > 70 y	Excretion of niacin metabolites

Pregnancy	
≤ 18 y through 50 y	Age-specific requirement + increased energy utilization and growth needs during pregnancy

Lactation

≤ 18 y through 50 y   Age-specific requirement + energy expenditure of human milk production

The UL

The Tolerable Upper Intake Level (UL) is the highest level of daily nutrient intake that is likely to pose no risk of adverse effects for almost all people. Members of the general population should not routinely consume more than the UL. The UL for niacin represents preformed niacin and is based on flushing as the critical adverse effect. The UL developed for niacin applies to all forms of niacin added to foods or taken as supplements (e.g., immediate-release, slow- or sustained-release nicotinic acid, and niacinamide [nicotinamide]). Individuals who take over-the-counter niacin to treat themselves, such as for high blood cholesterol, for example, might exceed the UL on a chronic basis. The UL is not meant to apply to individuals who are receiving niacin under medical supervision. Niacin intake data indicate that only a small percentage of the U.S. population is likely to exceed the UL for niacin.

Special Considerations

Individuals susceptible to adverse effects: People with the following conditions are particularly susceptible to the adverse effects of excess niacin intake: liver dysfunction or a history of liver disease, diabetes mellitus, active peptic ulcer disease, gout, cardiac arrhythmias, inflammatory bowel disease, migraine headaches, and alcoholism. Individuals with these conditions might not be protected by the UL for niacin for the general population.

DIETARY SOURCES

Foods

Data from the Continuing Survey of Food Intakes by Individuals (CSFII, 1994–1996) indicated that the greatest contribution to the niacin intake of the U.S. adult population came from mixed dishes high in meat, fish, or poultry; poultry as an entree; enriched and whole-grain breads and bread products; and fortified ready-to-eat cereals. Most flesh foods are rich sources of niacin.

Dietary Supplements

In the 1986 National Health Interview Survey (NHIS), approximately 26 percent of all adults reported taking a supplement containing niacin. For adults who took supplements and participated in the Boston Nutritional Status Survey (1981–1984), median supplemental niacin intakes were 20 mg/day for men and 30 mg/day for women. Supplements containing up to about 400 mg of niacin are available without a prescription in the United States.

Bioavailability

Niacin from meat, liver, beans, and fortified or enriched foods appears to be highly bioavailable, whereas niacin from unfortified cereal grains is bound and only about 30 percent available (although alkali treatment of the grains increases the percentage absorbed). Niacin added during enrichment or fortification is in the free form of niacin; foods that contain this free form include beans and liver.

The conversion efficiency of tryptophan to niacin, although assumed to be 60:1, varies depending on a number of dietary and metabolic factors. The efficiency of conversion is decreased by deficiencies in some other nutrients (see "Dietary Interactions"). Individual differences also account for a substantial difference in conversion efficiency.

Dietary Interactions

There is some evidence that inadequate iron, riboflavin, or vitamin B_6 status increases niacin needs by decreasing the conversion of tryptophan to niacin. Data were not available to quantitatively assess the effects of these nutrient–nutrient interactions on the niacin requirement.

INADEQUATE INTAKE AND DEFICIENCY

The classic disease of severe niacin deficiency is pellagra, which is characterized by the following signs and symptoms:

- Pigmented rash
- Vomiting, constipation, or diarrhea
- Bright red tongue
- Depression
- Apathy
- Headache
- Fatigue
- Memory loss

Pellagra was common in the United States and parts of Europe in the early 20th century in areas where corn or maize (low in both niacin and tryptophan) was the dietary staple. Now it is occasionally seen in developing nations, such as in India, China, and Africa. In industrialized nations, it is generally only associated with chronic alcoholism and in individuals with conditions that disrupt the metabolism of tryptophan. Deficiencies of other micronutrients, such as pyridoxine and iron, which are required to convert tryptophan to niacin, may also contribute to the appearance of pellagra.

EXCESS INTAKE

There is no evidence of adverse effects associated with the excess consumption of naturally occurring niacin in foods. But adverse effects may result from excess niacin intake from dietary supplements, pharmaceutical preparations, and fortified foods. Most of the data concerning adverse effects of niacin has come from studies and case reports involving patients with hyperlipidemia or other disorders who were treated with pharmacological preparations that contained immediate-release nicotinic acid or slow- or sustained-release nicotinic acid. The potential adverse effects of excess niacin intake include the following:

- Flushing (the first observed adverse effect observed; generally occurs at lower doses than do other adverse effects)
- Nausea and vomiting
- Liver toxicity
- Impaired glucose tolerance

KEY POINTS FOR NIACIN

✓   Niacin is involved in many biological reactions, including intracellular respiration and fatty acid synthesis. The amino acid tryptophan is converted in part into nicotinamide and thus can contribute to meeting the requirement for niacin.

✓   The requirements for niacin are based on the urinary excretion of niacin metabolites. The UL is based on flushing as the critical adverse effect.

✓   The requirements are expressed in niacin equivalents (NEs), allowing for some conversion of the amino acid tryptophan to niacin (1 mg niacin = 60 mg tryptophan).

✓   The UL for niacin represents preformed niacin (the UL is not expressed in NEs) and applies to synthetic forms obtained from supplements, fortified foods, or a combination of the two.

✓   Niacin intake data indicate that only a small percentage of the U.S. population is likely to exceed the UL for niacin.

✓   People with an increased need for niacin include those with Hartnup's disease, liver cirrhosis, carcinoid syndrome, and malabsorption syndrome, as well as those on long-term isoniazid treatment for tuberculosis or on hemodialysis or peritoneal dialysis. Also, pregnant females who are carrying more than one fetus or breastfeeding more than one infant may require additional niacin.

✓   Meat, liver, poultry, and fish are rich sources of niacin. Other contributors to niacin intake include enriched and whole-grain breads and bread products and fortified ready-to-eat cereals.

✓   The classic disease of severe niacin deficiency is pellagra, which in industrialized nations generally only occurs in people with chronic alcoholism or conditions that inhibit the metabolism of tryptophan.

✓   There is no evidence of adverse effects associated with the excess consumption of naturally occurring niacin in foods. But adverse effects may result from excess niacin intake from dietary supplements, pharmaceutical preparations, and fortified foods.

✓   The adverse effects of excess niacin intake include flushing, nausea and vomiting, liver toxicity, and impaired glucose tolerance. However, most of the data on adverse effects has come from research with patients with special conditions who were treated with pharmacological preparations.

TABLE 1 Dietary Reference Intakes for Pantothenic Acid by Life Stage Group

	DRI values (mg/day)	
	AI[a]	UL[b]
Life stage group[c]		
0 through 6 mo	1.7	
7 through 12 mo	1.8	
1 through 3 y	2	
4 through 8 y	3	
9 through 13 y	4	
14 through 18 y	5	
19 through 30 y	5	
31 through 50 y	5	
51 through 70 y	5	
> 70 y	5	
Pregnancy		
≤ 18 y	6	
19 through 50 y	6	
Lactation		
≤ 18 y	7	
19 through 50 y	7	

[a] **AI** = Adequate Intake.

[b] **UL** = Tolerable Upper Intake Level. Data were insufficient to set a UL. In the absence of a UL, extra caution may be warranted in consuming levels above the recommended intake.

[c] All groups except Pregnancy and Lactation represent males and females.

PANTOTHENIC ACID

Pantothenic acid functions as a component of coenzyme A (CoA), which is involved in fatty acid metabolism. Pantothenic acid is widely distributed in foods and is essential to almost all forms of life.

Since data were insufficient to set an Estimated Average Requirement (EAR) and thus calculate a Recommended Dietary Allowance (RDA) for pantothenic acid, an Adequate Intake (AI) was instead developed. The AIs for pantothenic acid are based on pantothenic acid intake sufficient to replace urinary excretion. Data were insufficient to set a Tolerable Upper Intake Level (UL). DRI values are listed by life stage group in Table 1.

Major food sources of pantothenic acid include chicken, beef, potatoes, oat cereals, tomato products, liver, kidney, yeast, egg yolk, broccoli, and whole grains. Pantothenic acid deficiency is rare, and no adverse effects have been associated with high intakes.

PANTOTHENIC ACID AND THE BODY

Function

Pantothenic acid is involved in the synthesis of coenzyme A (CoA), which is involved in the synthesis of fatty acids and membrane phospholipids, amino acids, steroid hormones, vitamins A and D, porphyrin and corrin rings, and neurotransmitters.

Absorption, Metabolism, Storage, and Excretion

Pantothenic acid is absorbed in the small intestine by active transport at low concentrations of the vitamin and by passive transport at higher concentrations. Because the active transport system is saturable, absorption is less efficient at higher concentrations of intake. However, the exact intake levels at which absorption decreases in humans are not known. Pantothenic acid is excreted in the urine in amounts that are proportional with dietary intake over a wide range of intake values.

DETERMINING DRIS

Determining Requirements

Since data were insufficient to set an EAR and thus calculate an RDA, an AI was instead developed. The AIs for pantothenic acid are based on pantothenic acid intake sufficient to replace urinary excretion.

Criteria for Determining Pantothenic Acid Requirements, by Life Stage Group

Life stage group	Criterion
0 through 6 mo	Human milk content
7 through 12 mo	Mean of extrapolation from younger infants and from adults
1 through 18 y	Extrapolation from adults
19 through > 70 y	Pantothenic acid intake sufficient to replace urinary excretion
Pregnancy	
≤ 18 y through 50 y	Mean intake of pregnant women
Lactation	
≤ 18 y through 50 y	Pantothenic acid sufficient to replace amount excreted in milk + amount needed to maintain concentration of maternal blood levels

The UL

The Tolerable Upper Intake Level (UL) is the highest level of daily nutrient intake that is likely to pose no risk of adverse effects for almost all people. Due to insufficient data on adverse effects of oral pantothenic acid consumption, a UL for pantothenic acid could not be determined.

DIETARY SOURCES

Foods

Data on the pantothenic acid content of food are very limited. Foods that are reported to be major sources include chicken, beef, potatoes, oat cereals, tomato products, liver, kidney, yeast, egg yolk, broccoli, and whole grains. Food processing, including the refining of whole grains and the freezing and canning of vegetables, fish, meat, and dairy products, lowers the pantothenic acid content of these foods.

Dietary Supplements

Results from the 1986 National Health Interview Survey (NHIS) indicated that 22 percent of U.S. adults took a supplement that contained pantothenic acid.

Bioavailability

Little information exists on the bioavailability of dietary pantothenic acid. Values of 40–61 percent (average of 50 percent) have been reported for absorbed food-bound pantothenic acid.

Dietary Interactions

This information was not provided at the time the DRI values for this nutrient were set.

INADEQUATE INTAKE AND DEFICIENCY

Pantothenic acid deficiency is rare and has only been observed in individuals who were fed diets devoid of the vitamin or who were given a pantothenic-acid metabolic antagonist. The signs and symptoms of deficiency may include the following:

- Irritability and restlessness
- Fatigue
- Apathy
- Malaise
- Sleep disturbances
- Nausea, vomiting, and abdominal cramps
- Neurobiological symptoms, such as numbness, paresthesias, muscle cramps, and staggering gait
- Hypoglycemia and increased sensitivity to insulin

EXCESS INTAKE

No adverse effects have been associated with high intakes of pantothenic acid.

KEY POINTS FOR PANTOTHENIC ACID

✓ Pantothenic acid functions as a component of coenzyme A (CoA), which is involved in fatty acid metabolism.

✓ Since data were insufficient to set an EAR and thus calculate an RDA for pantothenic acid, an AI was instead developed.

✓ The AIs for pantothenic acid are based on pantothenic acid intake sufficient to replace urinary excretion.

✓ Data were insufficient to set a UL.

✓ Major food sources of pantothenic acid include chicken, beef, potatoes, oat cereals, tomato products, liver, kidney, yeast, egg yolk, broccoli, and whole grains.

✓ Pantothenic acid deficiency is rare and has only been observed in individuals who were fed diets devoid of the vitamin or who were given a pantothenic acid metabolic antagonist.

✓ No adverse effects have been associated with high intakes of pantothenic acid.

TABLE 1 Dietary Reference Intakes for Riboflavin by Life Stage Group

| | DRI values (mg/day) | | | | | |
| | EAR[a] | | RDA[b] | | AI[c] | UL[d] |
	males	females	males	females		
Life stage group						
0 through 6 mo					0.3	
7 through 12 mo					0.4	
1 through 3 y	0.4	0.4	0.5	0.5		
4 through 8 y	0.5	0.5	0.6	0.6		
9 through 13 y	0.8	0.8	0.9	0.9		
14 through 18 y	1.1	0.9	1.3	1.0		
19 through 30 y	1.1	0.9	1.3	1.1		
31 through 50 y	1.1	0.9	1.3	1.1		
51 through 70 y	1.1	0.9	1.3	1.1		
> 70 y	1.1	0.9	1.3	1.1		
Pregnancy						
≤ 18 y		1.2		1.4		
19 through 50 y		1.2		1.4		
Lactation						
≤ 18 y		1.3		1.6		
19 through 50 y		1.3		1.6		

[a] **EAR** = Estimated Average Requirement.
[b] **RDA** = Recommended Dietary Allowance.
[c] **AI** = Adequate Intake.
[d] **UL** = Tolerable Upper Intake Level. Data were insufficient to set a UL. In the absence of a UL, extra caution may be warranted in consuming levels above the recommended intake.

RIBOFLAVIN

Riboflavin (vitamin B_2) functions as a coenzyme for numerous oxidation–reduction reactions in several metabolic pathways and in energy production. The rate of absorption is proportional to intake, and it increases when riboflavin is ingested along with other foods and in the presence of bile salts.

The requirements for riboflavin are based on intake in relation to a combination of indicators, including the excretion of riboflavin and its metabolites, blood values for riboflavin, and the erythrocyte glutathione reductase activity coefficient. Data were insufficient to set a Tolerable Upper Intake Level (UL). DRI values are listed by life stage group in Table 1.

Major food sources of riboflavin for the U.S. adult population include milk and milk drinks, bread products, and fortified cereals. Riboflavin deficiency (ariboflavinosis) is most often accompanied by other nutrient deficiencies, and it may lead to deficiencies of vitamin B_6 and niacin, in particular. Diseases such as cancer, cardiac disease, and diabetes mellitus are known to precipitate or exacerbate riboflavin deficiency. There is no evidence of adverse effects from excess riboflavin intake. Its apparent nontoxic nature may be due its limited absorption in the gut and its rapid excretion in the urine.

RIBOFLAVIN AND THE BODY

Function

Riboflavin functions as a coenzyme for numerous oxidation–reduction reactions in several metabolic pathways and in energy production. The primary form of the vitamin is as an integral component of the coenzymes flavin mononucleotide and flavin-adenine dinucleotide. It is in these bound coenzymes that riboflavin functions as a catalyst for redox reactions.

Absorption, Metabolism, Storage, and Excretion

Primary absorption of riboflavin occurs in the small intestine via a rapid, saturable transport system. A small amount is absorbed in the large intestine. The rate of absorption is proportional to intake, and it increases when riboflavin is ingested along with other foods and in the presence of bile salts. At low intake levels, most absorption of riboflavin occurs via an active or facilitated transport system. At higher levels of intake, riboflavin can be absorbed by passive diffusion.

In the plasma, a large portion of riboflavin associates with other proteins, mainly immunoglobulins, for transport. Pregnancy increases the level of carrier proteins available for riboflavin, which results in a higher rate of riboflavin uptake at the maternal surface of the placenta.

The metabolism of riboflavin is a tightly controlled process that depends on a person's riboflavin status. Riboflavin is converted to coenzymes within most tissues, but primarily in the small intestine, liver, heart, and kidneys.

When riboflavin is absorbed in excess, very little is stored in the body. The excess is excreted primarily in the urine. Urinary excretion of riboflavin varies with intake, metabolic events, and age. In healthy adults who consume well-balanced diets, riboflavin accounts for 60–70 percent of the excreted urinary flavins. In newborns, urinary excretion is slow; however, the cumulative amount excreted is similar to the amount excreted by older infants.

DETERMINING DRIS

Determining Requirements

The requirements for riboflavin are based on intake in relation to a combination of indicators, including the excretion of riboflavin and its metabolites, blood values for riboflavin, and the erythrocyte glutathione reductase activity coefficient.

Special Considerations

Individuals with increased needs: People undergoing hemodialysis or peritoneal dialysis and those with severe malabsorption are likely to require extra riboflavin. Women who are carrying more than one fetus or breastfeeding more than one infant are also likely to require more riboflavin. It is possible that individuals who are ordinarily extremely physically active may also have increased needs for riboflavin.

Criteria for Determining Riboflavin Requirements, by Life Stage Group

Life stage group	Criterion
0 through 6 mo	Human milk content
7 through 12 mo	Extrapolation from younger infants and from adults
1 through 18 y	Extrapolation from adults

| 19 through 70 y | Excretion of riboflavin and its metabolites, blood values for riboflavin, and the erythrocyte glutathione reductase activity coefficient |
| > 70 y | Extrapolation from younger adults |

Pregnancy

| ≤ 18 y through 50 y | Age-specific requirement + increased energy utilization and growth needs during pregnancy |

Lactation

| ≤ 18 y through 50 y | Age-specific requirement + energy expenditure of human milk production |

The UL

The Tolerable Upper Intake Level (UL) is the highest level of daily nutrient intake that is likely to pose no risk of adverse effects for almost all people. Due to insufficient data on adverse effects of excess riboflavin consumption, a UL for riboflavin could not be determined. Although no adverse effects have been associated with excess riboflavin intake, this does not mean that there is no potential for adverse effects to occur with high intakes. Because data on adverse effects are limited, caution may be warranted.

DIETARY SOURCES

Foods

Most plant and animal tissues contain at least small amounts of riboflavin. Data from the Continuing Survey of Food Intakes by Individuals (CSFII, 1994–1996) indicate that the greatest contribution to the riboflavin intake by the U.S. adult population came from milk and milk beverages, followed by bread products and fortified cereals. Organ meats are also good sources of riboflavin. (It should be noted that the riboflavin content of milk is decreased if the milk is exposed to light.)

Dietary Supplements

Approximately 26 percent of all adults reported taking a supplement containing riboflavin, according to the 1986 National Health Interview Survey (NHIS). For adults who took supplements and participated in the Boston Nutritional Status Survey (1981–1984), median supplemental riboflavin intakes were 1.9 mg/day for men and 2.9 mg/day for women.

Bioavailability

Approximately 95 percent of food flavin is bioavailable, up to a maximum of about 27 mg absorbed per single meal or dose. More than 90 percent of riboflavin is estimated to be in the form of readily digestible flavocoenzymes.

Dietary Interactions

Riboflavin interrelates with other B vitamins: notably niacin, which requires riboflavin for its formation from tryptophan, and vitamin B_6, which also requires riboflavin for a conversion to a coenzyme form. These interrelationships are not known to affect the requirement for riboflavin.

INADEQUATE INTAKE AND DEFICIENCY

Riboflavin deficiency (ariboflavinosis) has been documented in industrialized and developing nations and across various demographic groups. Riboflavin deficiency is most often accompanied by other nutrient deficiencies, and it may lead to deficiencies of vitamin B_6 and niacin, in particular. The signs and symptoms of riboflavin deficiency include the following:

- Sore throat
- Hyperemia and edema of the pharyngeal and oral mucous membranes
- Cheilosis
- Angular stomatitis
- Glossitis (magenta tongue)
- Seborrheic dermatitis (dandruff)
- Normocytic anemia associated with pure erythrocyte cytoplasia of the bone marrow

Special Considerations

Conditions that increase deficiency risk: Diseases such as cancer, cardiac disease, and diabetes mellitus are known to precipitate or exacerbate riboflavin deficiency.

EXCESS INTAKE

No adverse effects associated with excess riboflavin consumption from food or supplements have been reported. However, studies involving large doses of riboflavin have not been designed to systematically evaluate adverse effects. The apparent lack of harm resulting from high oral doses of riboflavin may be due to its limited solubility and limited capacity for absorption in the human gastrointestinal tract and its rapid excretion in the urine.

KEY POINTS FOR RIBOFLAVIN

✓   Riboflavin (vitamin B_2) functions as a coenzyme in numerous oxidation–reduction reactions in several metabolic pathways and in energy production.

✓   The metabolism of riboflavin is a tightly controlled process that depends on a person's riboflavin status.

✓   The requirements for riboflavin are based on intake in relation to a combination of indicators, including the excretion of riboflavin and its metabolites, blood values for riboflavin, and the erythrocyte glutathione reductase activity coefficient

✓   Data were insufficient to set a UL.

✓   Certain individuals may have an increased need for riboflavin, including those undergoing dialysis, those with severe malabsorption, and women who are carrying more than one fetus or breastfeeding more than one infant.

✓   Major food sources of riboflavin for the U.S. adult population include milk and milk beverages, bread products, and fortified cereals.

✓   Riboflavin deficiency is most often accompanied by other nutrient deficiencies, and it may lead to deficiencies of vitamin B_6 and niacin, in particular.

✓   The signs and symptoms of riboflavin deficiency include sore throat, hyperemia and edema of the pharyngeal and oral mucous membranes, cheilosis, angular stomatitis, glossitis, seborrheic dermatitis, and normocytic anemia associated with pure erythrocyte cytoplasia of the bone marrow.

✓   Diseases such as cancer, cardiac disease, and diabetes mellitus are known to precipitate or exacerbate riboflavin deficiency.

✓   There is no evidence of adverse effects from excess riboflavin intake. Its apparent nontoxic nature may be due to its limited absorption in the gut and rapid excretion in the urine.

TABLE 1 Dietary Reference Intakes for Thiamin by Life Stage Group

	DRI values (mg/day)					
	EAR[a]		RDA[b]		AI[c]	UL[d]
	males	females	males	females		
Life stage group						
0 through 6 mo					0.2	
7 through 12 mo					0.3	
1 through 3 y	0.4	0.4	0.5	0.5		
4 through 8 y	0.5	0.5	0.6	0.6		
9 through 13 y	0.7	0.7	0.9	0.9		
14 through 18 y	1.0	0.9	1.2	1.0		
19 through 30 y	1.0	0.9	1.2	1.1		
31 through 50 y	1.0	0.9	1.2	1.1		
51 through 70 y	1.0	0.9	1.2	1.1		
> 70 y	1.0	0.9	1.2	1.1		
Pregnancy						
≤ 18 y		1.2		1.4		
19 through 50 y		1.2		1.4		
Lactation						
≤ 18 y		1.2		1.4		
19 through 50 y		1.2		1.4		

[a] **EAR** = Estimated Average Requirement.
[b] **RDA** = Recommended Dietary Allowance.
[c] **AI** = Adequate Intake.
[d] **UL** = Tolerable Upper Intake Level. Data were insufficient to set a UL. In the absence of a UL, extra caution may be warranted in consuming levels above the recommended intake.

THIAMIN

hiamin, also known as vitamin B$_1$ and aneurin, functions as a coenzyme in the metabolism of carbohydrates and branched-chain amino acids. Only a small percentage of a high dose of thiamin is absorbed, and elevated serum values result in active urinary excretion of the vitamin.

The adult requirements for thiamin are based on the amount of the vitamin needed to achieve and maintain normal erythrocyte transketolase activity, while avoiding excessive thiamin excretion. Data were insufficient to set a Tolerable Upper Intake Level (UL). DRI values are listed by life stage group in Table 1.

Food sources of thiamin include grain products, pork, ham, and fortified meat substitutes. The classic disease of thiamin deficiency is beriberi, which is sometimes seen in developing countries. Severe thiamin deficiency in industrialized nations is often associated with chronic heavy alcohol consumption, where it presents as Wernicke-Korsakoff syndrome. Evidence of adverse effects from excess thiamin consumption is extremely limited. The apparent lack of toxicity of supplemental thiamin may be explained by the rapid decline in absorption that occurs at intakes above 5 mg and the rapid urinary excretion of the vitamin.

THIAMIN AND THE BODY

Function

Thiamin (also known as vitamin B$_1$ and aneurin) was the first B vitamin to be identified. It functions as a coenzyme in the metabolism of carbohydrates and branched-chain amino acids.

Absorption, Metabolism, Storage, and Excretion

Absorption of thiamin occurs mainly in the jejunum. At low concentrations of thiamin, absorption occurs by an active transport system that involves phosphorylation; at higher concentrations, absorption occurs by passive diffusion. Only a small percentage of a high dose of thiamin is absorbed, and elevated serum values result in active urinary excretion of the vitamin.

Total thiamin content of the adult human is approximately 30 mg, and the biological half-life of the vitamin is in the range of 9 to 18 days. Thiamin is transported in blood in both erythrocytes and plasma and is excreted in the urine.

DETERMINING DRIS

Determining Requirements

The adult requirements for thiamin are based on metabolic studies in which urinary thiamin was measured during depletion–repletion, along with the measurement of erythrocyte transketolase activity.

Special Considerations

Individuals with increased needs: People who may have increased needs for thiamin include those being treated with hemodialysis or peritoneal dialysis, individuals with malabsorption syndrome, and women who are carrying more than one fetus or breastfeeding more than one infant. It was concluded that under normal conditions, physical activity does not appear to influence thiamin requirements to a substantial degree. However, those who engage in physically demanding occupations or who spend much time training for active sports may require additional thiamin.

Criteria for Determining Thiamin Requirements, by Life Stage Group

Life stage group	Criterion
0 through 6 mo	Human milk content
7 through 12 mo	Extrapolation from adults
1 through 18 y	Extrapolation from adults
19 through 50 y	Maintenance of normal erythrocyte transketolase activity and urinary thiamin excretion
51 through > 70 y	Extrapolation from younger adults
Pregnancy	
≤ 18 y through 50 y	Age-specific requirement + increased energy utilization and growth needs during pregnancy
Lactation	
≤ 18 y through 50 y	Age-specific requirement + energy expenditure of human milk production

The UL

The Tolerable Upper Intake Level (UL) is the highest level of daily nutrient intake that is likely to pose no risk of adverse effects for almost all people. Due to insufficient data on adverse effects of excess thiamin consumption, a UL for thiamin could not be determined. Although no adverse effects have been associated with excess intake of thiamin from food or supplements, this does not mean that there is no potential for adverse effects resulting from high intakes.

DIETARY SOURCES
Foods

According to the Continuing Survey of Food Intakes by Individuals (CSFII, 1994–1996), the greatest contribution to thiamin intake by U.S. adults came from the following enriched, fortified, or whole-grain products: bread and bread products, mixed foods whose main ingredient is grain, and ready-to-eat cereals. Other dietary sources of thiamin included pork and ham products, as well as fortified cereals and fortified meat substitutes.

Dietary Supplements

Approximately 27 percent of adults surveyed took a thiamin-containing supplement, according to the 1986 National Health Interview Survey (NHIS). For adults over age 60 years who took supplements and participated in the Boston Nutritional Status Survey (1981–1984), median supplemental thiamin intakes were 2.4 mg/day for men and 3.2 mg/day for women.

Bioavailability

Data on the bioavailability of thiamin in humans were extremely limited. No adjustments for bioavailability were judged necessary for deriving the EAR for thiamin.

Dietary interactions

This information was not provided at the time the DRI values for this nutrient were set.

INADEQUATE INTAKE AND DEFICIENCY

Early stages of thiamin deficiency may be accompanied by nonspecific signs and symptoms that may be overlooked or easily misinterpreted. Signs and symptoms of thiamine deficiency include the following:

- Anorexia
- Weight loss

- Mental changes such as apathy, decreased short-term memory, confusion, and irritability
- Muscle weakness
- Cardiovascular effects such as enlarged heart

In developing nations, thiamin deficiency often manifests as beriberi. In "wet beriberi," edema occurs. In "dry beriberi," muscle wasting is obvious. In infants, cardiac failure may occur rather suddenly.

Severe thiamin deficiency in industrialized countries is likely to be related to heavy alcohol consumption with limited food consumption, where it presents as Wernicke-Korsakoff syndrome. In severe cases of this syndrome, renal and cardiovascular complications can become life threatening.

EXCESS INTAKE

There are no reports of adverse effects from the consumption of excess thiamin from food or supplements. Supplements that contain up to 50 mg/day of thiamin are widely available without a prescription, but the possible occurrence of adverse effects resulting from this level or more of intake has not been studied systematically.

The apparent lack of toxicity of supplemental thiamin may be explained by the rapid decline in absorption that occurs at intakes above 5 mg and the rapid urinary excretion of the vitamin.

KEY POINTS FOR THIAMIN

✓ Thiamin (also known as vitamin B_1 and aneurin) functions as a coenzyme in the metabolism of carbohydrates and branched-chain amino acids.

✓ The adult requirements for thiamin are based on the amount of the vitamin needed to achieve and maintain normal erythrocyte transketolase activity, while avoiding excessive thiamin excretion.

✓ Data were insufficient to set a UL.

✓ Food sources of thiamin include grain products, pork, ham, and fortified meat substitutes.

✓ The classic disease of thiamin deficiency is beriberi, which is sometimes seen in developing countries.

✓ Severe thiamin deficiency in industrialized nations is often associated with chronic heavy alcohol consumption and presents as Wernicke-Korsakoff syndrome.

✓ There are no reports of adverse effects from excess thiamin consumption from food or supplements.

✓ The apparent lack of toxicity of supplemental thiamin may be explained by the rapid decline in absorption that occurs at intakes above 5 mg and the rapid urinary excretion of the vitamin.

TABLE 1 Dietary Reference Intakes for Calcium by Life Stage Group

	DRI values (mg/day)	
	AI[a]	UL[b]
Life stage group[c]		
0 through 6 mo	210	ND[d]
7 through 12 mo	270	ND
1 through 3 y	500	2,500
4 through 8 y	800	2,500
9 through 13 y	1,300	2,500
14 through 18 y	1,300	2,500
19 through 30 y	1,000	2,500
31 through 50 y	1,000	2,500
51 through 70 y	1,200	2,500
> 70 y	1,200	2,500
Pregnancy		
≤ 18 y	1,300	2,500
19 through 50 y	1,000	2,500
Lactation		
≤ 18 y	1,300	2,500
19 through 50 y	1,000	2,500

[a] **AI** = Adequate Intake.

[b] **UL** = Tolerable Upper Intake Level. Unless otherwise specified, the UL represents total intake from food, water, and supplements.

[c] All groups except Pregnancy and Lactation represent males and females.

[d] **ND** = Not determinable. This value is not determinable due to the lack of data of adverse effects in this age group and concern regarding the lack of ability to handle excess amounts. Source of intake should only be from food to prevent high levels of intake.

Calcium

Calcium plays a key role in bone health. In fact, more than 99 percent of total body calcium is found in the bones and teeth. Calcium is also involved in vascular, neuromuscular, and glandular functions in the body.

Since data were inadequate to determine an Estimated Average Requirement (EAR) and thus calculate a Recommended Dietary Allowance (RDA) for calcium, an Average Intake (AI) was instead developed. The AIs for calcium are based on desirable rates of calcium retention (as determined from balance studies), factorial estimates of requirements, and limited data on changes in bone mineral density (BMD) and bone mineral content (BMC). The Tolerable Upper Intake Level (UL) is based on milk-alkali syndrome as the critical endpoint. DRI values are listed by life stage group in Table 1.

Foods rich in calcium include milk, yogurt, cheese, calcium-set tofu, calcium-fortified orange juice, Chinese cabbage, kale, and broccoli. Calcium may be poorly absorbed from foods that are rich in oxalic acid or phytic acid. The effects of calcium deficiency include osteopenia, osteoporosis, and an increased risk of bone fractures. The effects of excess intake include kidney stones, hypercalcemia with renal insufficiency, and a decreased absorption of certain minerals.

CALCIUM AND THE BODY

Function

Calcium's primary role in the body is to form the structure of bones and teeth. More than 99 percent of total body calcium is stored in the skeleton, where it exists primarily in the form of hydroxyapatite. The remainder is found in the blood, extracellular fluid, muscle, and other tissues, where it is involved in vascular contraction and vasodilation, muscle contraction, neural transmission, and glandular secretion.

Absorption, Metabolism, Storage, and Excretion

Calcium is absorbed by active transport and passive diffusion across the intestinal mucosa. Active transport of calcium into the intestine requires the active form of vitamin D (1,25-dihydroxyvitamin D) and accounts for most of the absorption of calcium at low and moderate intake levels, as well as at times of great need, such as growth, pregnancy, or lactation. Passive diffusion becomes more important at high calcium intakes.

As calcium intake decreases, the efficiency of calcium absorption increases (and vice versa). However, this increased efficiency of calcium absorption, or fractional calcium absorption, is generally not sufficient to offset the loss of absorbed calcium that occurs with a decrease in dietary calcium intake. Calcium absorption declines with aging in both men and women. Calcium is excreted in the urine and feces.

DETERMINING DRIS

Determining Requirements

There is no biochemical assay that reflects calcium nutritional status. Except in extreme circumstances, such as severe malnutrition or hyperparathyroidism, circulating levels of blood calcium can actually be normal during chronic calcium deficiency because calcium is resorbed from the skeleton to maintain a normal circulating concentration. Since data were inadequate to determine an EAR and thus calculate an RDA for calcium, an AI was instead developed. Therefore, the adult AIs for calcium are based on desirable rates of calcium retention (as determined from balance studies), factorial estimates of requirements, and limited data on changes in bone mineral density (BMD) and bone mineral content (BMC). These indicators were chosen as reasonable surrogate markers to reflect changes in skeletal calcium content and, therefore, calcium retention.

The AI represents the approximate calcium intake that appears sufficient to maintain calcium nutriture, while recognizing that lower intakes may be adequate for some. However, this evaluation must await additional studies on calcium balance over broad ranges of intakes or long-term measures of calcium sufficiency, or both.

During pregnancy, the maternal skeleton is not used as a reserve for fetal calcium needs. Calcium-regulating hormones adjust maternal calcium absorption efficiency so that the AI does not have to be increased during pregnancy. Although increased dietary calcium intake will not prevent the loss of calcium from the maternal skeleton during lactation, the calcium that is lost appears to be regained following weaning. Thus, the AI for calcium in lactating women is the same as that of nonlactating women.

Criteria for Determining Calcium Requirements, by Life Stage Group

Life stage group	Criterion[a]
0 through 6 mo	Human milk content
7 through 12 mo	Human milk + solid food
1 through 3 y	Extrapolation of data on desirable calcium retention from 4 through 8 year olds
4 through 8 y	Calcium accretion / Δ BMC / calcium balance
9 through 18 y	Desirable calcium retention / factorial / Δ BMC
19 through 30 y	Desirable calcium retention / factorial
31 through 50 y	Calcium balance
51 through 70 y	Desirable calcium retention / factorial / Δ BMD
> 70 y	Extrapolation of desirable calcium retention from 51 through 70 year age group / Δ BMD / fracture rate

Pregnancy

≤ 18 y through 50 y	Bone mineral mass

Lactation

≤ 18 y through 50 y	Bone mineral mass

[a] Δ BMC is the change in bone mineral mass. Δ BMD is the change in bone mineral density.

The UL

The Tolerable Upper Intake Level (UL) is the highest level of daily nutrient intake that is likely to pose no risk of adverse effects for almost all people. Members of the general population should not routinely exceed the UL. The UL value for calcium is based on milk-alkali syndrome (characterized by hypercalemia and renal insufficiency) as the critical endpoint and is derived from case studies of people who consumed large doses of calcium, mostly in the form of supplements. The UL for calcium represents total intake from food, water, and supplements.

Although the 95th percentile of daily intake did not exceed the UL for any age group in the Continuing Survey of Food Intakes by Individuals (CSFII, 1994–1996), people with very high caloric intakes, especially if intakes of dairy products are also high, may exceed the UL of 2,500 mg/day. Although users of dietary supplements of any kind tend to also have higher intakes of calcium from food than nonusers, it is unlikely that the same person would fall at the upper end of both ranges. Prevalence of usual intakes, from foods plus supplements, above the UL is well below 5 percent, even for age groups with relatively high intakes. However, with calcium-fortified foods becoming more common, it is important to maintain surveillance of these foods in the marketplace and to monitor their impact on calcium intake.

DIETARY SOURCES

Foods

Dairy products, such as milk, yogurt, and cheese, are the most calcium-rich foods in Western diets. Other calcium-rich foods include calcium-set tofu, calcium-fortified plant-based beverages, Chinese cabbage, kale, calcium-fortified fruit juices, and broccoli.

Although grains are not particularly rich in calcium, the use of calcium-containing additives in these foods accounts for a substantial proportion of the calcium ingested by people who consume a large amount of grains. Among Mexican Americans, corn tortillas are the second most important source of calcium, after milk. White bread is the second most important source among Puerto Rican adults.

Dietary Supplements

According to U.S. data from the 1986 National Health Interview Survey (NHIS), 14 percent of men, 25 percent of women, and 7.5 percent of children 2 to 6 years of age took supplements that contained calcium. Data from 11,643 adults who participated in the 1992 NHIS showed that calcium intakes were higher for men and women who took daily supplements with calcium (of any kind) compared with those who seldom or never took supplements. (This difference was only statistically significant for women.) However, adults who took calcium supplements did not have higher intakes of food calcium.

Bioavailability

With regard to food sources of calcium, bioavailability is generally less important than the overall calcium content of the food. Calcium absorption efficiency is fairly similar for most foods, including milk products and grains, both of which represent major sources of calcium in North American diets. Calcium may be poorly absorbed from foods rich in oxalic acid (such as spinach, sweet potatoes, rhubarb, and beans) and from foods rich in phytic acid (such as unleavened bread, raw beans, seeds, nuts, grains, and soy isolates). Although soybeans contain large amounts of phytic acid, calcium absorption from these legumes is relatively high compared with other foods rich in phytic acid. Compared with calcium absorption from milk, calcium absorption from dried beans is about half; from spinach it is about one-tenth.

As for dietary supplements, the bioavailability of calcium depends on the size of the dose, the form, and the presence or absence of a meal, with the former improving absorption. Tablet disintegration of supplements is crucial, and the efficiency of calcium absorption from supplements is greatest when calcium is taken in doses of 500 mg or less.

Dietary Interactions

There is evidence that calcium may interact with certain other nutrients and dietary substances (see Table 2).

INADEQUATE INTAKE AND DEFICIENCY

Chronic calcium deficiency can result from inadequate intake or poor intestinal absorption. During chronic calcium deficiency, the mineral is resorbed from the skeleton to maintain a normal circulating concentration, thereby compromising bone health. Consequently, chronic calcium deficiency is one of several important causes of reduced bone mass and osteoporosis. In the United States each year, approximately 1.5 million fractures are associated with osteoporosis; in Canada in 1993, there were approximately 76,000 such fractures. The potential effects of calcium deficiency include the following:

- Osteopenia (lower than normal bone-mineral density)
- Osteoporosis (very low bone-mineral density)
- An increased risk of fractures

Special Considerations

Amenorrhea: Induced by exercise or anorexia nervosa, amenorrhea results in reduced calcium retention and net calcium absorption, respectively, along with lower bone mass.

Menopause: Decreased estrogen production at menopause is associated with accelerated bone loss for about 5 years. Lower levels of estrogen are accompanied by decreased calcium absorption efficiency and increased rates of bone turnover. However, available evidence suggests that the calcium intake requirement for women does not appear to change acutely with menopause.

Lactose intolerance: People with lactose intolerance who avoid dairy products and do not consume calcium-rich lactose-free foods may be at risk for calcium deficiency. Although lactose intolerance may influence intake, lactose-intolerant individuals absorb calcium normally from milk.

TABLE 2 Potential Interactions with Other Dietary Substances

Substance	Potential Interaction	Notes
SUBSTANCES THAT AFFECT CALCIUM		
Caffeine	Caffeine may increase urinary loss of calcium and decrease calcium absorption. These effects are modest.	Accelerated bone loss associated with caffeine consumption has been seen only in postmenopausal women with low calcium intakes. Available evidence does not warrant different calcium intake recommendations for people with different caffeine intakes.
Magnesium	Magnesium deficiency may cause hypocalcemia.	In general, magnesium deficiency must become moderate to severe before symptomatic hypocalcemia develops. However, a 3-week study of dietary-induced experimental magnesium depletion in humans demonstrated that even a mild degree of magnesium depletion may result in a significant decrease in serum calcium concentration.
Oxalic acid	Oxalic acid may inhibit calcium absorption.	Foods rich in oxalic acid include spinach, sweet potatoes, rhubarb, and beans.
Phosphorus	Excess intake of phosphorus may interfere with calcium absorption.	This is less likely to pose a problem if calcium intake is adequate. Foods rich in phosphorus include dairy foods, colas or other soft drinks, and meats.
Phytic acid	Phytic acid may inhibit calcium absorption.	Foods rich in phytic acid include unleavened bread, raw beans, seeds, nuts, grains, and soy isolates.
Protein	Protein may increase urinary loss of calcium.	The effect of dietary protein on calcium retention is controversial. Available evidence does not warrant adjusting calcium intake recommendations based on dietary protein intake.
Sodium	Moderate and high sodium intake may increase urinary loss of calcium.	High sodium chloride (salt) intake results in an increased loss of urinary calcium. There is indirect evidence that dietary sodium chloride has a negative effect on the skeleton. However, direct evidence linking sodium intake with bone loss and fracture is lacking. Available evidence does not warrant different calcium intake requirements for individuals based on their salt consumption.

TABLE 2 Continued

Substance	Potential Interaction	Notes
CALCIUM AFFECTING OTHER SUBSTANCES		
Iron	Calcium may decrease iron absorption.	Calcium inhibits iron absorption in a dose-dependent and dose-saturable fashion. However, the available human data fail to show cases of iron deficiency or even reduced iron stores as a result of calcium intake.
Magnesium	High intakes of calcium may decrease magnesium absorption.	Most human studies of the effects of dietary calcium on magnesium absorption have shown no effect, but one has reported decreased magnesium absorption rates. Calcium intakes of as much as 2,000 mg/day (in adult men) did not affect magnesium absorption. Calcium intakes in excess of 2,600 mg/day have been reported to decrease magnesium balance. Several studies have found that high sodium and calcium intake may result in increased renal magnesium excretion. Overall, at the dietary levels recommended in this publication, the interaction of magnesium with calcium is not of concern.
Phosphorus	Pharmacological doses of calcium carbonate may interfere with phosphorus absorption.	Calcium in the normal adult intake range is not likely to pose a problem for phosphorus absorption.
Zinc	Calcium may decrease zinc absorption.	Dietary calcium may decrease zinc absorption, but there is not yet definitive evidence. Human studies have found that calcium phosphate (1,360 mg/day of calcium) decreased zinc absorption, whereas calcium in the form of a citrate–malate complex (1,000 mg/day of calcium) had no statistically significant effect on zinc absorption. Data suggest that consuming a calcium-rich diet does not lower zinc absorption in people who consume adequate zinc. The effect of calcium on zinc absorption in people with low zinc intakes has not been extensively studied.

Vegetarian diets: Vegetarian diets, which may have relatively high contents of oxalic acid and phytic acid (see Table 2), may reduce calcium bioavailability.

Mothers who breastfeed multiple infants: Due to the increased milk production of a mother while breastfeeding multiple infants, increased intakes of calcium during lactation, as with magnesium, should be considered.

EXCESS INTAKE

The available data on the adverse effects of excess calcium intake in humans have primarily come from the study of nutrient supplements. Of the many possible adverse effects of excessive calcium intake, the three most widely studied and biologically important are the following:

- Kidney stones
- Hypercalcemia and renal insufficiency (also known as milk-alkali syndrome)
- The interaction of calcium with absorption of other minerals (see Table 2)

Although these are not the only adverse effects associated with excess calcium intake, they do constitute the vast majority of reported effects.

Special Considerations

Individuals susceptible to adverse effects: Some people may be at greater risk for adverse effects related to calcium. They include those with renal failure, those who take thiazide diuretics, and those with low intakes of minerals that interact with calcium (see Table 2).

KEY POINTS FOR CALCIUM

✓ Calcium plays a key role in bone health. In fact, more than 99 percent of total body calcium found in the teeth and bones.

✓ As calcium intake decreases, the efficiency of calcium absorption increases (and vice versa). However, this increased efficiency of calcium absorption is generally not sufficient to offset the loss of absorbed calcium that occurs with a decrease in dietary calcium intake.

✓ There is no biochemical assay that reflects calcium nutritional status. During chronic calcium deficiency, the mineral is resorbed from the skeleton to keep the circulating concentration normal, thereby compromising bone health.

✓ Since data were inadequate to determine an EAR and thus calculate an RDA for calcium, an AI was instead developed.

✓ The adult AIs for calcium are based on desirable rates of calcium retention (as determined from balance studies), factorial estimates of requirements, and limited data on changes in bone mineral density (BMD) and bone mineral content (BMC). The UL is based on milk-alkali syndrome as the critical endpoint.

✓ Calcium absorption declines with aging in both men and women.

✓ Although increased dietary calcium intake will not prevent the loss of calcium from the maternal skeleton during lactation, the calcium that is lost appears to be regained following weaning. Thus, the AI for calcium in lactating women is the same as that of nonlactating women.

✓ The UL value is derived from case studies of people who consumed large doses of calcium, mostly in the form of supplements.

✓ Foods rich in calcium include milk, yogurt, cheese, calcium-set tofu, calcium-fortified orange juice, Chinese cabbage, kale, and broccoli. Calcium may be poorly absorbed from foods that are rich in oxalic acid or phytic acid.

✓ Calcium deficiency can result from inadequate intake or poor intestinal absorption and can cause osteopenia, osteoporosis, and an increased risk of fractures.

✓ Excessive calcium intake can cause kidney stones, hypercalcemia with renal insufficiency, and decreased absorption of certain other minerals.

TABLE 1 Dietary Reference Intakes for Chromium by Life Stage Group

| | DRI values (µg/day) | | |
| | AI[a] | | UL[b] |
	males	females	
Life stage group			
0 through 6 mo	0.2	0.2	
7 through 12 mo	5.5	5.5	
1 through 3 y	11	11	
4 through 8 y	15	15	
9 through 13 y	25	21	
14 through 18 y	35	24	
19 through 30 y	35	25	
31 through 50 y	35	25	
51 through 70 y	30	20	
> 70 y	30	20	
Pregnancy			
≤ 18 y		29	
19 through 50 y		30	
Lactation			
≤ 18 y		44	
19 through 50 y		45	

[a] **AI** = Adequate take.
[b] **UL** = Tolerable Upper Intake Level. Data were insufficient to set a UL. In the absence of a UL, extra caution may be warranted in consuming levels above the recommended intake.

CHROMIUM

Chromium potentiates the action of insulin and may improve glucose tolerance. The form of chromium found in foods is trivalent chromium, or chromium III, which is the form discussed in this chapter.

Since data were insufficient to set an Estimated Average Requirement (EAR) and thus calculate a Recommended Dietary Allowance (RDA) for chromium, an Average Intake (AI) was instead developed. Data were insufficient to set a Tolerable Upper Intake Level (UL). The AIs for chromium are based on estimated intakes of chromium derived from the average amount of chromium/1,000 kcal of balanced diets and average energy intake. DRI values are listed by life stage group in Table 1.

Rich sources of chromium include cereals, particularly some high-bran cereals. Whole grains have more chromium than do refined grains. Some beers and wines are also high in chromium. The clinical signs and symptoms of deficiency include impaired plasma glucose utilization and an increased need for insulin. Few serious adverse effects have been associated with excess intake of chromium from foods.

CHROMIUM AND THE BODY

Function

The form of chromium found in foods is trivalent chromium, or chromium III, which is the form discussed in this chapter. (Another form, hexavalent chromium, or chromium VI, is found in the environment as a chemical by-product and has been shown to be carcinogenic when inhaled.)

Dietary chromium potentiates the action of insulin. Early studies identified chromium as the element that restores glucose tolerance in rats. A number of studies have demonstrated beneficial effects of chromium on circulating glucose, insulin, and lipids, although the potential mechanisms of action are still being investigated. Progress in the field has been limited by the difficulty in producing chromium deficiency in animals and also by the lack of a simple, widely accepted method for identifying subjects who are chromium depleted and, thus, who would be expected to respond to chromium supplementation.

Absorption, Metabolism, Storage, and Excretion

Chromium absorption by the body is generally low, with absorption estimates ranging from 0.4 to 2.5 percent. Some studies suggest that chromium absorption increases with exercise, but further research is necessary. Chromium is stored in the liver, spleen, soft tissue, and bone. Most absorbed chromium is excreted rapidly in the urine, and most unabsorbed chromium is excreted in the feces.

DETERMINING DRIS

Determining Requirements

Since data were insufficient to set an EAR and thus calculate an RDA for chromium, an AI was instead developed. The AIs for chromium are based on estimated intakes of chromium derived from the average amount of chromium/1,000 kcal of balanced diets and average energy intake taken from the Third National Health and Nutrition Examination Survey (NHANES III, 1988–1994).

Criteria for Determining Chromium Requirements, by Life Stage Group

Life stage group	Criterion
0 through 6 mo	Average chromium intake from human milk
7 through 12 mo	Average chromium intake from human milk and complementary foods
1 through 18 y	Extrapolation from adult AI
19 through > 70 y	Average chromium intake based on the chromium content of foods/1,000 kcal and average energy intake[a]
Pregnancy	
≤ 18 y	Extrapolation from adolescent female AI based on body weight
19 through 50 y	Extrapolation from adult female AI based on body weight
Lactation	
≤ 18 y	Adolescent female intake plus average amount of chromium secreted in human milk
19 through 50 y	Adult female intake plus average amount of chromium secreted in human milk

---

[a] The average chromium content in well-balanced diets was determined to be 13.4 µg/1,000 kcal, and the average energy intake for adults was obtained from NHANES III.

The UL

The Tolerable Upper Intake Level (UL) is the highest level of daily nutrient intake that is likely to pose no risk of adverse effects for almost all people. Data were insufficient to set a UL for chromium. No adverse effects have been convincingly associated with excess intake from food or supplements, but this does not mean that there is no potential for adverse effects resulting from high intakes. Since data were limited, caution may be warranted.

DIETARY SOURCES

Foods

Chromium is widely distributed throughout the food supply, but many foods contribute less than 1–2 µg per serving. Determining the chromium content of foods requires rigorous contamination control because standard methods of sample preparation contribute substantial amounts of chromium to the foods being analyzed. In addition, the chromium content of individual foods widely varies and may be influenced by geochemical factors. Consequently, dietary chromium intakes cannot be determined using any existing databases.

The chromium content of foods may increase or decrease with processing. Refined grains have been shown to have less chromium than whole grains; conversely, acidic foods have been shown to gain chromium content during processing that involves the use of stainless steel containers or utensils.

Cereals tend to be a significant contributor of chromium to diets. High-bran cereals are generally, but not always, high in chromium. Most dairy products are low in chromium and provide less than 0.6 µg per serving. Meats, poultry, and fish generally contribute 1–2 µg per serving, but processed meats are higher in chromium and may acquire it from exogenous sources. Chromium concentrations of fruits and vegetables highly vary. Some brands of beer and some French wines, particularly red wines, are high in chromium. Wines have not been analyzed for chromium in the United States.

Dietary Supplements

According to U.S. data from the 1986 National Health Interview Survey (NHIS), 8 percent of adults consumed supplements that contained chromium. Based on data from NHANES III, the median supplemental intake of chromium was 23 µg/day for those who took supplements, an amount similar to the average dietary chromium intake.

Bioavailability

Most chromium compounds are soluble at the pH of the stomach, but less soluble hydroxides may form as pH is increased. The environment of the gastrointestinal tract and ligands provided by food and supplements are important for mineral absorption. Several dietary factors may affect the bioavailability of chromium (see "Dietary Interactions").

Dietary Interactions

There is evidence that chromium may interact with certain other nutrients and dietary substances (see Table 2).

TABLE 2 Potential Interactions with Other Dietary Substances

Substance	Potential Interaction	Notes
SUBSTANCES THAT AFFECT CHROMIUM		
Vitamin C	Vitamin C may enhance the absorption of chromium.	In one study, plasma chromium concentrations in three women were consistently higher when they were given 1 mg chromium as $CrCl_3$ with 100 mg ascorbic acid than when given chromium without ascorbic acid.
Simple sugars	Diets high in simple sugars (35 percent of total kcal) may increase urinary excretion of chromium.	Urinary chromium excretion was found to be related to the insulinogenic properties of carbohydrates.
Phytate	Phytate may decrease chromium absorption.	In rats, phytate at high levels had adverse effects on chromium absorption, but lower levels of phytate did not have detrimental effects on chromium status.
Medications	Antacids and other drugs that alter stomach acidity or gastrointestinal prostaglandins may affect chromium absorption.	When rats were dosed with physiological doses of chromium and prostaglandin inhibitors, such as aspirin, chromium levels in the blood, tissues, and urine markedly increased. Medications, such as antacids, reduced chromium absorption and retention.

INADEQUATE INTAKE AND DEFICIENCY

Chromium deficiency has been reported in three patients who did not receive supplemental chromium in their total parenteral nutrition (TPN) solutions. Their clinical signs and symptoms included unexplained weight loss, peripheral neuropathy, impaired plasma glucose removal, increased insulin requirements, elevated plasma free fatty acids, and low respiratory quotient.

Because chromium is known to potentiate the action of insulin and because these chromium-deficient TPN patients were observed to have impaired glucose utilization and increased insulin requirements, it has been hypothesized that poor chromium status contributes to the incidence of impaired glucose tolerance and Type II diabetes (prevalence of impaired glucose tolerance was 15.8 percent in adults aged 40 to 74 years in NHANES III). However, addressing this hypothesis is difficult because of the current lack of information about the variability in dietary chromium intakes and because there is not a simple, widely acceptable method that identifies potential study subjects with poor chromium status.

EXCESS INTAKE

Ingested chromium has a low level of toxicity that is partially due to its very poor absorption. Although no adverse effects have been convincingly associated with the excess intake of chromium from food or supplements, this does not mean that the potential for adverse effects does not exist. Because data on the adverse effects of chromium intake were limited, caution may be warranted.

Special Considerations

Individuals susceptible to adverse effects: Data suggest that people with preexisting renal and liver disease may be particularly susceptible to the adverse effects of excess chromium. These individuals should be particularly careful to limit their chromium intake.

KEY POINTS FOR CHROMIUM

✓ Chromium potentiates the action of insulin and may improve glucose tolerance.

✓ Since data were insufficient to set an EAR and thus calculate an RDA for chromium, an AI was instead developed.

✓ The AIs for chromium are based on estimated intakes of chromium derived from the average amount of chromium/1,000 kcal of balanced diets and average energy intake.

✓ Data were insufficient to set a UL.

✓ Although no adverse effects have been convincingly associated with the excess intake of chromium from food or supplements, this does not mean that the potential for adverse effects does not exist.

✓ The form of chromium found in the diet is trivalent chromium, or chromium III. Another form, hexavalent chromium, or chromium VI, is found in the environment as a chemical by-product and has been shown to be carcinogenic when inhaled.

✓ Dietary chromium intakes cannot be determined using any existing databases.

✓ Rich sources of chromium include cereals, particularly all-bran cereals. Whole grains have more chromium than do refined grains.

✓ Because chromium is known to potentiate the action of insulin and because some chromium-deficient TPN patients have been observed to have impaired glucose utilization and increased insulin requirements, it has been hypothesized that poor chromium status contributes to the incidence of impaired glucose tolerance and Type II diabetes. The potential relationship between chromium and Type II diabetes remains under study.

✓ Ingested chromium has a low level of toxicity that is partially due to its very poor absorption.

✓ Data suggest that people with preexisting renal and liver disease may be particularly susceptible to the adverse effects of excess chromium.

TABLE 1 Dietary Reference Intakes for Copper by Life Stage Group

	DRI values (µg/day)					
	EAR[a]		RDA[b]		AI[c]	UL[d]
	males	females	males	females		
Life stage group						
0 through 6 mo					200	ND[e]
7 through 12 mo					220	ND
1 through 3 y	260	260	340	340		1,000
4 through 8 y	340	340	440	440		3,000
9 through 13 y	540	540	700	700		5,000
14 through 18 y	685	685	890	890		8,000
19 through 30 y	700	700	900	900		10,000
31 through 50 y	700	700	900	900		10,000
51 through 70 y	700	700	900	900		10,000
> 70 y	700	700	900	900		10,000
Pregnancy						
≤ 18 y		785		1,000		8,000
19 through 50 y		800		1,000		10,000
Lactation						
≤ 18 y		985		1,300		8,000
19 through 50 y		1,000		1,300		10,000

[a] **EAR** = Estimated Average Requirement.
[b] **RDA** = Recommended Dietary Allowance.
[c] **AI** = Adequate Intake.
[d] **UL** = Tolerable Upper Intake Level. Unless otherwise specified, the UL represents total intake from food, water, and supplements.
[e] **ND** = Not determinable. This value is not determinable due to the lack of data of adverse effects in this age group and concern regarding the lack of ability to handle excess amounts. Source of intake should only be from food to prevent high levels of intake.

COPPER

Copper functions as a component of several metalloenzymes, which act as oxidases in the reduction of molecular oxygen. The activities of some copper metalloenzymes have been shown to decrease in human copper depletion.

The requirements for copper are based on a combination of indicators, including plasma copper and ceruloplasmin concentrations, erythrocyte superoxide dismutase activity, and platelet copper concentration in controlled human depletion/repletion studies. The Tolerable Upper Intake Level (UL) is based on protection from liver damage as the critical adverse event. DRI values are listed by life stage group in Table 1.

Sources of copper include organ meats, seafood, nuts, seeds, wheat-bran cereals, and whole-grain products. Frank copper deficiency in humans is rare. Symptoms associated with deficiency include normocytic, hypochromic anemia; leucopenia; and neutropenia; and, in copper-deficient infants and growing children, osteoporosis. Copper toxicity is generally rare except in individuals genetically susceptible to the increased risk of adverse effects from excess copper intake.

COPPER AND THE BODY

Function

Copper functions as a component of several metalloenzymes, which act as oxidases in the reduction of molecular oxygen. Some of the principal copper metalloenzymes found in humans include the following:

- Diamine oxidase, which inactivates the histamine released during allergic reactions
- Monoamine oxidase (MAO), which is important in serotonin degradation and in the metabolism of epinephrine, norepinephrine, and dopamine; MAO inhibitors are used as antidepressant drugs
- Ferroxidases, which are copper enzymes found in the plasma and function in ferrous iron oxidation that is needed to bind iron to transferrin
- Dopamine β-monooxygenase, which uses ascorbate, copper, and O_2 to convert dopamine to norepinephrine

- Copper/zinc superoxide dismutase (Cu/Zn SOD), which defends against oxidative damage; mutations in the Cu/Zn SOD gene, which alter the protein's redox behavior, produce amyotrophic lateral sclerosis (Lou Gehrig's disease)

Absorption, Metabolism, Storage, and Excretion

Copper absorption primarily occurs in the small intestine via both saturable-mediated and nonsaturable-nonmediated mechanisms. The Menkes P-type ATPase (MNK; ATP7A) is believed to be responsible for copper trafficking to the secretory pathway for efflux from cells, including enterocytes. A defective MNK gene causes Menkes' disease, which is characterized by reduced copper absorption and placental copper transport. The extent of copper absorption varies with dietary copper intake; it ranges from more than 50 percent at an intake of less than 1 mg/day to less than 20 percent at intakes above 5 mg/day. About 35 percent of a 2 mg/day intake is absorbed and transported via the portal vein to the liver, bound to albumin, for uptake by liver parenchymal cells.

Nearly two-thirds of body copper content is found in the skeleton and muscle, but the liver appears to be the key site in maintaining plasma copper concentration. Biliary copper excretion is adjusted to maintain balance. Copper is released via the plasma to extrahepatic sites, where up to 95 percent of the copper is bound to cerulosplasmin.

Urinary copper excretion is normally very low (< 0.1 mg/day) over a wide range of dietary intakes. As with other trace elements, renal dysfunction can lead to increased urinary losses.

DETERMINING DRIS

Determining Requirements

The primary criterion used to estimate the requirements for copper is based on a combination of indicators, including plasma copper and ceruloplasmin concentrations, erythrocyte superoxide dismutase activity, and platelet copper concentration in controlled human depletion/repletion studies.

Criteria for Determining Copper Requirements, by Life Stage Group

Life stage group	Criterion
0 through 6 mo	Average copper intake from human milk
7 through 12 mo	Average copper intake from human milk and complementary foods

1 through 18 y	Extrapolation from adult EAR
19 through 50 y	Plasma copper, serum ceruloplasmin, and platelet copper concentrations and erythrocyte superoxide dismutase activity
51 through > 70 y	Extrapolation from 19 through 50 y

Pregnancy

| ≤ 18 y | Adolescent female EAR plus fetal accumulation of copper |
| 19 through 50 y | Adult female EAR plus fetal accumulation of copper |

Lactation

| ≤ 18 y | Adolescent female EAR plus average amount of copper secreted in human milk |
| 19 through 50 y | Adult female EAR plus average amount of copper secreted in human milk |

The UL

The Tolerable Upper Intake Level (UL) is the highest level of daily nutrient intake that is likely to pose no risk of adverse effects for almost all people. Members of the general population should not routinely exceed the UL. The UL for copper is based on liver damage as the critical endpoint and represents intake from food, water, and supplements.

Based on data from the Third National Health and Nutrition Examination Survey (NHANES III, 1988–1994), the highest median intakes of copper from the diet and supplements for any gender and life stage group were approximately 1,700 µg/day for men aged 19 through 50 years and approximately 1,900 µg/day for lactating women. The highest reported intake from food and supplements at the 99th percentile was 4,700 µg/day, also in lactating women. The next highest reported intake at the 99th percentile was 4,600 µg/day in pregnant women and men aged 50 through 70 years. The risk of adverse effects resulting from excess intake of copper from food, water, and supplements appears to be low in the highest intakes noted above.

DIETARY SOURCES

Foods

Copper is widely distributed in foods. The accumulation of copper in plants is not affected by the copper content of the soil in which they are grown. Major contributors of copper include organ meats, seafood, nuts, and seeds. Wheat-bran cereals and whole-grain products are also sources of copper. Foods that contribute substantial amounts of copper to the U.S. diet include those high in copper, such as organ meats, grains, and cocoa products, as well as foods relatively low in copper, but which are consumed in substantial amounts, such as tea, potatoes, milk, and chicken.

Dietary Supplements

According to U.S. data from the 1986 National Health Interview Survey (NHIS) approximately 15 percent of adults in the United States consumed supplements that contained copper. Based on data from the NHANES III, the median dietary plus supplemental copper intake was similar to the intake from food alone. The mean intake of dietary and supplemental copper (1.3–2.2 mg/day) was approximately 0.3–0.5 mg/day greater for men and women than the mean intake from food (1.0–1.7 mg/day).

Bioavailability

The bioavailability of copper is markedly influenced by the amount of copper in the diet, rather than by the diet's composition. Bioavailability ranges from 75 percent of dietary copper absorbed by the body when the diet contains only 400 μg/day to 12 percent absorbed when the diet contains 7.5 mg/day. The absolute amount of copper absorbed is higher with increased intake. In addition, the excretion of copper into the gastrointestinal tract regulates copper retention. As more copper is absorbed, turnover is faster and more copper is excreted into the gastrointestinal tract. This excretion is probably the primary point of regulation of total body copper. This efficient homeostatic regulation of absorption and retention helps protect against copper deficiency and toxicity.

Dietary Interactions

Copper homeostasis is affected by interactions among zinc, copper, iron, and molybdenum. In addition, the level of dietary protein, interacting cations, and sulfate all can influence the absorption and utilization of copper. Some evidence that copper may interact with certain nutrients and dietary substances appears in Table 2.

INADEQUATE INTAKE AND DEFICIENCY

Frank copper deficiency in humans is rare, but it has been found in a number of special conditions. It has also been observed in premature infants fed milk formulas deficient in copper, infants recovering from malnutrition associated with chronic diarrhea and fed cow milk, and patients with prolonged total

TABLE 2 Potential Interactions with Other Dietary Substances

Substance	Potential Interaction	Notes
SUBSTANCES THAT AFFECT COPPER		
Zinc	Zinc (at very high intakes) may decrease copper absorption.	This usually only occurs at intakes well in excess of the amount of zinc normally found in the diet.
Iron	High iron may interfere with copper absorption in infants.	Infants fed a formula that contained low concentrations of iron absorbed more copper than infants who consumed the same formula with a higher iron concentration. Such an interaction has been reported to produce reduced copper status in infants.

parenteral nutrition (TPN). In these cases, serum copper and ceruloplasmin concentrations were as low as 0.5 μmol/L and 35 mg/L, respectively, compared with reported normal ranges of 10–25 μmol/L for serum copper concentration and 180–400 mg/L for ceruloplasmin concentration. Supplementation with copper resulted in rapid increases in serum copper and ceruloplasmin concentrations. The symptoms associated with copper deficiency include the following:

- Normocytic, hypochromic anemia
- Leukopenia
- Neutropenia
- Osteoporosis (in copper-deficient infants and growing children)

EXCESS INTAKE

The long-term toxicity of copper has not been well studied in humans, but it is rare in normal populations without some hereditary defect in copper homeostasis. Potential adverse effects have been associated with excess intake of soluble copper salts in both supplements and drinking water, although most have only been reported based on acute and not chronic intakes. The consumption of drinking water or other beverages containing high levels of copper has resulted mostly in gastrointestinal illness, including abdominal pain, cramps, nausea, diarrhea, and vomiting.

Special Considerations

Individuals susceptible to adverse effects: Liver damage in humans due to excess intake of copper is observed almost exclusively in individuals with Wilson's disease, idiopathic copper toxicosis (ICT), and children with Indian childhood cirrhosis (ICC). Thus, these individuals will be at an increased risk of adverse effects from excess copper intake.

KEY POINTS FOR COPPER

✓   Copper functions as a component of several metalloenzymes, which act as oxidases in the reduction of molecular oxygen.

✓   The requirements for copper are based on a combination of indicators, including plasma copper and ceruloplasmin concentrations, erythrocyte superoxide dismutase activity, and platelet copper concentration in controlled human depletion/repletion studies. The UL is based on protection from liver damage as the critical adverse event.

✓   The risk of adverse effects resulting from excess intake of copper from food, water, and supplements appears to be low.

✓   Good sources of copper include organ meats, seafood, nuts, seeds, wheat-bran cereals, and whole-grain products.

✓   Frank copper deficiency in humans is rare. The signs and symptoms of deficiency include normocytic, hypochromic anemia; leucopenia; and neutropenia; and, in copper-deficient children, osteoporosis.

✓   The long-term toxicity of copper has not been well studied in humans, but it is rare in normal populations without some hereditary defect in copper homeostasis. Potential adverse effects have been associated with excess intake of soluble copper salts in both supplements and drinking water, although most have only been reported based on acute and not chronic intakes.

✓   People at an increased risk of adverse effects from excess copper intake include individuals with Wilson's disease (homozygous and heterozygous), idiopathic copper toxicosis (ICT), and Indian childhood cirrhosis (ICC).

TABLE 1 Dietary Reference Intakes for Fluoride by Life Stage Group

	DRI values (mg/day)		
	AI[a]		UL[b]
	males	females	
Life stage group			
0 through 6 mo	0.01	0.01	0.7
7 through 12 mo	0.5	0.5	0.9
1 through 3 y	0.7	0.7	1.3
4 through 8 y	1	1	2.2
9 through 13 y	2	2	10
14 through 18 y	3	3	10
19 through 30 y	4	3	10
31 through 50 y	4	3	10
51 through 70 y	4	3	10
> 70 y	4	3	10
Pregnancy			
≤ 18 y		3	10
19 through 50 y		3	10
Lactation			
≤ 18 y		3	10
19 through 50 y		3	10

[a] **AI** = Adequate Intake.
[b] **UL** = Tolerable Upper Intake Level. Unless otherwise specified, the UL represents total intake from food, water, and supplements.

FLUORIDE

luoride is vital for the health of teeth and bones. About 99 percent of body fluoride is found in calcified tissues, where it protects against dental caries and can stimulate new bone formation.

Since data were inadequate to determine an Estimated Average Requirement (EAR) and thus calculate a Recommended Dietary Allowance (RDA) for fluoride, an Average Intake (AI) was instead developed. The AIs for fluoride (for people aged 7 months and older) are based on the prevention of dental caries. The Tolerable Upper Intake (UL) was derived using data on the risk of developing early signs of skeletal fluorosis. DRI values are listed by life stage group in Table 1.

Fluoridated water is a primary source of dietary fluoride intake. Average fluoride intakes tend to be higher in communities with fluoridated water compared with those with nonfluoridated water. The primary effect of inadequate fluoride intake is an increased risk of dental caries. The potential effects of excess intake are discolored or pitted teeth (in children who consume excess amounts of fluoride prior to the eruption of teeth) and skeletal fluorosis, a very rare effect characterized by elevated bone-ash fluoride concentrations. In the United States and Canada, it is unlikely that older children and adults are exceeding the UL for fluoride.

FLUORIDE AND THE BODY

Function

Fluoride is vital for the health of teeth and bones. Ingesting fluoride during the pre-eruptive phase of tooth development can help prevent dental caries. This is due to the uptake of fluoride in the dental enamel and the formation of fluorhydroxyapatite. Even after teeth have erupted, fluoride can protect against dental caries, but this protection requires frequent exposure to fluoride throughout a person's lifetime to achieve and maintain adequate concentrations of the ion in dental plaque and enamel.

Absorption, Metabolism, Storage, and Excretion

In general, 50 percent of dietary fluoride is absorbed from the gastrointestinal tract. In the absence of calcium, which may bind with fluoride, absorption typically increases to about 80 percent or more. Because of fluoride's affinity for calcium, about 99 percent of body fluoride is found in calcified tissues. Elimination of absorbed fluoride occurs through the kidneys.

The body's retention of fluoride changes throughout life. In young children, whose skeletons and teeth are still growing, as much as 80 percent of absorbed fluoride may be retained and only 20 percent excreted. In healthy young and middle-aged adults, approximately 50 percent of absorbed fluoride is retained in the skeleton and 50 percent is excreted in the urine. In older adults, it is likely that the fraction of fluoride excreted is greater than the fraction retained.

Under most dietary conditions, fluoride balance is positive. When fluoride intake is chronically insufficient to maintain plasma concentrations, fluoride excretion in both infants and adults can exceed the amounts ingested due to mobilization from calcified tissues.

DETERMINING DRIS

Determining Requirements

For fluoride, the data are strong on risk reduction, but the evidence upon which to base an actual requirement is scant. Since data were inadequate to determine an EAR and thus calculate an RDA, an AI was instead developed. The AIs for fluoride (for people aged 7 months and older), are based on the intake values that maximally reduce the occurrence of dental caries in a group of individuals without causing unwanted effects including moderate tooth enamel mottling known as dental fluorosis.

Special Considerations

Nonfluoridated water: Infants and children who live in areas with nonfluoridated water will not easily achieve the AI for fluoride. Therefore, the American Dental Association, the American Academy of Pediatrics, and the Canadian Paediatric Society have recommended fluoride supplements for these children, with daily doses based on a child's age and the fluoride concentration of his or her main drinking water source.

Criteria for Determining Fluoride Requirements, by Life Stage Group

Life stage group	Criterion
0 through 6 mo	Human milk content
For all other life stage groups	Caries prevention

The UL

The Tolerable Upper Intake Level (UL) is the highest level of daily nutrient intake that is likely to pose no risk of adverse effects for almost all people. Members of the general population should not routinely exceed the UL. The UL value for fluoride represents total intake from food, water, and supplements.

The UL for fluoride for individuals aged 9 years and older was derived using data on the risk of developing early signs of skeletal fluorosis, which is associated with a fluoride intake greater than 10 mg/day for a period of 10 years or longer. The UL for infants and children younger than 8 years old was based on a critical adverse effect of developing fluorosis of the anterior teeth, not skeletal fluorosis.

Data from studies of fluoride exposure from dietary sources or work environments showed that a UL of 10 mg/day for a period of 10 years or longer carries only a small risk for an individual to develop preclinical or stage 1 skeletal fluorosis (see "Excess Intake").

Although the prevalence of enamel fluorosis in both fluoridated and nonfluoridated communities in the United States and Canada is substantially higher than it was when the original epidemiological studies were done some 60 years ago, the severity remains largely limited to the very mild and mild categories. Based on several U.S. studies done in the 1980s, it is estimated that approximately 1 in 100 children exceed the UL in areas where the water fluoride concentration is 1.0 mg/L or slightly higher. Any additional intake by children who are at risk of enamel fluorosis is almost certainly derived from the use of fluoride-containing dental products, especially if they are inadvertently swallowed. The virtual absence of evidence showing skeletal changes consistent with a diagnosis of skeletal fluorosis indicates that the UL for older children and adults is not being exceeded in the United States and Canada.

DIETARY SOURCES

Foods and Water

Most foods have fluoride concentrations well below 0.05 mg/100 g. Exceptions to this include fluoridated water, beverages (including teas), some marine fish (especially if eating with bones, e.g., sardines), and some infant formulas that are made or reconstituted with fluoridated water. Because tea leaves can accumulate fluoride to concentrations exceeding 10 mg/100 g dry weight, brewed tea contains fluoride at concentrations of 1–6 mg/L, depending on the amount of dry tea used, the fluoride concentration of the water, and brewing time. Decaffeinated teas have roughly twice the fluoride concentration of caffeinated teas.

Dietary Supplements

Fluoride supplements are intended for use by children living in areas with low water fluoride concentrations so that their intake is similar to that of children with access to water fluoride concentrations of approximately 1.0 mg/L. Based on the 1986 National Health Interview Survey (NHIS) data, in the United States approximately 15 percent of children up to age 5 years and 8 percent of those aged 5 to 17 years are given dietary fluoride supplements. Supplements are rarely prescribed for adults.

Dental Products

Fluoride intake from dental products (such as toothpaste and mouth rinse) can add considerable fluoride content to the diet, often approaching or exceeding intake from foods and water. This is a particular concern in young children who may inadvertently swallow toothpaste or mouth rinses.

Bioavailability

The bioavailability of fluoride is generally high, but it can be affected by the method in which it is ingested. When a soluble compound such as sodium fluoride is ingested from fluoridated water, absorption is nearly complete. If it is ingested with milk, infant formula, or foods, particularly those with high concentrations of calcium or certain divalent or trivalent ions that form insoluble compounds, absorption may be reduced by 10–25 percent. The absorption of fluoride from ingested toothpaste, whether added as sodium fluoride or monofluorophosphate, is nearly 100 percent.

Dietary Interactions

There is evidence that fluoride may interact with certain nutrients and dietary substances (see Table 2).

TABLE 2 Potential Interactions with Other Dietary Substances

Substance	Potential Interaction	Notes
SUBSTANCES THAT AFFECT FLUORIDE		
Calcium	High concentrations of calcium ingested with fluoride may reduce fluoride absorption.	The rate and extent of fluoride absorption from the gastrointestinal tract are somewhat reduced by ingestion with solid foods and some liquids, particularly those rich in calcium, such as milk or infant formulas.

INADEQUATE INTAKE AND DEFICIENCY

The primary effect of inadequate fluoride intake is an increased risk of dental caries. The results of many studies conducted prior to the availability of fluoride-containing dental products showed that the prevalence of dental caries in communities with optimal water fluoride concentrations was 40–60 percent lower than in areas with low water fluoride concentrations. In a later survey conducted in 1986–1987, the National Caries Program of the National Institute of Dental Research found that the overall difference in caries prevalence between fluoridated and nonfluoridated regions in the United States was 18 percent. The exclusion of children with reported exposure to fluoride supplements increased the difference to 25 percent.

EXCESS INTAKE

The primary adverse effects associated with chronic excess fluoride intake are the following:

- Enamel fluorosis, which occurs during the pre-eruptive development of teeth and results in mainly cosmetic effects in the form of discolored or pitted teeth
- Skeletal fluorosis, which results in elevated bone-ash fluoride concentrations and potentially debilitating symptoms. The following are stages of skeletal fluorosis:

    Stage 1 skeletal fluorosis: Characterized by occasional stiffness or pain in the joints and some osteosclerosis of the pelvis and vertebrae. Bone-ash fluoride concentrations usually range from 6,000 to 7,000 mg/kg.

Stages 2 and 3 skeletal fluorosis: Symptoms are more severe and may include the calcification of ligaments, osteosclerosis, exostoses, possible osteoporosis of long bones, muscle wasting, and neurological defects due to the hypercalcification of vertebrae. Bone-ash fluoride concentrations typically exceed 7,500–8,000 mg/kg.

The development and severity of skeletal fluorosis directly relate to the level and duration of fluoride exposure. Most epidemiological evidence indicates that an intake of at least 10 mg/day for a period of 10 years or longer is needed to produce clinical signs of the condition's milder forms. Crippling skeletal fluorosis is extremely rare in the United States and Canada.

Special Considerations

Tropical climates: Reports of relatively marked osteofluorotic signs and symptoms have been associated with concentrations of fluoride in drinking water of approximately 3 mg/L in tropical climates. These adverse effects have been attributed to poor nutrition and hard manual labor leading to excessive sweat loss and compensatory high levels of water intake. Therefore, an increased risk for skeletal fluorosis from excess fluoride intake may exist for malnourished individuals who live in hot climates or tropical environments.

KEY POINTS FOR FLUORIDE

✓ Fluoride is vital for the health of teeth and bones. About 99 percent of body fluoride is found in calcified tissues, where it protects against dental caries and can stimulate new bone formation.

✓ Since data were inadequate to determine an EAR and thus calculate an RDA for fluoride, an AI was instead developed.

✓ The AIs for fluoride are based on the prevention of dental caries. The UL for adults was derived using data on the risk of developing early signs of skeletal fluorosis.

✓ Infants and children who live in nonfluoridated water areas will not easily achieve the AI for fluoride. Thus, fluoride supplements have been recommended based on life stage and level of water fluoridation.

✓ Fluoridated water is a primary source of dietary fluoride intake.

✓ The primary effect of inadequate intake is an increased risk of dental caries.

✓ The primary adverse effects associated with chronic excess fluoride intake are enamel fluorosis and skeletal fluorosis.

✓ Dental products such as toothpaste and mouth rinses can significantly increase fluoride intake, a particular concern in young children if they inadvertently swallow these products.

✓ In the United States and Canada, it is unlikely that older children and adults are exceeding the UL for fluoride.

TABLE 1 Dietary Reference Intakes for Iodine by Life Stage Group

	DRI values (µg/day)					
	EAR[a]		RDA[b]		AI[c]	UL[d]
	males	females	males	females		
Life stage group						
0 through 6 mo					110	ND[e]
7 through 12 mo					130	ND
1 through 3 y	65	65	90	90		200
4 through 8 y	65	65	90	90		300
9 through 13 y	73	73	120	120		600
14 through 18 y	95	95	150	150		900
19 through 30 y	95	95	150	150		1,100
31 through 50 y	95	95	150	150		1,100
51 through 70 y	95	95	150	150		1,100
≥ 70 y	95	95	150	150		1,100
Pregnancy						
≤ 18 y		160		220		900
19 through 50 y		160		220		1,100
Lactation						
≤ 18 y		209		290		900
19 through 50 y		209		290		1,100

[a] **EAR** = Estimated Average Requirement.
[b] **RDA** = Recommended Dietary Allowance.
[c] **AI** = Adequate Intake.
[d] **UL** = Tolerable Upper Intake Level. Unless otherwise specified, the UL represents total intake from food, water, and supplements.
[e] **ND** = Not determinable. This value is not determinable due to the lack of data of adverse effects in this age group and concern regarding the lack of ability to handle excess amounts. Source of intake should only be from food to prevent high levels of intake.

IODINE

I odine is an essential component of thyroid hormones that are involved in the regulation of various enzymes and metabolic processes. These hormones regulate many key biochemical reactions, including protein synthesis and enzymatic activity. Major organs that are affected by these processes include the brain, muscles, heart, pituitary gland, and kidneys.

The requirements for iodine are based on thyroid iodine accumulation and turnover. The Tolerable Upper Intake Level (UL) is based on serum thyroptropin concentration in response to varying levels of ingested iodine. DRI values are listed by life stage group in Table 1.

The iodine content of most food sources is low and can be affected by soil content, irrigation, and fertilizers. Seafood has high concentrations; processed foods may also have high levels due to the addition of iodized salt or additives that contain iodine. In North America where much of the iodine consumed is from salt iodized with potassium iodide, symptoms of iodine deficiency are rare. However, severe iodine deficiency can result in impaired cognitive development in children and goiter in adults. For the general population, high iodine intakes from food, water, and supplements have been associated with thyroiditis, goiter, hypothyroidism, hyperthyroidism, sensitivity reactions, thyroid papillary cancer, and acute responses in some individuals. However, most individuals are very tolerant of excess iodine intake from foods.

IODINE AND THE BODY

Function

Iodine is an essential component of the thyroid hormones thyroxine (T4) and triiodothyronine (T3), comprising 65 and 59 percent of their respective weights. These hormones regulate many key biochemical reactions, including protein synthesis and enzymatic activity. Major organs that are affected by these processes include the brain, muscles, heart, pituitary gland, and kidneys.

Absorption, Metabolism, Storage, and Excretion

Iodine is ingested in a variety of chemical forms. Most ingested iodine is reduced in the gut to iodide and absorbed almost completely. Some iodine-containing compounds (e.g., thyroid hormones) are absorbed intact. Iodate, widely used in many countries as an additive to salt, is rapidly reduced to iodide and completely absorbed. Once in the circulation, iodide is principally removed by the thyroid gland and kidneys. The thyroid selectively concentrates iodide in amounts required for adequate thyroid hormone synthesis; most of the remaining iodine is excreted in the urine.

A sodium/iodide transporter in the thyroidal basal membrane transfers iodide from the circulation into the thyroid gland at a concentration gradient of about 20 to 50 times that of the plasma. This ensures that the thyroid gland obtains adequate amounts of iodine for hormone synthesis. During iodine deficiency, the thyroid gland concentrates a majority of the iodine available from the plasma. The thyroid of an average adult from an iodine-sufficient geographical region contains about 15 mg of iodine. Most excretion of iodine occurs through the urine, with the remainder excreted in the feces.

DETERMINING DRIS

Determining Requirements

The requirements for iodine are based on thyroid iodine accumulation and turnover.

Special Considerations

Individuals susceptible to adverse effects: People with autoimmune thyroid disease (AITD) and iodine deficiency respond adversely to intakes that are considered safe for the general population. AITD is common in the U.S. population and particularly in older women. Individuals with AITD who are treated for iodine deficiency or nodular goiter may have an increased sensitivity to the adverse effects of iodine intake.

Criteria for Determining Iodine Requirements, by Life Stage Group

Life stage group	Criterion
0 through 6 mo	Average iodine intake from human milk
7 through 12 mo	Extrapolation from 0 to 6 mo AI
1 through 8 y	Balance data on children
9 through 18 y	Extrapolation from adult EAR
19 through 50 y	Thyroid iodine accumulation and turnover
51 through > 70 y	Extrapolation of iodine turnover studies from 19 through 50 y

Pregnancy

≤ 18 y through 50 y   Balance data during pregnancy

Lactation

≤ 18 y   Adolescent female EAR plus average amount of iodine secreted
          in human milk

19 through 50 y   Adult female EAR plus average amount of iodine secreted
          in human milk

The UL

The Tolerable Upper Intake Level (UL) is the highest level of daily nutrient intake that is likely to pose no risk of adverse effects for almost all healthy people. Members of the general population should not routinely exceed the UL. The UL for iodine is based on thyroid dysfunction, characterized by elevated serum thyroptropin (also known as TSH) concentrations in response to increasing levels of ingested iodine; it represents intake from food, water, and supplements. A high urinary iodine excretion distinguishes this hypothyroidism from that produced in iodine deficiency. The UL is not meant to apply to individuals who are receiving iodine under medical supervision.

Based on the Food and Drug Administration's Total Diet Study, the highest intake of dietary iodine for any life stage or gender group at the 95th percentile was approximately 1.14 mg/day, which is equivalent to the UL for adults. The iodine intake from the diet and supplements at the 95th percentile was approximately 1.15 mg/day. For most people, iodine intake from usual foods and supplements is unlikely to exceed the UL.

Special Considerations

Goiter: In certain regions of the world where goiter is present, therapeutic doses may exceed the UL.

AITD: The UL for iodine does not apply to individuals with AITD (see "Determining Requirements"). Due to inadequate data, a UL could not be set for these individuals.

DIETARY SOURCES

Foods

The iodine content of most food sources is low and can be affected by soil content, irrigation, and fertilizers. Most foods provide 3–75 µg per serving. Seafood has higher concentrations of iodine because marine animals can concentrate iodine from seawater. Processed foods may also have higher levels due to the addition of iodized salt or additives such as calcium iodate, potassium iodate, potassium iodide, and cuprous iodide. Both the United States and Canada iodize salt with potassium iodide at 100 ppm (76 mg iodine/kg salt). Iodized salt is mandatory in Canada and discretionary in the United States. Iodized salt is optionally used by about 50 percent of the U.S. population.

Dietary Supplements

According to the Third National Health and Nutrition Examination Survey (NHANES III, 1988–1994), the median intake of iodine from supplements was approximately 140 µg/day for adults. The 1986 National Health Interview Survey (NHIS) reported that approximately 12 percent of men and 15 percent of nonpregnant women took a supplement that contained iodine.

Bioavailability

Under normal conditions, the absorption of dietary iodine by the body is greater than 90 percent. The bioavailability of orally administered thyroxine is approximately 75 percent.

Soya flour has been shown to inhibit iodine absorption, and goiter and hypothyroidism were reported in several infants who consumed infant formula containing soya flour. However, if iodine was added to this formula, no goiter appeared.

Some foods contain goitrogens, which interfere with thyroid hormone production or utilization. These foods, which include cassava, millet, and cruciferous vegetables (e.g., cabbage), generally are of no clinical significance unless there is a coexisting iodine deficiency. Water from shallow or polluted streams and wells may also contain goitrogens. Deficiencies of vitamin A, selenium, or iron can each exacerbate the effects of iodine deficiency.

Some ingested substances contain large amounts of iodine that can interfere with proper thyroid function. They include radiocontrast media, food coloring, certain medications (e.g., amiodarone), water purification tablets, and skin and dental disinfectants.

Dietary Interactions

This information was not provided at the time the DRI values for this nutrient were set.

INADEQUATE INTAKE AND DEFICIENCY

In North America, where much of the iodine consumed is from salt iodized with potassium iodide, symptoms of iodine deficiency are rare. However, most countries currently have some degree of iodine deficiency, including some industrialized countries in Western Europe. Of historical note, during the early part of the 20th century iodine deficiency was a significant problem in the United States and Canada, particularly in the interior, the Great Lakes region, and the Pacific Northwest.

The clinical signs and symptoms of iodine deficiency that result from inadequate thyroid hormone production due to a lack of sufficient iodine, include the following:

- Goiter (thyroid enlargement; usually the earliest clinical feature of deficiency)
- Mental retardation
- Hypothyroidism (elevated thyroid stimulating hormone [TSH])
- Cretinism (extreme form of neurological damage from fetal hypothyroidism; can be reversed with iodine treatment, especially when begun early)
- Growth and developmental abnormalities

The most damaging effect of iodine deficiency involves the developing brain. Thyroid hormone is particularly important for myelination of the central nervous system, which is most active in the perinatal period and during fetal and early postnatal development. Numerous population studies have correlated an iodine-deficient diet with an increased incidence of mental retardation. The effects of iodine deficiency on brain development are similar to those of hypothyroidism from any other cause.

Other consequences of iodine deficiency across populations include impaired reproductive outcome, increased childhood mortality, decreased learning ability, and economic stagnation. Major international efforts have produced dramatic improvements in the correction of iodine deficiency, mainly through the use of iodized salt in iodine-deficient countries.

EXCESS INTAKE

Most people are very tolerant of excess iodine intake from food. For the general population, high iodine intakes (in excess of the UL) from food, water, and supplements have been associated with the following adverse effects:

- Thyroiditis
- Goiter
- Hypothyroidism (elevated thyroid stimulating hormone [TSH])
- Hyperthyroidism
- Sensitivity reactions
- Thyroid papillary cancer
- Acute effects of iodine poisoning, such as burning of the mouth, throat, and stomach; abdominal pain; fever; nausea; vomiting; diarrhea; weak pulse; cardiac irritability; coma; and cyanosis (These symptoms are quite rare and are usually associated with doses of many grams.)

KEY POINTS FOR IODINE

✓ Iodine is an essential component of thyroid hormones that are involved in the regulation of various enzymes and metabolic processes.

✓ The requirements for iodine are based on thyroid iodine accumulation and turnover. The UL is based on serum thyroptropin concentration in response to varying levels of ingested iodine.

✓ Certain subpopulations, such as those with autoimmune thyroid disease (AITD) and iodine deficiency, respond adversely to intakes that are considered safe for the general population. AITD is common in the U.S. population and particularly in older women.

✓ For most people, iodine intake from usual foods and supplements is unlikely to exceed the UL. In certain regions of the world where goiter is present, therapeutic doses may exceed the UL.

✓ The iodine content of most food sources is low and can be affected by soil content, irrigation, and fertilizers. Most foods provide 3–75 µg per serving. Seafood has higher concentrations of iodine because marine animals can concentrate iodine from seawater.

✓ Processed foods may also have higher levels due to the addition of iodized salt or additives that contain iodine. Iodized salt is mandatory in Canada and optionally used by about 50 percent of the U.S. population.

✓   In North America, where much of the iodine consumed is from salt iodized with potassium iodide, symptoms of iodine deficiency are rare. However, most countries currently have some degree of iodine deficiency, including some industrialized countries in Western Europe.

✓   The clinical signs and symptoms of iodine deficiency include goiter, mental retardation, hypothyroidism, cretinism, and growth and developmental abnormalities.

✓   The use of iodized salt has helped reduce iodine deficiency.

✓   Most people are very tolerant of excess iodine intake from food and supplements.

✓   The potential adverse effects of iodine intakes in excess of the UL include thyroiditis, goiter, hypothyroidism, hyperthyroidism, sensitivity reactions, thyroid papillary cancer, and acute responses in some individuals.

TABLE 1 Dietary Reference Intakes for Iron by Life Stage Group

| | DRI values (mg/day) | | | | | |
| | EAR[a] | | RDA[b] | | AI[c] | UL[d] |
	males	females	males	females		
Life stage group						
0 through 6 mo					0.27	40
7 through 12 mo	6.9	6.9	11	11		40
1 through 3 y	3.0	3.0	7	7		40
4 through 8 y	4.1	4.1	10	10		40
9 through 13 y	5.9	5.7	8	8		40
14 through 18 y	7.7	7.9	11	15		45
19 through 30 y	6.0	8.1	8	18		45
31 through 50 y	6.0	8.1	8	18		45
51 through 70 y	6.0	5.0	8	8		45
> 70 y	6.0	5.0	8	8		45
Pregnancy						
≤ 18 y		23		27		45
19 through 50 y		22		27		45
Lactation						
≤ 18 y		7		10		45
19 through 50 y		6.5		9		45

[a] **EAR** = Estimated Average Requirement.
[b] **RDA** = Recommended Dietary Allowance.
[c] **AI** = Adequate Intake.
[d] **UL** = Tolerable Upper Intake Level. Unless otherwise specified, the UL represents total intake from food, water, and supplements.

IRON

I ron is a critical component of several proteins, including enzymes, cytochromes, myoglobin, and hemoglobin, the latter of which transports oxygen throughout the body. Almost two-thirds of the body's iron is found in hemoglobin that is present in circulating erythrocytes and involved in the transport of oxygen from the environment to tissues throughout the body for metabolism. Iron can exist in various oxidation states, including the ferrous, ferric, and ferryl states.

The requirements for iron are based on factorial modeling using the following factors: basal iron losses; menstrual losses; fetal requirements in pregnancy; increased requirement during growth for the expansion of blood volume; and increased tissue and storage iron. The Tolerable Upper Intake Level (UL) is based on gastrointestinal distress as the critical adverse effect. DRI values are listed by life stage group in Table 1.

About half of the iron from meat, poultry, and fish is heme iron, which is highly bioavailable; the remainder is nonheme, which is less readily absorbed by the body. Iron in dairy foods, eggs, and all plant-based foods is entirely nonheme. Particularly rich sources of nonheme iron are fortified plant-based foods, such as breads, cereals, and breakfast bars.

Iron deficiency anemia is the most common nutritional deficiency in the world. Adverse effects associated with excessive iron intake include gastrointestinal distress, secondary iron overload, and acute toxicity.

IRON AND THE BODY

Function

Iron is a component of several proteins, including enzymes, cytochromes, myoglobin, and hemoglobin. Almost two-thirds of the body's iron is found in hemoglobin that is present in circulating erythrocytes and involved in the transport of oxygen from the environment to tissues throughout the body for metabolism. A readily mobilizable iron store contains another 25 percent. Most of the remaining 15 percent is in the myoglobin of muscle tissue. Iron can exist in various oxidation states, including the ferrous, ferric, and ferryl states.

Four major classes of iron-containing proteins exist in the mammalian system: iron-containing heme proteins (hemoglobin, myoglobin, cytochromes), iron-sulfur enzymes (flavoproteins, hemeflavoproteins), proteins for iron storage and transport (transferrin, lactoferrin, ferritin), and other iron-containing or activated enzymes (sulfur, nonheme enzymes).

Absorption, Metabolism, Storage, and Excretion

The iron content of the body is highly conserved and strongly influenced by the size of a person's iron stores. The greater the stores, the less iron that is absorbed.

Adult men need to absorb about 1 mg/day to maintain iron balance. Menstruating women need to absorb about 1.5 mg/day, with a small proportion of this group needing to absorb as much as 3.4 mg/day. Menstrual losses highly vary among women and explain why iron requirements in menstruating women are not symmetrically distributed. The median amount of iron lost through menstruation in adult women is approximately 0.51 mg/day; in adolescent girls it is approximately 0.45 mg/day. Women in the late stages of pregnancy must absorb 4–5 mg/day to maintain iron balance. Requirements are also higher in childhood, particularly during periods of rapid growth in early childhood (6 to 24 months of age) and adolescence.

Iron absorption occurs in the upper small intestine via pathways that allow the absorption of heme and nonheme iron. Heme iron is more highly bioavailable than nonheme iron (see "Bioavailability" and "Dietary Sources"). Many factors can affect iron absorption (see "Dietary Interactions"). Therefore, exact figures for absorption of heme and nonheme iron are unknown. A conservative estimate for heme iron absorption is 25 percent; for nonheme iron the mean percentage of absorption is estimated to be approximately 16.8 percent. Absorption of bioavailable iron occurs by an energy-dependent carrier-mediated process; the iron is then intracellularly transported and transferred into the plasma.

Iron that enters the cells may be incorporated into functional compounds, stored as ferritin, or used to regulate future cellular iron metabolism. The liver, spleen, and bone marrow are the primary sites of iron storage in the body. The majority of iron that is absorbed into enterocytes, but not taken up by transferrin, is excreted in the feces, since these intestinal cells are sloughed off every 3 to 5 days. Little iron is excreted into the urine. In the absence of bleeding (including menstruation) or pregnancy, only a small quantity of iron is lost each day. As stated above, iron is also lost through menstrual bleeding, and these losses can widely vary among premenopausal women.

DETERMINING REQUIREMENTS

Determining Requirements

The requirements for iron are based on factorial modeling using the following factors: basal iron losses; menstrual losses; fetal requirements in pregnancy; increased requirements during growth for the expansion of blood volume; and increased tissue and storage iron.

It is important to note that iron requirements are known to be skewed rather than normally distributed for menstruating women. Information on the distribution of iron requirements can be found in Appendix G.

Special Considerations

Individuals susceptible to iron deficiency: People with decreased stomach acidity, such as those who overconsume antacids, ingest alkaline clay, or have pathological conditions, such as achlorhydria or partial gastrectomy, may have impaired iron absorption and be at greater risk for deficiency.

Infants: Because cow milk is a poor source of bioavailable iron, it is not recommended for infants under the age of 1 year; in Canada, the recommendation is 9 months of age. Early inappropriate ingestion of cow milk is associated with a higher risk of iron deficiency anemia. U.S. and Canadian pediatric societies have concluded that infants who are not, or only partially, fed human milk should receive an iron-fortified formula. Supplementation is also recommended for preterm infants as their iron stores are low.

Age of menarche: The RDA for iron for girls increases from 8 mg/day to 15 mg/day at the age of 14 years to account for menstruation. For girls who have reached this age, but are not yet menstruating, the requirement is approximately 10.5 mg/day, rather than 15 mg/day.

Adolescent and preadolescent growth spurt: The rate of growth during the growth spurt can be more than double the average rate for boys and up to 50 percent higher for girls. The increased requirement for dietary iron for boys and girls in the growth spurt is 2.9 mg/day and 1.1 mg/day, respectively.

Use of oral contraceptives and hormone replacement therapy (HRT): The use of oral contraceptives lowers menstrual blood loss. As a result, adolescent girls and women using oral contraceptives may have lower iron requirements. HRT may cause some uterine bleeding in some women. In this situation, women who are on HRT may have higher iron requirements than postmenopausal women who are not.

Vegetarian diets: Because heme iron is more bioavailable than nonheme iron (milk products and eggs are of animal origin, but they contain only nonheme iron), it is estimated that the bioavailability of iron from a vegetarian diet is approximately 10 percent, rather than the 18 percent from a mixed Western diet. Hence, the requirement for iron is 1.8 times higher for vegetarians. It is important to emphasize that lower bioavailability diets (approaching 5 percent overall absorption) may be encountered with very strict vegetarian diets.

Intestinal parasitic infection: A common problem in developing nations, intestinal parasites can cause significant blood loss, thereby increasing an individual's iron requirement.

Blood donation: A 500 mL donation just once a year translates to an additional iron loss of approximately 0.6 mg/day over the year. People who frequently donate blood have higher iron requirements.

Regular, intense physical activity: Studies show that iron status is often marginal or inadequate in many individuals, particularly females, who engage in regular, intense physical activity. The requirement of these individuals may be as much as 30–70 percent greater than those who do not participate in regular strenuous exercise.

Criteria for Determining Iron Requirements, by Life Stage Group

Life stage group	Criterion
0 through 6 mo	Average iron intake from human milk
7 through 12 mo	Factorial modeling
1 through 70 y	Factorial modeling
> 70 y	Extrapolation of factorial analysis from 51 through 70 y

Pregnancy	
≤ 18 y through 50 y	Factorial modeling

Lactation	
≤ 18 y through 50 y	Adolescent female EAR minus menstrual losses plus average amount of iron secreted in human milk

The UL

The Tolerable Upper Intake Level (UL) is the highest level of daily nutrient intake that is likely to pose no risk of adverse effects for almost all healthy people. Members of the general population should not routinely exceed the UL. This value is based on gastrointestinal distress as the critical adverse effect and represents intake from food, water, and supplements.

According to the National Health and Nutrition Examination Survey (NHANES III, 1988–1994), the highest intake from food and supplements at the 90th percentile reported for any life stage and gender groups, excluding pregnancy and lactation, was approximately 34 mg/day for men 51 years of age and older. This value is below the UL of 45 mg/day. Between 50 and 75 percent of pregnant and lactating women consumed iron from food and supplements at a greater level than 45 mg/day, but iron supplementation is usually supervised in prenatal and postnatal care programs. Based on a UL of 45 mg/day of iron for adults, the risk of adverse effects from dietary sources appears to be low.

Special Considerations

Individuals susceptible to adverse effects: People with the following conditions are susceptible to the adverse effects of excess iron intake: hereditary hemochromatosis; chronic alcoholism; alcoholic cirrhosis and other liver diseases; iron-loading abnormalities, particularly thalassemias; congenital atransferrinemia; and aceruloplasminemia. These individuals may not be protected by the UL for iron. A UL for subpopulations such as persons with hereditary hemochromatosis cannot be determined until information on the relationship between iron intake and the risk of adverse effects from excess iron stores becomes available.

DIETARY SOURCES

Foods

About half of the iron from meat, fish, and poultry is a rich source of heme iron, which is highly bioavailable; the remainder is nonheme, which is less readily absorbed by the body. However, heme iron represents only 8–12 percent of dietary iron for boys and men and 7–10 percent of dietary iron for girls and women. Plant-based foods, such as vegetables, fruits, whole-grain breads, or whole-grain pasta contain 0.1–1.4 mg of nonheme iron per serving. Fortified products, including breads, cereals, and breakfast bars can contribute high amounts of nonheme iron to the diet. In the United States, some fortified cereals contain as much as 24 mg of iron (nonheme) per 1-cup serving, while in Canada most cereals are formulated to contain 4 mg per serving.

Dietary Supplements

The 1986 National Health Interview Survey (NHIS) reported that approximately 21–25 percent of women and 16 percent of men consumed a supplement containing iron. According to NHANES III, the median intake of iron from supplements was approximately 1 mg/day for men and women. The median iron intake from food plus supplements by pregnant women was approximately 21 mg/day.

Bioavailability

Heme iron, from meat, poultry, and fish, is generally very well absorbed by the body and only slightly influenced by other dietary factors. The absorption of nonheme iron, present in all foods, including meat, poultry, and fish, is strongly influenced by its solubility and interaction with other meal components that promote or inhibit its absorption (see "Dietary Interactions").

Because of the many factors that influence iron bioavailability, 18 percent bioavailability was used to estimate the average requirement of iron for nonpregnant adults, adolescents, and children over the age of 1 year consuming typical North American diets. The intake was assumed to contain some meat-based foods. Because the diets of children under the age of 1 year contain little meat and are rich in cereal and vegetables, a bioavailability of 10 percent was assumed in setting the requirements. During pregnancy, iron absorption was assumed to be 25 percent.

Dietary Interactions

There is evidence that iron may interact with other nutrients and dietary substances (see Table 2).

TABLE 2 Potential Interactions with Other Dietary Substances

Substance	Potential Interaction	Notes
SUBSTANCES THAT AFFECT IRON		
Ascorbic acid	Ascorbic acid strongly enhances the absorption of nonheme iron.	There appears to be a linear relation between ascorbic acid intake and iron absorption up to at least 100 mg of ascorbic acid per meal. Because ascorbic acid improves iron absorption through the release of nonheme iron bound to inhibitors, the enhanced iron absorption effect is most marked when ascorbic acid is consumed with foods containing high levels of inhibitors, including phytate and tannins.

TABLE 2 Continued

Substance	Potential Interaction	Notes
Animal muscle tissue	Meat, fish, and poultry improve nonheme iron absorption.	The mechanism of this enhancing effect is poorly studied, but is likely to involve low molecular weight peptides that are released during digestion.
Phytate	Phytate inhibits nonheme iron absorption.	The absorption of iron from foods high in phytate, such as soybeans, black beans, lentils, mung beans, and split peas, has been shown to be very low (0.84–0.91 percent) and similar to each other. Unrefined rice and grains also contain phytate.
Polyphenols	Polyphenols inhibit nonheme iron absorption.	Polyphenols, such as those in tea, inhibit iron absorption through the binding of iron to tannic acids in the intestine. The inhibitory effects of tannic acid are dose-dependent and reduced by the addition of ascorbic acid. Polyphenols are also found in many grain products, red wine, and herbs such as oregano.
Vegetable proteins	Vegetable proteins inhibit nonheme iron absorption.	This effect is independent of the phytate content of the food.
Calcium	Calcium inhibits the absorption of both heme and nonheme iron.	This interaction is not well understood; however, it has been suggested that calcium inhibits heme and nonheme iron absorption during transfer through the mucosal cell. Despite the significant reduction of iron absorption by calcium in single meals, little effect has been observed on serum ferritin concentrations in supplementation trials with calcium supplementation at levels of 1,000–1,500 mg/day.

IRON AFFECTING OTHER SUBSTANCES

Substance	Potential Interaction	Notes
Zinc	High iron intakes may reduce zinc absorption.	In general, data indicate that supplemental iron may inhibit zinc absorption if both are taken without food, but does not inhibit zinc absorption if it is consumed with food.

INADEQUATE INTAKE AND DEFICIENCY

Iron deficiency anemia is the most common nutritional deficiency in the world. The most important functional indicators of iron deficiency are reduced physical work capacity, delayed psychomotor development in infants, impaired cognitive function, and adverse effects for both the mother and the fetus (such as maternal anemia, premature delivery, low birth weight, and increased perinatal infant mortality).

A series of laboratory indicators can be used to precisely characterize iron status and to categorize the severity of iron deficiency. Three levels of iron deficiency are customarily identified:

- Depleted iron stores, but where there appears to be no limitation in the supply of iron to the functional compartment
- Early functional iron deficiency (iron-deficient erythropoiesis), where the supply of iron to the functional compartment is suboptimal but not sufficiently reduced to cause measurable anemia
- Iron deficiency anemia, where there is a measurable deficit in the most accessible functional compartment, the erythrocyte

Available laboratory tests can be used in combination with each other to identify the evolution of iron deficiency through these three stages (see Table 3).

TABLE 3 Laboratory Measurements Commonly Used in the Evaluation of Iron Status

Stage of Iron Deficiency	Indicator	Diagnostic Range
Depleted stores	Stainable bone marrow iron	Absent
	Total iron binding capacity	> 400 µg/dL
	Serum ferritin concentration	< 12 µg/L
Early functional iron deficiency	Transferrin saturation	< 16%
	Free erythrocyte protoporphyrin	> 70 µg/dL erythrocyte
	Serum transferrin receptor	> 8.5 mg/L
Iron deficiency anemia	Hemoglobin concentration	< 130 g/L (male)
		< 120 g/L (female)
	Mean cell volume	< 80 fL

EXCESS INTAKE

The risk of adverse effects of excessive iron intake from dietary sources appears to be low in the general population. Adverse effects may include the following:

- Acute toxicity with vomiting and diarrhea, followed by cardiovascular, central nervous system, kidney, liver, and hematological effects.
- Gastrointestinal effects associated with high-dose supplements, such as constipation, nausea, vomiting, and diarrhea
- Secondary iron overload, which occurs when body iron stores are increased as a consequence of parenteral iron administration, repeated blood transfusions, or hematological disorders that increase the rate of iron absorption

Special Considerations

Men and postmenopausal women: Currently the relationship between excessive iron intake and measure of iron status (e.g., serum ferritin concentrations) and both coronary heart disease and cancer is unclear. Nevertheless, the association between a high iron intake and iron overload in sub-Saharan Africa makes it prudent to recommend that men and postmenopausal women avoid iron supplements and highly fortified foods.

KEY POINTS FOR IRON

✓   Iron is a critical component of several proteins, including cytochromes, myoglobin, and hemoglobin, the latter of which transports oxygen throughout the body.

✓   The requirements for iron are based on factorial modeling using the following factors: basal iron losses; menstrual losses; fetal requirements in pregnancy; increased requirement during growth for the expansion of blood volume; and increased tissue and storage iron. The UL is based on gastrointestinal distress as the critical adverse effect.

✓   Special populations and situations in which iron requirements may vary include infants who do not receive human milk (0–6 months), preterm infants, teens/preteens in the growth spurt, oral contraceptive users, postmenopausal women using cyclic HRT, vegetarians, athletes, and blood donors.

✓   People with the following conditions are susceptible to the adverse effects of excess iron intake: hereditary hemochromatosis; chronic alcoholism; alcoholic cirrhosis, and other liver diseases; iron-loading abnormalities, particularly thalassemias; congenital atransferrinemia; and aceruloplasminemia. These individuals may not be protected by the UL for iron.

✓   About half of the iron from meat, poultry, and fish is heme iron, which is highly bioavailable; the remainder is nonheme, which is less readily absorbed by the body.

✓   Particularly rich sources of nonheme iron are fortified plant-based foods, such as breads, cereals, and breakfast bars. The absorption of nonheme iron is enhanced when it is consumed with foods that contain ascorbic acid (vitamin C) or meat, poultry, and fish.

✓   Iron deficiency anemia is the most common nutritional deficiency in the world.

✓   The most important functional indicators of iron deficiency are reduced physical work capacity, delayed psychomotor development in infants, impaired cognitive function, and adverse effects for both the mother and the fetus (such as maternal anemia, premature delivery, low birth weight, and increased perinatal infant mortality).

✓   Three levels of iron deficiency are customarily identified: depleted iron stores, early functional iron deficiency, and iron deficiency anemia.

✓   Adverse effects associated with excessive iron intake include acute toxicity, gastrointestinal distress, and secondary iron overload.

✓   Currently the relationship between excessive iron intake and high serum ferritin concentrations and both coronary heart disease and cancer is unclear. Nevertheless, the association between a high iron intake and iron overload in sub-Saharan Africa makes it prudent to recommend that men and post-menopausal women avoid iron supplements and highly fortified foods.

TABLE 1 Dietary Reference Intakes for Magnesium by Life Stage Group

	DRI values (mg/day)						
	EAR[a]		RDA[b]		AI[c]		UL[d,e]
	males	females	males	females	males	females	
Life stage group							
0 through 6 mo					30	30	ND[f]
7 through 12 mo					75	75	ND
1 through 3 y	65	65	80	80			65
4 through 8 y	110	110	130	130			110
9 through 13 y	200	200	240	240			350
14 through 18 y	340	300	410	360			350
19 through 30 y	330	255	400	310			350
31 through 50 y	350	265	420	320			350
51 through 70 y	350	265	420	320			350
> 70 y	350	265	420	320			350
Pregnancy							
≤ 18 y		335		400			350
19 through 30 y		290		350			350
31 through 50 y		300		360			350
Lactation							
≤ 18 y		300		360			350
19 through 30 y		255		310			350
31 through 50 y		265		320			350

[a] **EAR** = Estimated Average Requirement.

[b] **RDA** = Recommended Dietary Allowance.

[c] **AI** = Adequate Intake.

[d] **UL** = Tolerable Upper Intake Level. Unless otherwise specified, the UL represents total intake from food, water, and supplements.

[e] The ULs for magnesium represent intake from pharmacological agents only and do not include intake from food and water.

[f] **ND** = Not determinable. This value is not determinable due to the lack of data of adverse effects in this age group and concern regarding the lack of ability to handle excess amounts. Source of intake should only be from food to prevent high levels of intake.

MAGNESIUM

Magnesium is involved in more than 300 enzymatic processes in the body, as well as in bone health and in the maintenance of intracellular levels of potassium and calcium. Magnesium also plays a role in the development and maintenance of bone and other calcified tissues.

Magnesium requirements for adults are based primarily on balance studies. The Tolerable Upper Intake Level (UL) is based on diarrhea as the critical endpoint and was derived from several studies on adults evaluating the effect of vitamin D intake on serum calcium in humans. DRI values are listed by life stage group in Table 1.

Foods rich in magnesium include green leafy vegetables, whole grains, and nuts. Magnesium may be poorly absorbed from foods that are high in fiber and phytic acid. Magnesium deficiency may result in muscle cramps, hypertension, and coronary and cerebral vasospasms. Adverse effects from excess intake of magnesium from food sources are rare, but the use of pharmacological doses of magnesium from nonfood sources can result in magnesium toxicity, which is characterized by diarrhea, metabolic alkalosis, hypokalemia, paralytic ileus, and cardiorespiratory arrest.

MAGNESIUM AND THE BODY

Function

Magnesium is involved in more than 300 enzymatic processes in the body, as well as in the maintenance of intracellular levels of potassium and calcium. Magnesium also plays a role in the development and maintenance of bone and other calcified tissues.

Absorption, Metabolism, Storage, and Excretion

Magnesium is absorbed along the entire intestinal tract, with maximal absorption likely occurring at the distal jejunum and ileum. In both children and adults, fractional magnesium absorption is inversely proportional to the amount of magnesium consumed. That is, the more magnesium consumed, the lower the proportion that is absorbed (and vice versa). This may be explained by how magnesium is absorbed in the intestine, which is via an unsaturable passive and saturable active transport system.

To a small extent, vitamin D appears to enhance intestinal magnesium absorption. The body's level of magnesium is maintained primarily by the kidneys, where magnesium is filtered and reabsorbed. Approximately 50–60 percent of total body magnesium is stored in bone. Magnesium intake in excess of need is efficiently excreted in urine.

DETERMINING DRIS

Determining Requirements

The adult requirements for magnesium are based on dietary balance studies of magnesium. Although several magnesium balance studies have been performed, not all have met the requirements of a well-designed investigation. The minimum requirements for the balance studies used to determine the EAR included either an adaptation period of at least 12 days or a determination of balance made while subjects consume self-selected diets. The disadvantage of the latter is that they do not provide the two levels of intakes needed to determine the dose–response relationship.

Criteria for Determining Magnesium Requirements, by Life Stage Group

Life stage group	Criterion
0 through 6 mo	Human milk content
7 through 12 mo	Human milk + solid food
1 through 8 y	Extrapolation of balance studies in older children
9 through 70 y	Balance studies
> 70 y	Intracellular studies; decreases in absorption; balance studies in other adult ages
Pregnancy	
≤ 18 y through 50 y	Age-specific requirement + gain in lean mass
Lactation	
≤ 18 y through 50 y	Balance studies

The UL

The Tolerable Upper Intake Level (UL) is the highest level of magnesium taken acutely without food that is likely to pose no risk of adverse effects for almost all people. Members of the general population should not routinely exceed the UL.

When ingested as a naturally occurring substance in foods, magnesium has not been shown to exert any adverse effects. However, adverse effects of excessive magnesium intake have been observed with intakes from nonfood sources, such as various magnesium salts used for pharmacological purposes. Therefore, the UL for magnesium represents acute intake from pharmacological agents and does not include intake from food and water. The UL for adults is based on diarrhea as the critical endpoint and was derived from several studies on adults that evaluated the effects of excessive magnesium intake from nonfood sources.

Although a few studies have noted mild diarrhea and other mild gastrointestinal complaints in a small percentage of patients at levels of 360–380 mg/day, it is noteworthy that many other individuals have not encountered such effects, even when receiving substantially more than this amount of supplementary magnesium.

Using data from the 1986 National Health Interview Survey (NHIS), it is estimated that almost 1 percent of all adults in the United States took a nonfood magnesium supplement that exceeded the UL of 350 mg/day. The data on supplement use also indicated that at least 5 percent of young children who used magnesium supplements exceeded the UL for magnesium at 5 mg/kg/day. However, based on the reported frequency of intake in children, fewer than 1 percent of all children would be at risk for adverse effects. More information on supplement use by specific ages is needed.

Special Considerations

Individuals with certain conditions: People with neonatal tetany, hyperuricemia, hyperlipidemia, lithium toxicity, hyperthyroidism, pancreatitis, hepatitis, phlebitis, coronary artery disease, arrhythmia, and digitalis intoxication may benefit from the clinically prescribed use of magnesium in quantities exceeding the UL.

DIETARY SOURCES

Foods

Foods rich in magnesium include green leafy vegetables, whole grains, and nuts. Meats, starches, and milk are intermediate in magnesium content, and refined foods generally have the lowest magnesium content. According to the 1989 Total Diet Study of the U.S. Food and Drug Administration, approximately 45 percent of dietary magnesium was obtained from vegetables, fruits, grains, and nuts, whereas approximately 29 percent was obtained from milk, meat, and eggs.

With the increased consumption of refined and processed foods, dietary magnesium intake appears to have decreased over the years. Total magnesium intake usually depends on calorie intake, which explains the higher intake levels generally seen in young children and adult males and the lower intake levels seen in women and the elderly. Water is a variable source of magnesium intake. Typically, "hard" water has a higher concentration of magnesium salts than "soft" water.

Dietary Supplements

According to the 1986 NHIS, about 14 percent of men and 17 percent of women took supplements that contained magnesium, while approximately 8 percent of young children (2 to 6 years of age) did so. Women and men who used magnesium supplements took similar doses, about 100 mg/day, although the 95th percentile of intake was somewhat higher for women (400 mg/day) than it was for men (350 mg/day). Children who took magnesium had a median daily intake of 23 mg and a 95th-percentile daily supplemental intake of 117 mg.

Bioavailability

In a typical diet, approximately 50 percent of the magnesium consumed will be absorbed. High levels of dietary fiber from fruits, vegetables, and grains decrease magnesium absorption or retention, or both.

Dietary Interactions

There is evidence that magnesium may interact with certain other nutrients and dietary substances (see Table 2).

TABLE 2 Potential Interactions with Other Dietary Substances

Substance	Potential Interaction	Notes
SUBSTANCES THAT AFFECT MAGNESIUM		
Phytic acid and fiber	Phytic acid, or phytate, may decrease magnesium absorption.	Foods high in fiber, which contain phytic acid, may decrease intestinal magnesium absorption, likely by binding magnesium to phosphate groups on phytic acid.
Phosphorus	Phosphorus may decrease magnesium absorption.	Studies of subjects on high-phosphate diets have shown that phosphate binding to magnesium may explain decreases in intestinal magnesium absorption.

TABLE 2 Continued

Substance	Potential Interaction	Notes
Calcium	High intakes of calcium may decrease magnesium absorption.	Most human studies of the effects of dietary calcium on magnesium absorption have shown no effect. Calcium intakes of as much as 2,000 mg/day (in adult men) did not affect magnesium balance. However, calcium intakes in excess of 2,600 mg/day have been reported to decrease magnesium balance. Several studies have found that high sodium and calcium intake may result in increased renal magnesium excretion. Overall, at the dietary levels recommended in this report, the interaction of magnesium with calcium is not a concern.
Protein	Protein may affect magnesium absorption.	Magnesium absorption has been shown to be lower when protein intake is less than 30 g/day. A higher protein intake may increase renal magnesium excretion, perhaps because an increased acid load increases urinary magnesium excretion. Studies in adolescents have shown improved magnesium absorption and retention when protein intakes were higher (93 vs. 43 mg/day).

MAGNESIUM AFFECTING OTHER SUBSTANCES

Substance	Potential Interaction	Notes
Calcium	Magnesium deficiency may cause hypocalcemia.	In general, magnesium deficiency must become moderate to severe before symptomatic hypocalcemia develops. However, a 3-week study of dietary-induced experimental magnesium depletion in humans demonstrated that even a mild degree of magnesium depletion may result in a significant decrease in serum calcium concentration.
Vitamin D	Magnesium deficiency may affect the body's response to pharmacological vitamin D.	Individuals with hypocalcemia and magnesium deficiency are resistant to pharmacological doses of vitamin D, $1,\alpha$-hydroxyvitamin D, and 1,25-dihydroxyvitamin D.

INADEQUATE INTAKE AND DEFICIENCY

Severe magnesium depletion leads to specific biochemical abnormalities and clinical manifestations that can be easily detected. The potential effects of inadequate magnesium intake or deficiency include the following:

- Symptomatic hypocalcemia (A prominent manifestation of magnesium deficiency in humans, symptomatic hypocalcemia develops when magnesium deficiency becomes moderate to severe. See Table 2.)
- Muscle cramps
- Interference with vitamin D metabolism (see Table 2)
- Neuromuscular hyperexcitability (often the initial problem cited in individuals who have or are developing magnesium deficiency)
- Latent tetany
- Spontaneous carpal-pedal spasm
- Seizures

Magnesium depletion may be found in several cardiovascular and neuromuscular diseases, malabsorption syndromes, diabetes mellitus, renal wasting syndromes, osteoporosis, and chronic alcoholism.

Special Considerations

Excessive alcohol intake: Excessive alcohol intake has been shown to cause renal magnesium wasting. Individuals who consume marginal amounts of magnesium and who excessively consume alcohol could be at risk for magnesium depletion. However, current evidence does not support the suggestion that magnesium deficiency causes alcoholism.

Medications: A growing number of medications have been found to result in increased renal magnesium excretion. Diuretics, which are commonly used to treat hypertension, heart failure, and edema, may cause hypermagnesuria.

Mothers who breastfeed multiple infants: Due to the increased milk production of a mother while breastfeeding multiple infants, increased intakes of magnesium during lactation, as with calcium, should be considered.

The elderly: Several studies have found that elderly people have relatively low dietary intakes of magnesium. This may be due to several factors. With aging, intestinal magnesium absorption tends to decrease and urinary magnesium excretion tends to increase. Other factors include poor appetite, diminished senses of taste or smell (or both), poorly fitting dentures, and difficulty in shopping for and preparing meals. It should also be noted that meals served by some long-term care facilities may provide less than the recommended levels of magnesium.

EXCESS INTAKE

Excess intake of magnesium from food sources is not associated with adverse effects. However, adverse effects have been observed with excessive intake from nonfood sources that are used acutely for pharmacological purposes, such as magnesium salts. They include the following:

- Diarrhea (primary symptom)
- Nausea
- Abdominal cramps

More severe adverse effects may occur with very large pharmacological doses of magnesium. They include the following:

- Metabolic alkalosis
- Hypokalemia
- Paralytic ileus

Special Considerations

Impaired renal function: Individuals with impaired renal function are at greater risk of magnesium toxicity (from nonfood sources).

KEY POINTS FOR MAGNESIUM

✓   Magnesium is involved in more than 300 enzymatic processes in the body, as well as in bone health and in the maintenance of intracellular levels of potassium and calcium.

✓   The more magnesium consumed, the lower the proportion that is absorbed (and vice versa).

✓   The adult requirements for magnesium are based primarily on balance studies. The UL for adults was based on diarrhea as the critical endpoint and was derived from several studies on adults evaluating the effect of vitamin D intake on serum calcium in humans. The UL is based on intake from pharmacological sources of magnesium, rather than from food and water.

✓   Foods rich in magnesium include green leafy vegetables, whole grains, and nuts; population intakes of magnesium have declined with decreased intakes of these foods.

✓   Magnesium deficiency can result in hypocalcemia, muscle cramps, and seizures, as well as interfere with vitamin D metabolism.

✓   No adverse effects of magnesium intake from food sources have been demonstrated.

✓   Acute excessive intake of magnesium from nonfood sources, such as pharmacological doses of magnesium salts, can cause metabolic alkalosis, hypokalemia, and paralytic ileus.

TABLE 1 Dietary Reference Intakes for Manganese by Life Stage Group

	DRI values (mg/day)		
	AI[a]		UL[b]
	males	females	
Life stage group			
0 through 6 mo	0.003	0.003	ND[c]
7 through 12 mo	0.6	0.6	ND
1 through 3 y	1.2	1.2	2
4 through 8 y	1.5	1.5	3
9 through 13 y	1.9	1.6	6
14 through 18 y	2.2	1.6	9
19 through 30 y	2.3	1.8	11
31 through 50 y	2.3	1.8	11
51 through 70 y	2.3	1.8	11
> 70 y	2.3	1.8	11
Pregnancy			
≤ 18 y		2.0	9
19 through 50 y		2.0	11
Lactation			
≤ 18 y		2.6	9
19 through 50 y		2.6	11

[a] **AI** = Adequate Intake.

[b] **UL** = Tolerable Upper Intake Level. Unless otherwise specified, the UL represents total intake from food, water, and supplements.

[c] **ND** = Not determinable. This value is not determinable due to the lack of data of adverse effects in this age group and concern regarding the lack of ability to handle excess amounts. Source of intake should only be from food to prevent high levels of intake.

MANGANESE

Manganese is involved in the formation of bone and in specific reactions related to amino acid, cholesterol, and carbohydrate metabolism. Manganese metalloenzymes include arginase, glutamine synthetase, phosphoenolpyruvate decarboxylase, and manganese superoxide dismutase.

Since data were insufficient to set an Estimated Average Requirement (EAR) and thus calculate a Recommended Dietary Allowance (RDA) for manganese, an Average Intake (AI) was instead developed. The AIs for manganese are based on intakes in healthy individuals, using the median manganese intakes reported from the Food and Drug Administration's (FDA's) Total Diet Study (1991–1997). The Tolerable Upper Intake Level (UL) is based on elevated blood manganese concentrations and neurotoxicity as the critical adverse effects. DRI values are listed by life stage group in Table 1.

The highest contributors of manganese to the diet are grains, beverages (tea), and vegetables. Although a manganese deficiency may contribute to one or more clinical symptoms, a clinical deficiency has not been clearly associated with poor dietary intakes of healthy individuals. Neurotoxicity of orally ingested manganese at relatively low doses is controversial, but evidence suggests that elevated blood manganese levels and neurotoxicity are possible.

MANGANESE AND THE BODY

Function

Manganese is an essential nutrient involved in the formation of bone and in specific reactions related to amino acid, cholesterol, and carbohydrate metabolism. Manganese metalloenzymes include arginase, glutamine synthetase, phosphoenolpyruvate decarboxylase, and manganese superoxide dismutase.

Absorption, Metabolism, Storage, and Excretion

Only a small percentage of dietary manganese is absorbed by the body. Some studies indicate that manganese is absorbed via active transport mechanisms, while other studies suggest that passive diffusion via a nonsaturable process occurs. Much of absorbed manganese is excreted very rapidly into the gut via the bile, and only a small amount is retained.

Manganese is taken up from the blood by the liver and transported to extrahepatic tissues by transferrin and possibly α_2-macroglobulin and albumin. Excretion primarily occurs in the feces. Urinary excretion of manganese is low and has not been found to be sensitive to dietary intake. Therefore, the potential risk for manganese toxicity is highest when bile excretion is low, such as in the neonate or in liver disease.

DETERMINING DRIS

Determining Requirements

Since data were insufficient to set an EAR and thus calculate an RDA for manganese, an AI was instead developed. The AIs for manganese are based on intakes in healthy individuals, using the median manganese intake from the FDA's Total Diet Study (1991–1997).

Special Considerations

Gender: Men have been shown to absorb significantly less manganese compared to women. This may be related to iron status, as men generally have higher serum ferritin concentrations than do women (see "Dietary Interactions").

Criteria for Determining Manganese Requirements, by Life Stage Group

Life stage group	Criterion
0 through 6 mo	Average manganese intake from human milk
7 through 12 mo	Extrapolation from adult AI
1 through > 70 y	Median manganese intake from the Total Diet Study
Pregnancy	
≤ 18 y	Extrapolation from adolescent female AI based on body weight
19 through 50 y	Extrapolation from adult female AI based on body weight
Lactation	
< 18 y through 50 y	Median manganese intake from the Total Diet Study

The UL

The Tolerable Upper Intake Level (UL) is the highest level of daily nutrient intake that is likely to pose no risk of adverse effects for almost all healthy people. Members of the general population should not routinely exceed the UL. This value is based on elevated blood manganese and neurotoxicity as the critical adverse effects and represents intake from food, water, and supplements.

Based on the Total Diet Study, the highest dietary manganese intake at the 95th percentile was 6.3 mg/day, which was the level consumed by men aged 31 to 50 years. Data from the Third National Health and Nutrition Examination Survey (NHANES III, 1988–1994) indicated that the highest supplemental intake of manganese at the 95th percentile was approximately 5 mg/day, which was consumed by adults, including pregnant women. The risk of an adverse effect resulting from excess intake of manganese from food and supplements appears to be low at these intakes.

DIETARY SOURCES

Foods

Based on the Total Diet Study, grain products contributed 37 percent of dietary manganese, while beverages (tea) and vegetables contributed 20 and 18 percent, respectively, to the adult male diet.

Dietary Supplements

According to U.S. data from the 1986 National Health Interview Survey (NHIS), 12 percent of adults consumed supplements that contained manganese. Based on data from NHANES III, the median supplemental intake of manganese was 2.4 mg/day for those adults who took supplements, an amount similar to the average dietary manganese intake.

Bioavailability

Several factors may affect the bioavailability of manganese (see "Dietary Interactions").

Dietary Interactions

There is evidence that manganese may interact with certain other nutrients and dietary substances (see Table 2).

INADEQUATE INTAKE AND DEFICIENCY

Although a manganese deficiency may contribute to one or more clinical symptoms, a clinical deficiency has not been clearly associated with poor dietary intakes of healthy individuals. In limited studies on induced manganese depletion in humans, subjects developed scaly dermatitis and hypocholesterolemia. Studies in various animal species observed signs and symptoms of deficiency, including impaired growth and skeletal development, impaired reproductive

TABLE 2 Potential Interactions with Other Dietary Substances

Substance	Potential Interaction	Notes
SUBSTANCES THAT AFFECT MANGANESE		
Calcium	Calcium may reduce manganese absorption.	In one study, adding calcium to human milk reduced the absorption of manganese from 4.9 percent to 3.0 percent.
Iron	Iron status may affect manganese absorption: low serum ferritin concentration may increase manganese absorption.	Low ferritin concentrations are associated with increased manganese absorption, thereby having a gender effect on manganese bioavailability (because women tend to have lower ferritin concentrations compared with men).
Phytate	Phytate may decrease manganese absorption.	In a study of infant formula, the soy-based formula without phytate produced manganese absorption of 1.6 percent, whereas a formula with phytate produced an absorption of 0.7 percent.

function, impaired glucose tolerance, and alterations in carbohydrate and lipid metabolism.

EXCESS INTAKE

Manganese toxicity, which causes central nervous system effects similar to those of Parkinson's disease, is a well-recognized occupational hazard for people who inhale manganese dust. The totality of evidence in animals and humans supports a causal association between elevated blood manganese concentrations and neurotoxicity.

Special Considerations

Individuals susceptible to adverse effects: People with chronic liver disease may be distinctly susceptible to the adverse effects of excess manganese intake, probably because elimination of manganese in bile is impaired. Also, manganese in drinking water and supplements may be more bioavailable than food manganese. Therefore, individuals who take manganese supplements, particularly those who already consume large amounts of manganese from diets high in plant products, should take extra caution.

Plasma manganese concentrations can become elevated in infants with choleostatic liver disease who are given supplemental manganese in total parenteral nutrition (TPN).

KEY POINTS FOR MANGANESE

✓   Manganese is an essential nutrient involved in the formation of bone and in specific reactions related to amino acid, cholesterol, and carbohydrate metabolism.

✓   Since data were insufficient to set an EAR and thus calculate an RDA for manganese, an AI was instead developed.

✓   The AIs for manganese are based on the intakes of healthy individuals, using median manganese intakes reported from the FDA's Total Diet Study. The UL is based on elevated blood manganese concentrations and neurotoxicity as the critical adverse effects.

✓   The risk of an adverse effect resulting from excess intake of manganese from food and supplements appears to be low.

✓   The highest contributors of manganese to the diet are grain products, beverages (tea), and vegetables.

✓   Although a manganese deficiency may contribute to one or more clinical symptoms, a clinical deficiency has not been clearly associated with poor dietary intakes of healthy individuals. In limited studies on induced manganese depletion in humans, subjects developed scaly dermatitis and hypocholesterolemia.

✓   Manganese toxicity, which causes central nervous system effects similar to those of Parkinson's disease, is a well-recognized occupational hazard for people who inhale manganese dust. Neurotoxicity of orally ingested manganese at relatively low doses is more controversial, but evidence suggests that elevated blood manganese levels and neurotoxicity are possible.

✓   Plasma manganese concentrations can become elevated in infants with choleostatic liver disease who are given supplemental manganese in total parenteral nutrition.

TABLE 1 Dietary Reference Intakes for Molybdenum by Life Stage Group

	DRI values (µg /day)					
	EAR[a]		RDA[b]		AI[c]	UL[d]
	males	females	males	females		
Life stage group						
0 through 6 mo					2	ND[e]
6 through 12 mo					3	ND
1 through 3 y	13	13	17	17		300
4 through 8 y	17	17	22	22		600
9 through 13 y	26	26	34	34		1,100
14 through 18 y	33	33	43	43		1,700
19 through 30 y	34	34	45	45		2,000
31 through 50 y	34	34	45	45		2,000
51 through 70 y	34	34	45	45		2,000
> 70 y	34	34	45	45		2,000
Pregnancy						
≤ 18 y		40		50		1,700
19 through 50 y		40		50		2,000
Lactation						
≤ 18 y		35		50		1,700
19 through 50 y		36		50		2,000

[a] **EAR** = Estimated Average Requirement.

[b] **RDA** = Recommended Dietary Allowance.

[c] **AI** = Adequate Intake.

[d] **UL** = Tolerable Upper Intake Level. Unless otherwise specified, the UL represents total intake from food, water, and supplements.

[e] **ND** = Not determinable. This value is not determinable due to the lack of data of adverse effects in this age group and concern regarding the lack of ability to handle excess amounts. Source of intake should only be from food to prevent high levels of intake.

MOLYBDENUM

Molybdenum functions as a cofactor for several enzymes, including sulfite oxidase, xanthine oxidase, and aldehyde oxidase. The requirements for molybdenum are based on controlled balance studies with specific amounts of molybdenum consumed. Adjustments were made for the bioavailability of molybdenum. The Tolerable Upper Intake Level (UL) is based on impaired reproduction and growth in animals. DRI values are listed by life stage group in Table 1.

Legumes, grain products, and nuts are the major contributors of dietary molybdenum. Molybdenum deficiency has not been observed in healthy people. Molybdenum compounds appear to have low toxicity in humans.

MOLYBDENUM AND THE BODY

Function

Molybdenum, in a form called molybdopterin, acts as a cofactor for several enzymes, including sulfite oxidase, xanthine oxidase, and aldehyde oxidase. These enzymes are involved in catabolism of sulfur amino acids and heterocylic compounds such as purines and pyrimidines. A clear molybdenum deficiency syndrome that produces physiological signs of molybdenum restriction has not been achieved in animals, despite major reduction in the activity of these molybdoenzymes. Rather, the essential nature of molybdenum is based on a genetic defect that prevents sulfite oxidase synthesis. Because sulfite is not oxidized to sulfate, severe neurological damage leading to early death occurs with this inborn error of metabolism.

Absorption, Metabolism, Storage, and Excretion

The absorption of molybdenum is highly efficient over a wide range of intakes, which suggests that the mechanism of action is a passive (nonmediated) diffusion process. However, the exact mechanism and location within the gastrointestinal tract of molybdenum absorption have not been studied. Protein-bound molybdenum constitutes 83–97 percent of the total molybdenum in erythrocytes. Potential plasma molybdenum transport proteins include α-macroglobulin.

Evidence suggests that the kidneys are the primary site of molybdenum homeostatic regulation. Excretion is primarily through the urine and is directly related to dietary intake. When molybdenum intake is low, about 60 percent of ingested molybdenum is excreted in the urine, but when molybdenum intake is high, more than 90 percent is excreted in the urine. Although related to dietary intake, urinary molybdenum alone does not reflect status.

DETERMINING DRIS

Determining Requirements

The requirements for molybdenum are based on controlled balance studies with specific amounts of molybdenum consumed. Adjustments were made for the bioavailability of molybdenum. Information on dietary intake of molybdenum is limited because of lack of a simple and reliable analytical method for determining molybdenum in foods.

Criteria for Determining Molybdenum Requirements, by Life Stage Group

Life stage group	Criterion
0 through 6 mo	Average molybdenum intake from human milk
7 through 12 mo	Extrapolation from 0 through 6 mo AI
1 through 18 y	Extrapolation from adult EAR
19 through 30 y	Balance data
31 through > 70 y	Extrapolation of balance data from 19 through 30 y
Pregnancy	
≤ 18 y	Extrapolation of adolescent female EAR based on body weight
19 through 50 y	Extrapolation of adult female EAR based on body weight
Lactation	
≤ 18 y	Adolescent female EAR plus average amount of molybdenum secreted in human milk
19 through 50 y	Adult female EAR plus average amount of molybdenum secreted in human milk

The UL

The Tolerable Upper Intake Level (UL) is the highest level of daily nutrient intake that is likely to pose no risk of adverse effects for almost all people. Members of the general population should not routinely exceed the UL. Inadequate data exist to identify a causal association between excess molybdenum intake in normal, apparently healthy individuals and any adverse health outcomes. In addition, studies have identified levels of dietary molybdenum intake that appear to be associated with no harm. Thus, the UL is based on adverse reproductive effects in rats fed high levels of molybdenum. The UL applies to all forms of molybdenum from food, water, and supplements. More soluble forms of molybdenum have greater toxicity than insoluble or less soluble forms.

National surveys do not provide percentile data on the dietary intake of molybdenum. Data available from the Third National Health and Nutrition Examination Survey (NHANES III, 1988–1994) indicate that the average U.S. intakes from molybdenum supplements at the 95th percentile were 80 µg/day for men and 84 µg/day for women. Because there was no information from national surveys on percentile distribution of molybdenum intakes, the risk of adverse effects could not be characterized.

DIETARY SOURCES
Foods

The molybdenum content of plant-based foods depends on the content of the soil in which the foods were grown. Legumes, grain products, and nuts are the major contributors of dietary molybdenum. Animal products, fruits, and many vegetables are generally low in molybdenum.

Dietary Supplements

Data from NHANES III indicated that the median intakes of molybdenum from supplements were 23 µg/day for men and 24 µg/day for women.

Bioavailability

Little is known about the bioavailability of molybdenum, except that it has been demonstrated to be less efficiently absorbed from soy than from other food sources (as is the case with other minerals). It is unlikely that molybdenum in other commonly consumed foods would be less available than the molybdenum in soy. The utilization of absorbed molybdenum appears to be similar regardless of food source.

Dietary Interactions

This information was not provided at the time the DRI values for this nutrient were set.

INADEQUATE INTAKE AND DEFICIENCY

Molybdenum deficiency has not been observed in healthy people. A rare metabolic defect called molybdenum cofactor deficiency results from the deficiency of molybdoenzymes. Few infants with this defect survive the first days of life, and those who do have severe neurological and other abnormalities.

EXCESS INTAKE

Molybdenum compounds appear to have a low toxicity in humans. Possible reasons for the presumed low toxicity of molybdenum include its rapid excretion in the urine, especially at higher intake levels. More soluble forms of molybdenum have greater toxicity than insoluble or less soluble forms.

There are limited toxicity data for molybdenum in humans; most of the data apply to animals. In the absence of adequate human studies, it is impossible to determine which adverse effects might be considered most relevant to humans.

Special Considerations

Individuals susceptible to adverse effects: People who are deficient in dietary copper or who have some dysfunction in copper metabolism that makes them copper-deficient could be at increased risk of molybdenum toxicity. However, the effect of molybdenum intake on copper status in humans remains to be clearly established.

KEY POINTS FOR MOLYBDENUM

✓   Molybdenum functions as a cofactor for certain enzymes, including sulfite oxidase, xanthine oxidase, and aldehyde oxidase.

✓   The requirements for molybdenum are based on controlled balance studies with specific amounts of molybdenum consumed. The UL is based on impaired reproduction and growth in animals.

✓   Information on dietary intake of molybdenum is limited because of lack of a simple and reliable analytical method for determining molybdenum in food. Usual intake is well above the dietary molybdenum requirement.

✓   The molybdenum content of plant-based foods depends on the content of the soil in which the foods were grown. Legumes, grain products, and nuts are the major contributors of dietary molybdenum.

✓   Molybdenum deficiency has not been observed in healthy people. A rare and usually fatal metabolic defect called molybdenum cofactor deficiency results from the deficiency of molybdoenzymes.

✓   Molybdenum compounds appear to have a low toxicity in humans.

✓   There are limited toxicity data for molybdenum in humans; most of the data apply to animals.

✓   Possible reasons for the presumed low toxicity of molybdenum include its rapid excretion in the urine, especially at higher intake levels.

TABLE 1 Dietary Reference Intakes for Phosphorus by Life Stage Group

	DRI values (mg /day)					
	EAR[a]		RDA[b]		AI[c]	UL[d]
	males	females	males	females		
Life stage group						
0 through 6 mo					100	ND[e]
7 through 12 mo					275	ND
1 through 3 y	380	380	460	460		3,000
4 through 8 y	405	405	500	500		3,000
9 through 13 y	1,055	1,055	1,250	1,250		4,000
14 through 18 y	1,055	1,055	1,250	1,250		4,000
19 through 30 y	580	580	700	700		4,000
31 through 50 y	580	580	700	700		4,000
51 through 70 y	580	580	700	700		4,000
> 70 y	580	580	700	700		3,000
Pregnancy						
≤ 18 y		1,055		1,250		3,500
19 through 50 y		580		700		3,500
Lactation						
≤ 18 y		1,055		1,250		4,000
19 through 50 y		580		700		4,000

[a] **EAR** = Estimated Average Requirement.
[b] **RDA** = Recommended Dietary Allowance.
[c] **AI** = Adequate Intake.
[d] **UL** = Tolerable Upper Intake Level. Unless otherwise specified, the UL represents total intake from food, water, and supplements.
[e] **ND** = Not determinable. This value is not determinable due to the lack of data of adverse effects in this age group and concern regarding the lack of ability to handle excess amounts. Source of intake should only be from food to prevent high levels of intake.

PHOSPHORUS

The element phosphorus is found in nature (e.g., foods, water, and living tissues) primarily as phosphate (PO_4). It is a major component of bones and teeth. In fact, 85 percent of total body phosphorus is found in bone. Phosphorus helps maintain a normal pH in the body and is involved in metabolic processes.

The adult requirements for phosphorus are based on studies of serum inorganic phosphate concentration in adults. The Tolerable Upper Intake Level (UL) was derived using data on the normal adult range for serum inorganic phosphate concentration. DRI values are listed by life stage group in Table 1.

Nearly all foods contain phosphorus, and it is also common in food additives. Phosphorus deficiency is generally not a problem; the average adult diet contains about 62 mg phosphorus per 100 kcal. Excess phosphorus intake is expressed as hyperphosphatemia, and essentially all adverse effects of phosphorus excess are due to the elevated inorganic phosphorus in the extracellular fluid (ECF).

PHOSPHORUS AND THE BODY

Function

Phosphorus is a major component of bones and teeth. Its main functions are to maintain a normal pH (by buffering excesses of acid or alkali), temporarily store and transfer energy derived from metabolic fuels, and activate catalytic proteins via phosphorylation. Structurally, phosphorus occurs in the body as phospholipids (a major component of biological membranes) and as nucleotides and nucleic acids. Dietary phosphorus supports tissue growth and replaces phosphorus stores that are lost through excretion and the shedding of skin cells.

Absorption, Metabolism, Storage, and Excretion

Phosphorus found in foods is a mixture of organic and inorganic forms, and most phosphorus absorption occurs as inorganic phosphate. Approximately 55–70 percent of dietary phosphorus is absorbed in adults and about 65–90 percent in infants and children. The majority of phosphorus absorption occurs through passive concentration-dependent processes.

The amount of phosphorus ingested does not appear to affect absorption efficiency, which suggests that this efficiency does not improve with low intakes (unlike calcium absorption). By the same token, when serum phosphorus is abnormally high, even dangerously so, phosphorus continues to be absorbed from the diet at a rate only slightly lower than normal. Phosphorus absorption is reduced by aluminum-containing antacids and pharmacological doses of calcium carbonate. However, when consumed at intakes in the typical adult range, calcium does not significantly interfere with phosphorus absorption.

In adults, 85 percent of phosphorus is found in bone, with the remaining 15 percent distributed through the soft tissues. Excretion is achieved mainly through the kidneys. In healthy adults, the amount of phosphorus excreted in the urine is essentially equal to the amount absorbed through diet, less small amounts lost in the shedding of skin cells and intestinal mucosa.

DETERMINING DRIS

Determining Requirements

The adult requirements for phosphorus are based on studies of serum inorganic phosphate concentration. The EAR, and hence the RDA, for healthy adolescents aged 9 through 18 years is based on a factorial approach and is higher than the adult value. This is because this age range brackets a period of intense growth, with growth rate, absorption efficiency, and normal values of inorganic phosphorus in the extracellular fluid changing during this time.

Criteria for Determining Phosphorus Requirements, by Life Stage Group

Life stage group	Criterion
0 through 12 mo	Human milk content
1 through 18 y	Factorial approach
19 through 50 y	Serum P_i (serum inorganic phosphate concentration)
51 through > 70 y	Extrapolation of serum P_i from 19 through 50 years
Pregnancy	
≤ 18 y	Factorial approach
19 through 50 y	Serum P_i
Lactation	
≤ 18 y	Factorial approach
19 through 50 y	Serum P_i

The UL

The Tolerable Upper Intake Level (UL) is the highest level of daily nutrient intake that is likely to pose no risk of adverse effects for almost all people. Members of the general population should not routinely exceed the UL. The UL value for phosphorus was derived using data on the normal adult range for serum inorganic phosphate concentration and represents total intake from food, water, and supplements.

Phosphorus exposure data, based on data from the Continuing Survey of Food Intakes by Individuals (CSFII, 1994–1996) and the 1986 National Health Interview Survey (NHIS), indicated that only a small percentage of the population was likely to routinely exceed the UL for phosphorus; however, because food composition data do not always indicate phosphorus from food additives, the full extent of phosphorus intake is not known.

DIETARY SOURCES

Foods

Phosphorus is found naturally in many foods in the form of phosphate (PO_4) and as a food additive in the form of various phosphate salts, which are used for nonnutrient functions during food processing, such as moisture retention, smoothness, and binding.

According to data from the National Health Survey (1976–1980), the phosphorus content of the average adult diet for both men and women is about 62 mg/100 kcal. Dietary intake of phosphorus appears to be affected more by total food intake and less by differences in food composition. People with a high intake of dairy products will have diets with higher phosphorus density values because the phosphorus density of cow milk is higher than for most other foods. People who consume several servings per day of colas or a few other soft drinks that contain phosphoric acid also tend to have high phosphorus intake. A 12-ounce serving of such beverages contains about 50 mg, which is only 5 percent of the typical intake by an adult woman. However, when consumed in a quantity of 5 or more servings per day, such beverages may contribute substantially to total phosphate intake.

Dietary Supplements

Phosphorus supplements are not widely used in the United States. Based on the 1986 NHIS study, about 10 percent of adults and 6 percent of children aged 2 to 6 years took supplements containing phosphorus. Supplement usage and dosage was similar for men and women, with a median intake from supplements of 120 mg/day.

Bioavailability

Most foods exhibit good phosphorus bioavailability. However, foods derived from plant seeds (e.g., beans, peas, cereals, and nuts) contain phytic acid (also called phytate), a stored form of phosphorus that is not directly available to humans. Absorption of this form requires the presence of phytase, an enzyme found in some foods and in some colonic bacteria. Because yeasts can hydrolyze phytate, whole grains that are incorporated into leavened bread products have higher phosphorus bioavailability than do grains used in unleavened bread or breakfast cereals. Also, unabsorbed calcium in the digestive tract combines with phytic acid and interferes with its digestion and absorption. This may partly explain why calcium interferes with phosphorus absorption.

In infants, phosphorus bioavailability is highest from human milk (85–90 percent), intermediate from cow milk (72 percent), and lowest from soy formulas, which contain phytic acid (59 percent). However, the higher amounts of phosphorus contained in cow milk and soy formulas offset this decreased bioavailability.

Dietary Interactions

There is evidence that phosphorus may interact with certain nutrients and dietary substances (see Table 2).

INADEQUATE INTAKE AND DEFICIENCY

Phosphorus deficiency is generally not a problem. This is because phosphorus is so ubiquitous in the diet that near total starvation is required to produce dietary phosphorus deficiency. However, if inadequate phosphorus intake does occur, such as in individuals recovering from alcoholic bouts, from diabetic ketoacidosis, and from refeeding with calorie-rich sources without paying attention to phosphorus needs, it is realized as hypophosphatemia. The effects of hypophosphatemia include the following:

- Anorexia
- Anemia
- Muscle weakness
- Bone pain
- Rickets (in children) and osteomalacia (in adults)
- General debility

TABLE 2 Potential Interactions with Other Dietary Substances

Substance	Potential Interaction	Notes
SUBSTANCES THAT AFFECT PHOSPHORUS		
Calcium	Pharmacological doses of calcium carbonate may interfere with phosphorus absorption.	Calcium in the normal adult intake range is not likely to pose a problem for phosphorus absorption.
Aluminum	When taken in large doses, antacids that contain aluminum may interfere with phosphorus absorption.	
PHOSPHORUS AFFECTING OTHER SUBSTANCES		
Calcium	Excess intake of phosphorus may interfere with calcium absorption.	This is less likely to pose a problem if calcium intake is adequate.

- Increased susceptibility to infection
- Paresthesias
- Ataxia
- Confusion
- Possible death

Special Considerations

Antacids: Antacids that contain aluminum can bind with dietary phosphorus and, when consumed in large doses, produce hypophosphatemia.

Treating malnutrition: The refeeding of energy-depleted individuals, either orally or parenterally, must supply adequate inorganic phosphate. Otherwise, severe and perhaps fatal hypophosphatemia may occur.

EXCESS INTAKE

Excess phosphorus intake from any source can result in hyperphosphatemia, the adverse effects of which are due to an elevated concentration of inorganic phosphate in the extracellular fluid. Hyperphosphatemia from dietary causes becomes a problem mainly in individuals with end-stage renal disease or in such conditions as vitamin D intoxication. The potential effects of hyperphosphatemia include the following:

- Reduced calcium absorption (less problematic with adequate calcium intake)
- Calcification of nonskeletal tissues, particularly the kidneys

Concern about high phosphorus intake has been raised because of a probable population-level increase in phosphorus intake through colas and a few other soft drinks that contain phosphoric acid and processed foods containing phosphate additives. High intakes of polyphosphates found in additives may interfere with the absorption of iron, copper, and zinc. However, further research is necessary in this area.

KEY POINTS FOR PHOSPHORUS

✓   The element phosphorus is found in nature primarily as phosphate (PO_4). It is a major component of bones and teeth. In fact, 85 percent of total body phosphorus is found in bone.

✓   Phosphorus helps maintain a normal pH in the body and is involved in metabolic processes. Dietary phosphorus supports tissue growth and replaces phosphorus stores that are lost through excretion and the shedding of skin cells.

✓   The adult requirements for phosphorus are based on studies of serum inorganic phosphate concentration. The UL was derived using data on the normal adult range for serum inorganic phosphate concentration.

✓   Nearly all foods contain phosphorus; dairy products are a particularly rich source.

✓   Foods derived from plant seeds (e.g., beans, peas, cereals, and nuts) contain phytic acid (also called phytate), a stored form of phosphorus that is poorly absorbed in humans.

✓   Phosphorus deficiency is generally not a problem; the average adult diet contains about 62 mg phosphorus per 100 kcal.

✓   Excess phosphorus intake from any source can result in hyperphosphatemia, the adverse effects of which are due to an elevated concentration of inorganic phosphate in the extracellular fluid. Hyperphosphatemia from dietary causes becomes a problem mainly in individuals with end-stage renal disease or in such conditions as vitamin D intoxication.

✓   There is concern about the population-level increase in phosphorus intake through colas and a few other soft drinks that contain phosphoric acid and processed foods containing phosphates. High intakes of polyphosphates found in additives may interfere with the absorption of iron, copper, and zinc. However, further research is necessary in this area.

TABLE 1 Dietary Reference Intakes for Potassium by Life Stage Group

	DRI values (g/day)	
	AI[a]	UL[b]
Life stage group[c]		
0 through 6 mo	0.4	
7 through 12 mo	0.7	
1 through 3 y	3.0	
4 through 8 y	3.8	
9 through 13 y	4.5	
14 through 18 y	4.7	
19 through 30 y	4.7	
31 through 50 y	4.7	
51 through 70 y	4.7	
> 70 y	4.7	
Pregnancy		
≤18 y	4.7	
19 through 50 y	4.7	
Lactation		
≤18 y	5.1	
19 through 50 y	5.1	

[a] **AI** = Adequate Intake.

[b] **UL** = Tolerable Upper Intake Level. Data were insufficient to set a UL. In the absence of a UL, extra caution may be warranted in consuming levels above the recommended intake.

[c] All groups except Pregnancy and Lactation represent males and females.

POTASSIUM

The mineral potassium is the main intracellular cation in the body and is required for normal cellular function. The ratio of extracellular to intracellular potassium affects nerve transmission, muscle contraction, and vascular tone.

Since data were inadequate to determine an Estimated Average Requirement (EAR) and thus calculate a Recommended Dietary Allowance (RDA) for potassium, an Average Intake (AI) was instead developed. The AIs for potassium are based on a level of dietary intake that should maintain lower blood pressure levels, reduce the adverse effects of sodium chloride intake on blood pressure, reduce the risk of recurrent kidney stones, and possibly decrease bone loss. In healthy people, excess potassium above the AI is readily excreted in the urine; therefore a UL was not set. DRI values are listed by life stage group in Table 1.

Fruits and vegetables, particularly leafy greens, vine fruit, and root vegetables, are good food sources of potassium. Although uncommon in the general population, the main effect of severe potassium deficiency is hypokalemia. Hypokalemia can cause cardiac arrhythmias, muscle weakness, and glucose intolerance. Moderate potassium deficiency, which typically occurs without hypokalemia, is characterized by elevated blood pressure, increased salt sensitivity, an increased risk of kidney stones, and increased bone turnover. An inadequate intake of potassium may also increase the risk of cardiovascular disease, particularly stroke.

There is no evidence that a high intake of potassium from foods has adverse effects in healthy people. However, for individuals whose urinary excretion of potassium is impaired, a potassium intake below the AI is appropriate because adverse cardiac effects (arrhythmias) can occur as a result of hyperkalemia (markedly elevated serum potassium concentration). Such individuals are typically under medical supervision.

POTASSIUM AND THE BODY

Function

Potassium is the major intracellular cation in the body. Although the mineral is found in both the intracellular and the extracellular fluids, it is more concentrated in the intracellular fluid (about 145 mmol/L). Even small changes in the concentration of extracellular potassium can greatly affect the ratio between extracellular and intracellular potassium. This, in turn, affects neural transmission, muscle contraction, and vascular tone.

Absorption, Metabolism, Storage, and Excretion

In unprocessed foods, potassium occurs mainly in association with bicarbonate-generating precursors like citrate and, to a lesser extent, phosphate. When potassium is added to foods during processing or to supplements, it is in the form of potassium chloride.

Healthy people absorb about 85 percent of the dietary potassium that they consume. The high intracellular concentration of potassium is maintained by the sodium-potassium-ATPase pump. Because insulin stimulates this pump, changes in the plasma insulin concentration can affect extracellular potassium concentration and thus plasma concentration of potassium.

About 77–90 percent of dietary potassium is excreted in the urine. This is because, in a steady state, the correlation between dietary potassium intake and urinary potassium content is high. The rest is excreted mainly in the feces, and much smaller amounts are lost through sweat.

DETERMINING DRIS

Determining Requirements

In unprocessed foods, the conjugate anions of potassium are organic anions, such as citrate, which are converted in the body to bicarbonate. Bicarbonate acts as a buffer, neutralizing diet-derived acids such as sulfuric acid generated from sulfur-containing amino acids found in meats and other high-protein foods. When the intake of bicarbonate precursors is inadequate, buffers in the bone matrix neutralize excess diet-derived acids. Bone becomes demineralized in the process. The resulting adverse consequences are increased bone turnover and calcium-containing kidney stones. In processed foods to which potassium has been added, and in supplements, the conjugate anion is typically chloride, which does not act as a buffer.

Because the demonstrated effects of potassium often depend on the accompanying anion and because it is difficult to separate the effects of potassium from the effects of its accompanying anion, this publication focuses on nonchloride forms of potassium naturally found in fruits, vegetables, and other potassium-rich foods.

Since data were inadequate to determine an EAR and thus calculate an RDA for potassium, an AI was instead developed. The AIs for potassium are based on a level of dietary intake that should maintain lower blood pressure levels, reduce the adverse effects of sodium chloride intake on blood pressure, reduce the risk of recurrent kidney stones, and possibly decrease bone loss.

Special Considerations

African Americans: Because African Americans have lower intakes of potassium and a higher prevalence of elevated blood pressure and salt sensitivity, this population subgroup would especially benefit from an increased intake of potassium. (In general terms, salt sensitivity is expressed as either the reduction in blood pressure in response to a lower salt intake or the rise in blood pressure in response to sodium loading.)

Individuals with certain conditions: Individuals with Type I diabetes and individuals taking cyclo-oxygenase-2 (COX-2) inhibitors or other nonsteroidal anti-inflammatory (NSAID) drugs should consume levels of potassium recommended by their health care professional. These levels may well be lower than the AI.

Impaired urinary potassium excretion: Common drugs that can substantially impair potassium excretion are angiotensin converting enzyme (ACE) inhibitors, angiotensin receptor blockers (ARB), and potassium-sparing diuretics. Medical conditions associated with impaired urinary potassium excretion include diabetes, chronic renal insufficiency, end-stage renal disease, severe heart failure, and adrenal insufficiency. Elderly individuals are at an increased risk of hyperkalemia because they often have one or more of these conditions or are treated with one of these medications.

Because arrhythmias due to hyperkalemia can be life-threatening, the AI does not apply to people with the above medical conditions or to those taking drugs that impair potassium excretion. In such cases, a potassium intake below the AI is often appropriate. In addition, salt substitutes containing potassium chloride should be cautiously used by these individuals, for whom medical supervision is also advised.

Criteria for Determining Potassium Requirements, by Life Stage Group

Life Stage Group	Criterion
0 through 6 months	Average consumption from human milk
7 through 12 months	Average consumption from human milk + complementary foods
1 through 18 y	Extrapolation of adult AI based on energy intake
19 through 70 y	Intake level to lower blood pressure, reduce the extent of salt sensitivity, and minimize the risk of kidney stones in adults

Pregnancy

≤ 18 through 50 y   Age-specific value

Lactation

≤ 18 through 50 y   Age-specific values + average amount of potassium estimated in breast milk during the first 6 months (0.4 g/day)

The UL

The Tolerable Upper Intake Level (UL) is the highest level of daily nutrient intake that is likely to pose no risk of adverse effects for almost all people. In otherwise healthy individuals (i.e., individuals without impaired urinary potassium excretion due to a medical condition or drug therapy), there is no evidence that a high level of potassium from foods has adverse effects. Therefore, a UL for potassium from foods has not been set. However, supplemental potassium can lead to acute toxicity, as well as adverse effects due to chronic consumption (see "Excess Intake"). Although no UL for potassium was set, potassium supplements should only be provided under medical supervision.

SOURCES OF POTASSIUM

Foods

Fruits and vegetables, particularly leafy greens, vine fruit (such as tomatoes, cucumbers, zucchini, eggplant, and pumpkin), and root vegetables, are good sources of potassium and bicarbonate precursors. Although meat, milk, and cereal products contain potassium, they do not contain enough bicarbonate precursors to adequately balance their acid-forming precursors, such as sulfur-containing amino acids. Nutrient tables of the citrate and bicarbonate content of foods are lacking, making it difficult to estimate the amount consumed of these other food components.

Dietary Supplements

The maximum amount of potassium found in over-the-counter, multivitamin-mineral supplements is generally less than 100 mg.

Bioavailability

This information was not provided at the time the DRI values for this nutrient were set.

TABLE 2 Potential Interactions with Other Dietary Substances

Substance	Potential Interaction	Notes
POTASSIUM AFFECTING OTHER SUBSTANCES		
Sodium chloride	Potassium bicarbonate mitigates the pressor effect of sodium chloride. Dietary potassium increases the urinary excretion of sodium chloride.	Supplemental potassium bicarbonate mitigates the effects of dietary sodium chloride. The effects seem to be more prominent in African Americans, who have a higher prevalence of hypertension and of salt sensitivity and a lower intake of potassium than non-African Americans.
Sodium: potassium ratio	The sodium:potassium ratio is typically more closely associated with blood pressure than with the intake of either substance alone. The incidence of kidney stones has been shown to increase with an increased sodium:potassium ratio.	Although blood pressure is inversely associated with potassium intake and directly associated with sodium intake and the sodium:potassium ratio, the ratio typically is more influential. Given the interrelatedness of sodium and potassium, the requirement for potassium may depend on dietary sodium intake. However, currently there are not enough data on which to make recommendations.

Dietary Interactions

There is evidence that potassium may interact with certain other nutrients and dietary substances (see Table 2).

INADEQUATE INTAKE AND DEFICIENCY

The adverse effects of inadequate potassium intake can result from a deficiency of potassium per se, a deficiency of the anion that accompanies it (e.g., citrate), or both. Severe potassium deficiency is characterized by hypokalemia, a condition marked by a serum potassium concentration of less than 3.5 mmol/L. The adverse consequences of hypokalemia include cardiac arrhythmias, muscle weakness, and glucose intolerance. Moderate potassium deficiency, which typically occurs without hypokalemia, is characterized by increased blood pressure, increased salt sensitivity, an increased risk of kidney stones, increased bone turnover, and a possible increased risk of cardiovascular disease, particularly stroke.

Processed foods and unprocessed foods differ in their composition of conjugate anions, which in turn, can affect bone mineralization. In unprocessed foods, the conjugate anions of potassium are mainly organic anions, such as citrate, which are converted in the body to bicarbonate. Consequently, an inadequate intake of potassium is also associated with a reduced intake of bicarbonate precursors. Bicarbonate acts as a buffer, neutralizing diet-derived noncarbonic acids such as sulfuric acid generated from sulfur-containing amino acids found in meats and other high-protein foods. If the intake of bicarbonate precursors is inadequate, buffers in the bone matrix neutralize the excess diet-derived acids. Bone becomes demineralized in the process. In processed foods to which potassium has been added, and in supplements, the conjugate anion is typically chloride, which does not act as a buffer.

Excess diet-derived acid titrates bone, leading to increased urinary calcium and reduced urinary citrate excretion. The possible adverse consequences are increased bone demineralization and an increased risk of calcium-containing kidney stones.

Special Considerations

Climate and physical activity: Heat exposure and exercise can increase potassium loss, primarily through sweat, thereby increasing potassium requirements.

Diuretics: Often used to treat hypertension and congestive heart failure, thiazide-type diuretics increase urinary potassium excretion and can lead to hypokalemia. For this reason, potassium supplements are often prescribed. Potassium-sparing diuretics prevent diuretic-induced potassium loss and are often concurrently used with thiazide-type diuretics. Individuals who take diuretics should have their serum potassium levels regularly checked by their health care providers.

Very low-carbohydrate, high-protein diets: Low-grade metabolic acidosis occurs with the consumption of very low-carbohydrate, high-protein diets to promote and maintain weight loss. These diets, which may be adequate in potassium due to their high protein content, are inadequate as a source of alkali because fruits are often excluded from them.

EXCESS INTAKE

For healthy individuals, there is no evidence that a high level of potassium intake from foods can have adverse effects. However, potassium supplements can cause acute toxicity in healthy people. Chronic consumption of high levels of supplemental potassium can lead to hyperkalemia (markedly elevated serum potassium) in people with an impaired ability to excrete potassium. The most serious potential effect of hyperkalemia is cardiac arrhythmia.

Gastrointestinal discomfort has been reported with some forms of potassium supplements. The specific product or vehicle in which the potassium supplement is provided is the critical determinant of the risk of gastrointestinal side effects.

Special Considerations

Problem pregnancy: High levels of potassium should be consumed with care by pregnant women with preeclampsia. The hormone progesterone, which is elevated during pregnancy, may make women with undetected kidney problems or decreased glomerular filtration rate (a side effect of preeclampsia) more likely to develop hyperkalemia when potassium intake is high.

KEY POINTS FOR POTASSIUM

✓ Potassium is the main intracellular cation in the body and is required for normal cellular function. The ratio of extracellular to intracellular potassium levels affects neural transmission, muscle contraction, and vascular tone.

✓ The AIs for potassium are based on a level of dietary intake that should maintain lower blood pressure levels, reduce the adverse effects of sodium chloride intake on blood pressure, reduce the risk of recurrent kidney stones, and possibly decrease bone loss.

✓ Since data were inadequate to determine an EAR and thus calculate an RDA for potassium, an AI was instead developed.

✓ Individuals with Type I diabetes; individuals with chronic renal insufficiency, who may certain medications; and individuals taking cyclo-oxygenase-2 (COX-2) inhibitors or other nonsteroidal anti-inflammatory (NSAID) drugs should consume levels of potassium recommended by their health care professional. These levels may well be lower than the AI.

✓ Because African Americans have lower intakes of potassium and a higher prevalence of elevated blood pressure and salt sensitivity, this population subgroup would especially benefit from an increased intake of potassium.

✓ In healthy individuals, excess potassium above the AI is readily excreted in the urine; therefore, a UL was not set.

✓ Good food sources of potassium include fruits and vegetables, particularly leafy greens, vine fruit, and root vegetables.

✓ Although uncommon in the general population, the main effect of severe potassium deficiency is hypokalemia, which can cause cardiac arrhythmias, muscle weakness, and glucose intolerance.

✓ Moderate potassium deficiency, which typically occurs without hypokalemia, is characterized by elevated blood pressure, increased salt sensitivity, an increased risk of kidney stones, and increased bone turnover.

✓   Chronic consumption of high levels of potassium can lead to hyperkalemia in people with an impaired ability to excrete potassium, The most serious potential effect of hyperkalemia is cardiac arrhythmia.

✓   Elderly individuals are often at increased risk of hyperkalemia.

TABLE 1 Dietary Reference Intakes for Selenium by Life Stage Group

	DRI values (µg/day)			
	EAR[a]	RDA[b]	AI[c]	UL[d]
Life stage group[e]				
0 through 6 mo			15	45
7 through 12 mo			20	60
1 through 3 y	17	20		90
4 through 8 y	23	30		150
9 through 13 y	35	40		280
14 through 18 y	45	55		400
19 through 30 y	45	55		400
31 through 50 y	45	55		400
51 through 70 y	45	55		400
> 70 y	45	55		400
Pregnancy				
≤ 18 y	49	60		400
19 through 50 y	49	60		400
Lactation				
≤ 18 y	59	70		400
19 through 50 y	59	70		400

[a] **EAR** = Estimated Average Requirement.
[b] **RDA** = Recommended Dietary Allowance.
[c] **AI** = Adequate Intake.
[d] **UL** = Tolerable Upper Intake Level. Unless otherwise specified, the UL represents total intake from food, water, and supplements.
[e] All groups except Pregnancy and Lactation represent males and females.

SELENIUM

Selenium is an antioxidant nutrient involved in the defense against oxidative stress. Selenoproteins regulate thyroid hormone actions and the redox status of vitamin C and other molecules. Most selenium found in animal tissue is in the form of selenomethionine (the major dietary form of selenium) or selenocysteine, both of which are well absorbed.

The method used to estimate the requirements for selenium relates to the intake needed to maximize the activity of the plasma selenoprotein glutathione peroxidase, an oxidant defense enzyme. The Tolerable Upper Intake Level (UL) is based on the adverse effect of selenosis, and pertains to intakes from food and supplements. Although some studies indicate a potential anticancer effect of selenium, the data were inadequate to set dietary selenium requirements based on this potential effect. DRI values are listed by life stage group in Table 1.

Food sources of selenium include meat, seafood, grains, dairy products, fruits, and vegetables, and the major dietary forms of selenium appear to be highly bioavailable. However, the selenium content of foods greatly varies depending on the selenium content of the soil where the animal was raised or where the plant was grown. Neither selenium deficiency nor toxicity appears to be common in U.S. and Canadian populations.

SELENIUM AND THE BODY

Function

Selenium functions through selenoproteins, several of which defend against oxidative stress; and as such, it plays a role as a dietary antioxidant. Although the function of all selenoproteins has not yet been characterized, selenium has been found to regulate both thyroid hormone actions and the redox status of vitamin C and other molecules.

Absorption, Metabolism, Storage, and Excretion

Most dietary selenium is in the form of selenomethionine (the major dietary form of selenium) or selenocysteine, both of which are well absorbed. Other forms of selenium include selenate and selenite, which are not major dietary constituents, but are commonly used in fortified foods and dietary supplements. Two pools of reserve selenium are present in the body. The first is as selenomethionine, which is not known to have a physiological function separate from that of methionine. The second reserve pool is the selenium found in liver glutathione peroxidase.

Ingested selenite, selenate, and selenocysteine are all metabolized directly to selenide, the reduced form of selenium. Selenomethionine can also be metabolized to selenide. Selenide can be metabolized to a precursor of other reactions or be converted into an excretory metabolite. Selenium is excreted mainly through the urine. The breath may also contain volatile metabolites when large amounts of selenium are being excreted.

DETERMINING DRIS

Determining Requirements

The adult requirements for selenium are based on the criterion of maximizing plasma glutathione peroxidase activity, as assessed by plateau concentration of plasma selenoproteins. Although some studies indicate a potential anticancer effect of selenium, the data were inadequate to set dietary selenium requirements based on this potential effect. Further large-scale trials are necessary.

Criteria for Determining Selenium Requirements, by Life Stage Group

Life stage group	Criterion
0 through 6 mo	Human milk content
7 through 12 mo	Human milk + solid food
1 through 18 y	Extrapolation from adult
19 through 30 y	Maximizing plasma glutathione peroxidase activity
31 through >70 y	Extrapolation of plasma glutathione peroxidase activity from 19 through 30 y

Pregnancy	
≤ 18 y through 50 y	Age-specific requirement + saturation of fetal selenoprotein

Lactation	
≤ 18 y through 50 y	Age-specific requirement + human milk content requirement

The UL

The Tolerable Upper Intake Level (UL) is the highest level of daily nutrient intake that is likely to pose no risk of adverse effects for almost all people. Members of the general population should not routinely exceed the UL. The

UL for selenium is based on selenosis as the adverse effect and represents total intake from food, water, and supplements. The most frequently reported features of selenosis (chronic toxicity) are hair and nail brittleness and loss and thus were selected as the critical endpoints on which to base a UL.

The extensive food distribution systems in Canada and the U.S. ensure that individuals do not eat diets that originate solely from one locality. This moderates the selenium content of diets, even in high-selenium areas. The risk of selenium intake above the UL for U.S. and Canadian populations appears to be small, and there is no known seleniferous area in the United States and Canada with recognized cases of selenosis.

DIETARY SOURCES

Foods

Dietary sources of selenium include meat, seafood, cereals and grains, dairy products, and fruits and vegetables. (Drinking water does not supply nutritionally significant amounts of selenium.)

However, the selenium content of food can greatly vary depending on the selenium content of the soil where the animal was raised or where the plant was grown. Food animals in the United States and Canada usually have controlled diets to which selenium is added, and thus, the amounts found in muscle meats, milk, and eggs are more consistent than for plant-based foods.

Dietary intake of selenium in the United States and Canada varies by geographical origin, based on the selenium content of the soil and meat content of the diet. This variation is buffered by a large food-distribution system, in which the extensive transport of food throughout North America prevents decreased intakes in people living in low-selenium areas. Although the food distribution systems in the United States and Canada ensure a mix of plant- and animal-based foods originating from a broad range of soil selenium conditions, local foods (e.g., from farmers' markets) may considerably vary from the mean values in food composition databases.

The content of selenium in plants depends on the availability of the element in the soil where the plant was grown. Unlike plants, animals require selenium, and so meat and seafood are reliable dietary sources of selenium. Therefore, the lowest selenium intakes are in populations that eat vegetarian diets comprising plants grown in low-selenium areas.

Dietary Supplements

Selenium is widely available in a variety of supplements and multivitamin preparations. In the 1986 National Health Interview Survey (NHIS), 9 percent of all adults reported the use of supplements containing selenium.

Bioavailability

Most dietary selenium is highly bioavailable, although its bioavailability from fortified foods and supplements is lower than for naturally occurring dietary forms of selenium.

Dietary Interactions

This information was not provided at the time the DRI values for this nutrient were set.

INADEQUATE INTAKE AND DEFICIENCY

Selenium deficiency in otherwise well-nourished individuals is not likely to cause overt symptoms. However, selenium deficiency may lead to biochemical changes that can predispose a person to illness associated with other stresses, such as:

- Keshan disease, a cardiomyopathy found only in selenium-deficient children that appears to be triggered by an additional stress, possibly an infection or chemical exposure
- Kashin-Beck disease, an endemic disease of cartilage that occurs in preadolescence or adolescence, has been reported in some of the low-selenium areas of Asia, although the pathogenesis remains uncertain

EXCESS INTAKE

The limited data available on humans suggest that chronic toxicities from inorganic and organic forms of selenium have similar clinical features, but differ in the rapidity of onset and the relationship to tissue selenium concentrations. Inorganic selenium can cause toxicity at tissue levels of selenium that are much lower than those seen with similar intakes of dietary selenium as selenomethionine. The signs and symptoms of chronic selenosis, or selenium toxicity, are the following:

- Hair and nail brittleness and loss (most frequently reported symptoms)
- Gastrointestinal disturbances

- Skin rash
- Garlic breath odor
- Fatigue
- Irritability
- Nervous system abnormalities

Special Considerations

Soil variations: There are high-selenium regions in the United States, such as western South Dakota and eastern Wyoming, but the U.S. Department of Agriculture has identified them and proscribed their use for raising animals for food. No evidence of selenosis has been found in these areas of high selenium content, even in the subjects consuming the most selenium.

KEY POINTS FOR SELENIUM

✓ Selenium functions through selenoproteins, several of which defend against oxidative stress and as such, plays a role as a dietary antioxidant.

✓ The requirements for selenium are based on the criterion of maximizing plasma glutathione peroxidase activity. The UL is based on the critical endpoints of hair and nail brittleness and loss.

✓ Although some studies indicate a potential anticancer effect of selenium, the data were inadequate to set dietary selenium requirements based on this potential effect.

✓ Food sources of selenium include meat, seafood, cereals and grains, dairy products, and fruits and vegetables.

✓ The lowest selenium intakes are in populations that eat vegetarian diets comprising plants grown in low-selenium geographic areas.

✓ The selenium content of foods can greatly vary depending on the selenium content of the soil where the animal was raised or where the plant was grown.

✓ Selenium deficiency in otherwise well-nourished individuals is not likely to cause overt symptoms.

✓ The limited data available on humans suggest that chronic toxicities from inorganic and organic forms of selenium have similar clinical features but differ in rapidity of onset and relationship to tissue selenium concentrations.

TABLE 1 Dietary Reference Intakes for Sodium and Chloride by Life Stage Group

| | DRI values (g/day) | | | |
| | Sodium | | Chloride | |
	AI[a]	UL[b]	AI	UL
Life stage group[c]				
0 through 6 mo	0.12	ND[d]	0.18	ND
7 through 12 mo	0.37	ND	0.57	ND
1 through 3 y	1.0	1.5	1.5	2.3
4 through 8 y	1.2	1.9	1.9	2.9
9 through 13 y	1.5	2.2	2.3	3.4
14 through 18 y	1.5	2.3	2.3	3.6
19 through 30 y	1.5	2.3	2.3	3.6
31 through 50 y	1.5	2.3	2.3	3.6
51 through 70 y	1.3	2.3	2.0	3.6
> 70 y	1.2	2.3	1.8	3.6
Pregnancy				
≤18 y	1.5	2.3	2.3	3.6
19 through 50 y	1.5	2.3	2.3	3.6
Lactation				
≤18 y	1.5	2.3	2.3	3.6
19 through 50 y	1.5	2.3	2.3	3.6

[a] **AI** = Adequate Intake.

[b] **UL** = Tolerable Upper Intake Level. Unless otherwise specified, the UL represents total intake from food, water, and supplements.

[c] All groups except Pregnancy and Lactation represent males and females.

[d] **ND** = Not determinable. This value is not determinable due to the lack of data of adverse effects in this age group and concern regarding the lack of ability to handle excess amounts. Source of intake should only be from food to prevent high levels of intake.

SODIUM AND CHLORIDE

S odium and chloride are necessary to maintain extracellular fluid volume and plasma osmolality. The cation sodium and the anion chloride are normally found in most foods together as sodium chloride (salt). For this reason, this publication presents data on the requirements for and the effects of sodium and chloride together.

Since data were inadequate to determine Estimated Average Requirements (EARs) and thus calculate Recommended Dietary Allowances (RDAs) for sodium and chloride, Adequate Intakes (AIs) were instead developed. The AIs for sodium are set at an intake that ensures that the overall diet provides an adequate intake of other important nutrients and covers sodium sweat losses in unacclimated individuals who are exposed to high temperatures or who become physically active. The AIs for chloride are set at a level equivalent on a molar basis to that of sodium, since almost all dietary chloride comes with sodium added during the processing or consumption of foods. The AIs for sodium do not apply to individuals who lose large volumes of sodium in sweat, such as competitive athletes and workers exposed to extreme heat stress (e.g., foundry workers and firefighters).

The adverse effects of higher levels of sodium intake on blood pressure provide the scientific rationale for setting the Tolerable Upper Intake Level (UL) for sodium and chloride. DRI values are listed by life stage group in Table 1.

In the United States, sodium chloride accounts for about 90 percent of total sodium intake in the United States. Most of the sodium chloride found in the typical diet is added to food during processing. Examples of high-sodium processed foods include luncheon meats and hot dogs, canned vegetables, processed cheese, potato chips, Worcestershire sauce, and soy sauce.

Overall, there is little evidence of any adverse effect of low dietary sodium intake on serum or plasma sodium concentrations in healthy people. Likewise, chloride deficiency is rarely seen because most foods that contain sodium also provide chloride. The primary adverse effect related to increased sodium chloride intake is elevated blood pressure, which is directly related to cardiovascular disease and end-stage renal disease. Individuals with hypertension, diabetes, and chronic kidney disease, as well as African Americans and older people, tend to be more sensitive than others to the blood pressure–raising effect of sodium chloride intake.

SODIUM AND CHLORIDE AND THE BODY

Function

About 95 percent of the body's sodium content is found in the extracellular fluid, where it serves as the primary cation. Sodium regulates extracellular fluid volume and plasma volume and also plays an important role in the membrane potential of cells (the electrical potential difference across a cell's plasma membrane) and the active transport of molecules across cell membranes.

Chloride, in association with sodium, is the primary osmotically active anion in the extracellular fluid. It plays a key role in maintaining fluid and electrolyte balance. In addition, chloride, in the form of hydrochloric acid, is an important component of gastric juice.

Absorption, Metabolism, Storage, and Excretion

Sodium and chloride ions are typically consumed as sodium chloride. About 98 percent of ingested sodium chloride is absorbed, mainly in the small intestine. Absorbed sodium and chloride remain in the extracellular compartments, which include the plasma, interstitial fluid, and plasma water. As long as sweating is not excessive, most of this sodium chloride is excreted in the urine. In people with "steady-state" sodium and fluid balance, and minimal sweat loss, the amount of sodium excreted in urine is roughly equal to the amount consumed, when other obligatory sodium losses are small.

A number of systems and hormones influence sodium and chloride balance, some of which are shown in Table 2.

DETERMINING DRIS

Determining Requirements

Since data were inadequate to determine EARs and thus calculate RDAs for sodium and chloride, AIs were instead developed. The AIs for sodium are set at an intake that ensures that the overall diet provides an adequate intake of other important nutrients and also covers sodium sweat losses in unacclimated individuals who are exposed to high temperatures or who become physically active (as recommended in Part II, "Physical Activity"). The AIs for chloride are set at a level equivalent on a molar basis to that of sodium, since almost all dietary chloride comes with the sodium added during processing or consumption of foods.

Concerns have been raised that a low level of sodium intake adversely affects blood lipids, insulin resistance, and cardiovascular disease risk. However, at the level of the AI, the preponderance of evidence does not support this

TABLE 2 Major Systems and Hormones That Influence Sodium Chloride Balance

System or Hormones	Activators	Effect
Renin-angiotensin-aldosterone axis	• Reduced salt intake • Reduced blood volume • Reduced blood pressure[a]	• Promotes retention of sodium and chloride by the kidneys • Promotes renal reabsorption of sodium
Atrial natriuretic peptide (counter-regulatory system to renin-angiotensin-aldosterone axis)	• Elevated blood volume • Increased salt intake • Increased blood pressure	• Increases glomerular filtration rate • Reduces blood volume • Reduces blood pressure • Increases sodium excretion
Sympathetic nervous system	• Reduced salt intake • Reduced blood volume • Reduced blood pressure	• Reduces sodium reabsorption • Reduces water reabsorption in the kidneys

[a] When the renin-angiotensin-aldosterone system is less responsive, as with advanced age, a greater decrease in blood pressure results from reduced sodium chloride intake.

contention. A potential indicator of an adverse effect of inadequate sodium is an increase in plasma renin activity. However, in contrast to the well-accepted benefits of blood pressure reduction, the clinical relevance of modest rises in plasma renin activity as a result of sodium reduction is uncertain.

It is well recognized that the current intake of sodium for most individuals in the United States and Canada greatly exceeds both the AI and the UL. Progress in achieving a reduced sodium intake will likely be gradual, requiring changes in personal behavior toward salt consumption, which includes the replacement of high sodium foods with lower sodium alternatives, as well as increased collaboration between the food industry and public health officials. Also required will be a broad spectrum of additional research that includes the development of reduced sodium foods that maintain flavor, texture, consumer acceptability, and low cost.

Special Considerations

Excessive sweat loss: The AI for sodium does not apply to individuals who lose large volumes of sodium in sweat, such as competitive athletes and workers exposed to extreme heat stress (e.g., foundry workers and firefighters).

Criteria for Determining Sodium and Chloride Requirements, by Life Stage Group

Life stage group	Criterion
0 through 6 months	Average consumption of sodium from human milk
7 through 12 months	Average consumption of sodium from human milk + complementary foods
1 through 18 y	Extrapolation of adult AI based on median energy intake level from CSFII
19 though 50 y	Intake level to cover possible daily losses, provide adequate intakes of other nutrients, and maintain normal function
> 50 y	Extrapolation from younger adults based on median energy intake level from CSFII

Pregnancy

≤ 18 through 50 y	Age-specific AI

Lactation

≤ 18 through 50 y	Age-specific AI

The UL

The Tolerable Upper Intake Level (UL) is the highest level of daily nutrient intake that is likely to pose no risk of adverse effects for almost all people. Members of the general population should not routinely exceed the UL. The major adverse effect of increased sodium chloride intake is elevated blood pressure. High blood pressure has been shown to be a risk factor for heart disease, stroke, and kidney disease.

The scientific rationale for setting the UL is based on the impact of sodium on blood pressure and represents total intake from food, water, and supplements. However, because the relationship between sodium intake and blood pressure is progressive and continuous without an apparent threshold, it is difficult to precisely set a UL, especially since other environmental factors (weight, exercise, potassium intake, dietary pattern, and alcohol intake) and genetic factors also affect blood pressure. There was inadequate evidence to support a different upper level of sodium intake in pregnant women from that of nonpregnant women as a means to prevent hypertensive disorders of pregnancy.

Data from the Third National Health and Nutrition Examination Survey (NHANES III, 1988–1994) indicated that more than 95 percent of men and 75 percent of women in the United States consumed sodium chloride in excess of the UL. According to NHANES III, 24.7 percent of men and 24.3 percent of women aged 18 years and older had hypertension, indicating that a substantial number of individuals appear to experience this adverse effect.

Data on Canadian consumption indicated that 90–95 percent of younger men (aged 19 to 50 years) and between 50 and 75 percent of younger women in the same age range had usual intakes above the UL. Neither of these surveys included discretionary salt usage (e.g., from the salt shaker).

Special Considerations:

Sensitive individuals: The UL may be even lower for people whose blood pressure is most sensitive to increased sodium intake (e.g., older people; African Americans; and individuals with hypertension, diabetes, or chronic kidney disease) and who also have an especially high incidence of heart disease related to high blood pressure.

Physical activity and temperature: In contrast, people unaccustomed to prolonged strenuous physical activity in a hot environment may have sodium needs that exceed the UL because of sodium loss through sweat.

DIETARY SOURCES OF SODIUM AND CHLORIDE

Foods

Sodium chloride (salt) accounts for about 90 percent of total sodium intake in the United States. As Table 3 shows, most of the sodium chloride found in the typical diet is added to food during processing.

Because salt is naturally present in only a few foods, such as celery and milk, the reduction of dietary salt does not cause diets to be inadequate in other nutrients. Although sodium chloride is the primary source of dietary sodium, other forms often found in foods as food additives include monosodium

TABLE 3 Sources of Dietary Sodium Chloride

Source of Salt	Percent of Total Sodium Chloride Intake
Added to food during processing	77
Naturally occurring in foods	12
Added while eating	6
Added during cooking	5
Tap water	< 1

glutamate, sodium benzoate, sodium nitrite, and sodium acid pyrophosphate. Sodium bicarbonate and sodium citrate are found in many antacids, which are sometimes consumed in large amounts.

Foods that are processed or canned tend to have high levels of additives that contain sodium. Examples include luncheon meats and hot dogs, canned vegetables, processed cheese, and potato chips. Condiments such as Worcestershire sauce, soy sauce, and ketchup also contain substantial amounts of sodium.

Dietary Supplements

This information was not provided at the time the DRI values for this nutrient were set.

Bioavailability

This information was not provided at the time the DRI values for this nutrient were set.

Dietary Interactions

There is evidence that sodium and chloride may interact with certain other nutrients and dietary substances (see Table 4).

INADEQUATE INTAKE AND DEFICIENCY

Overall, there is little evidence of any adverse effect of low dietary sodium intake on serum or plasma sodium concentrations in healthy people. Chloride loss usually accompanies sodium loss. Excess chloride depletion causes hypochloremic metabolic alkalosis, a syndrome seen in individuals with significant vomiting. In such cases, the chloride depletion is mainly due to the loss of hydrochloric acid. However, chloride deficiency is rarely seen in healthy people because most foods that contain sodium also provide chloride.

Special Considerations

Physical activity and temperature: Extremely vigorous physical activity performed in high temperatures can potentially affect sodium chloride balance due to the loss of sodium through sweat. The loss depends on a number of factors, including overall diet, sodium intake, sweating rate, hydration status, and one's degree of acclimation to the heat. People who are accustomed to heat exposure lose less sodium through their sweat than those unaccustomed to high temperatures.

TABLE 4 Potential Interactions with Other Dietary Substances

Substance	Potential Interaction	Notes
SUBSTANCES THAT AFFECT SODIUM AND CHLORIDE		
Potassium	Increased potassium intake increases urinary excretion of sodium chloride and blunts the rise in blood pressure resulting from excess sodium intake.	Potassium may inhibit sodium reabsorption in the kidneys, thereby reducing extracellular fluid and plasma volumes. This is considered to be an important aspect of the antihypertensive effect of potassium.
SODIUM AND CHLORIDE AFFECTING OTHER SUBSTANCES		
Sodium: potassium ratio	Sodium:potassium ratio is typically more closely associated with blood pressure than the intake of either substance alone, especially in older adults.	Clinical trials have shown that increased potassium intake lowers blood pressure, and the effects of potassium in reducing blood pressure appear to be greatest when sodium is concurrently high. Increased potassium intake also reduces the sensitivity of blood pressure changes to sodium intake.
	The incidence of kidney stones has been shown to increase with an increased sodium:potassium ratio.	Currently, there are not enough data to set different intake recommendations based on the sodium:potassium ratio.

Diuretics: Diuretics increase urinary excretion of water, sodium, and chloride, sometimes causing low blood levels of sodium (hyponatremia) and chloride (hypochloremia). Some people have experienced severe hyponatremia as a result of taking thiazide-type diuretics. However, this appears to be due to impaired water excretion rather than excessive sodium loss since it can be corrected by water restriction.

Cystic fibrosis: This genetic disorder is characterized by the body's production of abnormally thick, viscous mucus due to the faulty membrane transport of sodium chloride. As a result, the sodium and chloride content of sweat is very high. Although the increased amount of sodium and chloride required by people with cystic fibrosis is unknown, the needs are particularly high for those who exercise and therefore lose additional sodium and chloride through sweat.

Diabetes: High blood glucose levels increase renal excretion of sodium and water. In instances of acute hyperglycemia (e.g., diabetic ketoacidosis), low blood levels of sodium may occur and can generally be treated with intravenous sodium chloride and water along with insulin. Some hypoglycemic medications, such as chlorpropramide, have been associated with low blood sodium levels. In some elderly people with diabetes, hyporeninemic hypoaldosteronism may increase renal sodium loss.

EXCESS INTAKE

The major adverse effect of increased sodium chloride intake is elevated blood pressure, which has been shown to be an etiologically related risk factor for cardiovascular and renal diseases. On average, blood pressure rises progressively with increased sodium chloride intake. The dose-dependent rise in blood pressure appears to occur throughout the spectrum of sodium intake. However, the relationship is nonlinear in that the blood pressure response to changes in sodium intake is greater at sodium intakes below 2.3 g/day than above this level. The strongest dose–response evidence comes from clinical trials that specifically examined the effects of at least three levels of sodium intake on blood pressure. The range of sodium intake in these studies varied from 0.23 to 34.5 g/day. Several trials included sodium intake levels close to 1.5 g/day and 2.3 g/day.

Special Considerations

Special populations: Although blood pressure, on average, rises with increased sodium intake, there is well-recognized heterogeneity in the blood pressure response to changes in sodium chloride intake. Individuals with hypertension, diabetes, and chronic kidney disease, as well as older people and African Americans, tend to be more sensitive to the blood-pressure-raising effects of sodium chloride intake (defined as salt sensitivity) than others. Genetic factors also influence the blood pressure response to sodium chloride.

There is considerable evidence that salt sensitivity is modifiable. In research studies, different techniques and quantitative criteria have been used to define salt sensitivity. In general terms, salt sensitivity is expressed as either the reduction in blood pressure in response to a lower salt intake or the rise in blood pressure in response to sodium loading. Salt sensitivity differs among population subgroups and among individuals within a subgroup.

The rise in blood pressure from increased sodium chloride intake is blunted in the setting of a diet that is high in potassium or low in fat, and rich in minerals. Nonetheless, a dose–response relationship between sodium intake and blood pressure still persists. In nonhypertensive individuals, a reduced salt intake can decrease the risk of developing hypertension (typically defined as systolic blood pressure ≥140 mm Hg or diastolic blood pressure ≥ 90 mm Hg).

KEY POINTS FOR SODIUM AND CHLORIDE

✓   Sodium and chloride are necessary to maintain extracellular fluid volume and plasma osmolality. The cation sodium and the anion chloride are normally found in most foods together as sodium chloride (salt). About 98 percent of the sodium chloride consumed is absorbed.

✓   Since data were inadequate to determine EARs and thus calculate RDAs for sodium and chloride, AIs were instead developed.

✓   The AIs for sodium are set at an intake that ensures that the overall diet provides an adequate intake of other important nutrients and also covers sodium sweat losses in unacclimated individuals who are exposed to high temperatures or who become physically active. The AIs for chloride are set at a level equivalent on a molar basis to that of sodium. The UL is set based on the impact of sodium on blood pressure.

✓   It is well recognized that the current intake of sodium for most individuals in the United States and Canada greatly exceeds both the AI and the UL.

✓   There is inadequate evidence to support a different upper intake level of sodium intake in pregnant women from that of nonpregnant women as a means to prevent hypertensive disorders of pregnancy.

✓   The UL may be even lower among people whose blood pressure is most sensitive to increased sodium intake (e.g., older persons; African Americans; and individuals with hypertension, diabetes, or chronic kidney disease) and who also have an especially high incidence of heart disease related to high blood pressure.

✓   In contrast, people who are not accustomed to prolonged strenuous physical activity in a hot environment may have sodium needs that exceed the UL because of sodium losses through sweat.

✓   Sodium chloride (salt) accounts for about 90 percent of total sodium intake in the United States. Most of the sodium chloride found in the typical diet is added to food during processing. Examples include luncheon meats and hot dogs, canned vegetables, processed cheese, and potato chips. Condiments such as Worcestershire sauce, soy sauce, and ketchup also contain substantial amounts of sodium.

✓ There is little evidence of any adverse effect of low dietary sodium intake. Chloride deficiency is rarely seen because most foods that contain sodium also provide chloride.

✓ Diuretics increase urinary excretion of water, sodium, and chloride, sometimes causing low blood levels of sodium (hyponatremia) and chloride (hypochloremia).

✓ The primary adverse effect related to excessive sodium chloride intake is high blood pressure, which is a risk factor for heart disease, stroke, and kidney disease.

✓ On average, blood pressure rises progressively with increased sodium chloride intake. However, this relationship is nonlinear.

SULFATE

One of sulfate's key roles in the body is in the synthesis of 3'-phosphoadenosine-5'-phosphosulfate (PAPS), also known as active sulfate. In the body, active sulfate is used in the synthesis of many essential compounds, some of which are not absorbed intact when consumed in foods.

Sulfate requirements are met when intakes include recommended levels of sulfur amino acids. Therefore, neither an Estimated Average Requirement (EAR), and thus a Recommended Dietary Allowance (RDA), nor an Adequate Intake (AI) has been established for sulfate. Overall, there were insufficient data to set a Tolerable Upper Intake Level (UL) for sulfate.

About 19 percent of total sulfate intake comes from inorganic sulfate in foods and another 17 percent comes from inorganic sulfate in drinking water and beverages. Foods found to be high in sulfate include dried fruits, certain commercial breads, soya flour, and sausages. Beverages found to be high in sulfate include select juices, beers, wines, and ciders. Sulfate is also present in many other sulfur-containing compounds in foods, providing the remaining approximately 64 percent of total sulfate available for bodily needs.

Sulfate deficiency is not found in people who consume normal protein intakes containing adequate sulfur amino acids. Adverse effects have been noted in individuals whose drinking water source contains high levels of inorganic sulfate. Osmotic diarrhea that results from unabsorbed sulfate has been described and may be of particular concern in infants who consume fluids derived from water sources with high levels of sulfate.

SULFATE AND THE BODY

Function

Sulfate (inorganic sulfate [SO_4^{2-}]) is required by the body for the biosynthesis of 3'-phosphoadenosine-5'-phosphosulfate (PAPS), also known as active sulfate. PAPS is used in the biosynthesis of chondroitin sulfate, cerebroside sulfate, and many other important sulfur-containing compounds, some of which are not absorbed intact when consumed in foods.

Absorption, Metabolism, Storage, and Excretion

Sulfate can be absorbed in the stomach, small intestine, and colon. Absorption is a sodium-dependent active process. When sulfate is consumed in the form of soluble sulfate salts, such as potassium sulfate or sodium sulfate, more than 80 percent is absorbed. When sulfate is consumed as insoluble salts, such as barium sulfate, almost no absorption occurs. Unabsorbed sulfate is excreted in the feces, reabsorbed in the colon, or reduced by anaerobic bacteria to metabolites. The primary route of excretion is through the urine.

In addition to dietary sulfate intake from food and water, sulfate is derived in the body from methionine and cysteine found in dietary protein and the cysteine component of glutathione. In fact, most body sulfate is produced from the amino acids methionine and cysteine, both of which contain sulfur and are obtained from dietary protein and body protein turnover.

DETERMINING DRIS

Determining Requirements

Dietary inorganic sulfate in food and water, together with sulfate derived from methionine and cysteine found in dietary protein, as well as the cysteine component of glutathione, provide sulfate for use in PAPS biosynthesis. Sulfate requirements are thus met when intakes include recommended levels of sulfur amino acids. For this reason, neither an EAR, and thus an RDA, nor an AI for sulfate has been established.

The UL

The Tolerable Upper Intake Level (UL) is the highest level of daily nutrient intake that is likely to pose no risk of adverse effects for almost all people. Overall, there was insufficient information available to set a UL for sulfate.

Because there is no information from national surveys on sulfate intakes or on supplement usage, the risk of adverse effects within the United States or Canada cannot be characterized.

DIETARY SOURCES

Foods and Water

About 19 percent of total sulfate intake comes from inorganic sulfate in foods and another 17 percent comes from inorganic sulfate in drinking water and beverages. The remaining approximately 64 percent comes from organic compounds such as methionine, cysteine, glutathione, and taurine. Foods found to be high in inorganic sulfate include dried fruits, certain commercial breads, soya flour, and sausages. Beverages found to be high in sulfate include select juices, beers, wines, and ciders. An analysis of the sulfate content of various diets using foods purchased at supermarkets suggested a large variation in daily inorganic sulfate intake, ranging from 0.2–1.5 g (2.1–15.8 mmol)/day.

The sulfate content of drinking water highly varies depending on where in the country it was obtained. Distilled water contains very little, if any, sulfate, and deionized water contains no sulfate. However, an intake of inorganic sulfate as high as 1.3 g/day can be obtained from water and other beverages (0.5 g/L × 2.6 L/day).

Dietary Supplements

Some people self-prescribe sulfur-containing compounds such as chondroitin sulfate, glucosamine sulfate, and methylsulfonylmethane as possible aids to bones and joints. Evidence has been presented suggesting that the beneficial effects of glucosamine sulfate for osteoarthritis may be due more to the sulfate than to the glucosamine contained in the compound. No data were available on the intake of sulfur-containing compounds.

Bioavailability

This information was not provided at the time the DRI values for this nutrient were set.

Dietary Interactions

This information was not provided at the time the DRI values for this nutrient were set.

INADEQUATE INTAKE AND DEFICIENCY

Unlike most other nutrients, the body's need for sulfate can be met by consuming other required nutrients that contain sulfur amino acids. Thus, a deficiency of sulfate is not found in people who consume normal protein intakes containing adequate sulfur amino acids. Ingestion of methionine, cysteine, and glutathione in foods, along with consumption of other sulfated compounds in both food and beverages, is sufficient to meet the body's requirement for sulfate.

Research with animals has shown that growth is stunted when dietary sulfate is removed from the food and water supply, and when sulfur amino acids, particularly cysteine, are provided at levels that result in deficiency signs. Reintroducing sulfate to the diet prompts growth to resume.

EXCESS INTAKE

Adverse effects have been noted in individuals whose drinking-water source contains high levels of inorganic sulfate. Osmotic diarrhea resulting from unabsorbed sulfate has been reported and may be of particular concern in infants who consume fluids that are derived from water sources with high levels of sulfate.

Sulfate and undigested sulfur compounds have been implicated in the etiology of ulcerative colitis. High levels of hydrogen sulfide, produced in the colon from sulfate by sulfate-reducing bacteria, are thought to overburden mucosal detoxification systems, causing the colonic epithelial inflammation of ulcerative colitis. However, the possible link between dietary sulfate, colonic hydrogen sulfide levels, and ulcerative colitis has not been adequately evaluated.

Special Considerations

Kidney failure: Increased blood sulfate levels are a common feature of kidney failure. High serum sulfate levels may play a role in parathyroid stimulation and homocysteinemia, both of which commonly occur in people with chronic kidney disease.

KEY POINTS FOR SULFATE

✓   Sulfate is used in the biosynthesis of many essential compounds, some of which are not absorbed intact when consumed in foods. Inorganic sulfate is needed for the synthesis of 3'-phosphoadenosine-5'-phosphosulfate (PAPS), or active sulfate.

✓   Neither an EAR, and thus an RDA, nor an AI has been established for sulfate because most people consume adequate sulfate from foods and from sulfate produced in the body.

✓   Overall, there were insufficient data to set a UL for sulfate.

✓   About 19 percent of total sulfate intake comes from inorganic sulfate in foods and another 17 percent comes from inorganic sulfate in drinking water and beverages. Foods found to be high in inorganic sulfate include dried fruits, certain commercial breads, soya flour, and sausages. Beverages found to be high in sulfate include select juices, beers, wines, and ciders. Sulfate is also present in many other sulfur-containing compounds in foods, providing the remaining approximately 64 percent of total sulfate available for bodily needs.

✓   Unlike most other nutrients, the body's need for sulfate can be met by consuming other required nutrients that contain sulfur amino acids. Thus, a deficiency of sulfate is not found in people who consume normal protein intakes containing adequate sulfur amino acids.

✓   Osmotic diarrhea has been reported in people whose drinking water contains high levels of inorganic sulfate.

✓   Some association between increased hydrogen sulfide production and the risk of ulcerative colitis has been noted; however, this possible link has not been adequately evaluated.

TABLE 1 Dietary Reference Intakes for Zinc by Life Stage Group

	DRI values (mg/day)					
	EAR[a]		RDA[b]		AI[c]	UL[d]
	males	females	males	females		
Life stage group						
0 through 6 mo					2	4
7 through 12 mo	2.5	2.5	3	3		5
1 through 3 y	2.5	2.5	3	3		7
4 through 8 y	4.0	4.0	5	5		12
9 through 13 y	7.0	7.0	8	8		23
14 through 18 y	8.5	7.3	11	9		34
19 through 50 y	9.4	6.8	11	8		40
≥ 51 y	9.4	6.8	11	8		40
Pregnancy						
14 through 18 y		10.5		12		34
19 through 50 y		9.5		11		40
Lactation						
14 through 18 y		10.9		13		34
19 through 50 y		10.4		12		40

[a] **EAR** = Estimated Average Requirement.
[b] **RDA** = Recommended Dietary Allowance.
[c] **AI** = Adequate Intake.
[d] **UL** = Tolerable Upper Intake Level. Unless otherwise specified, the UL represents total intake from food, water, and supplements.

ZINC

Z inc is crucial for growth and development. It facilitates several enzymatic processes related to the metabolism of protein, carbohydrates, and fats. Zinc also helps form the structure of proteins and enzymes, and is involved in the regulation of gene expression.

The adult requirements for zinc are based on metabolic studies of zinc absorption, defined as the minimum amount of dietary zinc necessary to offset total daily losses of the nutrient. The Tolerable Upper Intake Level (UL) is based on a zinc-induced decrease in copper absorption that is manifest as a reduction in erythrocyte copper–zinc superoxide dismutase activity. DRI values are listed by life stage group in Table 1.

Foods rich in zinc include meat, some shellfish, legumes, fortified cereals, and whole grains. Overt human zinc deficiency is rare, and the signs and symptoms of mild deficiency are diverse due to zinc's ubiquitous involvement in metabolic processes. There is no evidence of adverse effects from intake of naturally occurring zinc in food. The adverse effects associated with chronic intake of supplemental zinc include acute gastrointestinal effects and headaches, impaired immune function, changes in lipoprotein and cholesterol levels, reduced copper status, and zinc–iron interactions.

ZINC AND THE BODY

Function

Zinc is essential for proper growth and development. Its biological functions can be divided into catalytic, structural, and regulatory. Zinc serves as a catalyst for nearly 100 specific enzymes, including alcohol dehydrogenase, alkaline phosphatase, and RNA polymerases. It is necessary for the structure of certain proteins, some of which are involved in gene expression as deoxyribonucleic acid–binding transcription factors. Examples include retinoic acid receptors and vitamin D receptors. Zinc also provides a structural function for some enzymes, the most notable of which is copper–zinc superoxide dismutase. Additionally, zinc plays a role in gene expression and has been shown to influence both apoptosis and protein kinase C activity.

Absorption, Metabolism, Storage, and Excretion

During digestion, zinc is absorbed by the small intestine through a transcellular process, with the jejunum being the site with the greatest transport rate. The mechanism of absorption appears to be saturable and there is an increase in transport velocity with zinc depletion. The absorbed zinc is bound to albumin and transferred from the intestine via the portal system.

More than 85 percent of the body's total zinc is stored in the skeletal muscle and bone; only about 0.1 percent of total body zinc is found in the plasma. However, the body tightly regulates plasma zinc concentrations to keep them steady at about 10–15 μmol/L. Factors such as stress, acute trauma, and infection can cause plasma zinc levels to drop. In humans, plasma zinc concentrations will remain relatively stable when zinc intake is restricted or increased, unless these changes in intake are severe and prolonged. This tight regulation also means that small amounts of zinc are more efficiently absorbed than large amounts and that people in poor zinc status can absorb the nutrient more efficiently than those in good status.

Zinc is excreted from the body primarily through the feces. Normal zinc losses may range from less than 1 mg/day with a zinc-poor diet to greater than 5 mg/day with a zinc-rich diet. Zinc loss through the urine represents only a fraction (less than 10 percent) of normal zinc losses, although urinary losses may increase with conditions such as starvation or trauma. Other modes of zinc loss from the body include skin cell turnover, sweat, semen, hair, and menstruation.

DETERMINING DRIS

Determining Requirements

The adult requirements for zinc are based on factorial analysis of metabolic studies of zinc absorption. Zinc absorption is defined for this purpose as the minimum amount of absorbed zinc necessary to match total daily zinc losses. The dietary intake corresponding to this average minimum quantity of absorbed zinc is the EAR.

Special Considerations

Children aged 3 years and under: The absorption of zinc from human milk is higher than from cow milk–based infant formula and cow milk. The zinc bioavailability from soy formulas is significantly lower than from milk-based formulas. Zinc nutriture in later infancy is quite different from that in the younger infant. Human milk provides only 0.5 mg/day of zinc by 7 months postpartum, and the concentration declines even further by 12 months. It is apparent, therefore, that human milk alone is an inadequate source of zinc after the first 6 months.

Vegetarian diets: Cereals are the primary source of dietary zinc for vegetarian diets. The bioavailability of zinc in vegetarian diets is reduced if phytate content in the diet is high, resulting in low zinc status (see "Dietary Interactions"). Zinc intake from vegetarian diets has been found to be similar to or lower than intake from nonvegetarian diets. Among vegetarians, zinc concentrations in the serum, plasma, hair, urine, and saliva are either the same as or lower than in individuals consuming nonvegetarian diets.

The variations found in these status indicators are most likely due in part to the amount of phytate, fiber, calcium, or other zinc absorption inhibitors in vegetarian diets. Even so, individuals consuming vegetarian diets were found to be in positive zinc balance. Yet, the requirement for dietary zinc may be as much as 50 percent greater for vegetarians, particularly for strict vegetarians whose major food staples are grains and legumes and whose dietary phytate:zinc molar ratio exceeds 15:1. This is due to poor absorption of zinc from vegetarian sources.

Alcohol intake: Long-term alcohol consumption is associated with impaired zinc absorption and increased urinary zinc excretion. Low zinc status is observed in approximately 30–50 percent of people with alcoholism. Thus, with long-term alcohol consumption, the daily requirement for zinc will be greater than that estimated by the factorial approach.

Criteria for Determining Zinc Requirements, by Life Stage Group

Life stage group	Criterion
0 through 6 mo	Average zinc intake from human milk
7 through 12 mo	Factorial analysis
1 through 50 y	Factorial analysis
≥ 51 y	Extrapolation of factorial data from 19 through 50 y
Pregnancy	
14 through 18 y	Adolescent female EAR plus fetal accumulation of zinc
19 through 50 y	Adult female average requirement plus fetal accumulation of zinc

Lactation

14 through 18 y   Adolescent female EAR plus average amount of zinc
                     secreted in human milk

19 through 50 y   Adult female EAR plus average amount of zinc secreted
                     in human milk

The UL

The Tolerable Upper Intake Level (UL) is the highest level of daily nutrient intake that is likely to pose no risk of adverse effects for almost all healthy people. Members of the general population should not routinely exceed the UL. The adverse effect of excess zinc on copper metabolism (i.e., reduced copper status) was chosen as the critical effect on which to base a UL for total daily intake of zinc from food, water, and supplements. The UL for zinc represents total intake from food, water, and supplements.

According to data from the Third National Health and Nutrition Examination Survey (NHANES III, 1988–1994), the highest reported zinc intake (from food) at the 95th percentile for all adults was 24 mg/day in men aged 19 to 30 years, which is lower than the UL. The 95th percentile of intake from food and supplements for adult men and nonpregnant women was approximately 25–32 mg/day; for pregnant and lactating women the 95th percentile of intake was 40 mg/day and 47 mg/day, respectively. The risk of adverse effects resulting from excess zinc intake appears to be low at these intake levels.

DIETARY SOURCES

Foods

Zinc is widely distributed in foods. Zinc-rich foods include red meat, some seafood, whole grains, and some fortified breakfast cereals. Because zinc is mainly found in the germ and bran portions of grain, as much as 80 percent of total zinc is lost during milling. This is why whole grains tend to be richer in zinc than unfortified refined grains.

Dietary Supplements

According to U.S. data from the 1986 National Health Interview Survey (NHIS), approximately 16 percent of Americans took supplements containing zinc. The median total (food plus supplements) zinc intakes by adults who took the supplements were similar to those adults who did not. However, the use of zinc supplements greatly increased the intakes of those in the upper quartile of intake level compared with those who did not take supplements.

TABLE 2 Qualitative Bioavailability of Zinc According to Diet Characteristics[a]

Bioavailability	Dietary Characteristics
High	Refined diets low in cereal fiber and phytic acid, with adequate protein primarily from meats and fish
	Phytate/zinc molar ratio < 5
Medium	Mixed diets containing animal or fish protein
	Vegetarian diets not based primarily on unrefined, unfermented cereal grains
	Phytate/zinc molar ratio 5–15
Low	Diets high in unrefined, unfermented, and ungerminated cereal grains, especially when animal protein intake is negligible
	High-phytate soy protein products are the primary protein source
	Diets in which ≥ 50 percent of energy is provided by high-phytate foods (high extraction rate [90 percent] flours and grains, legumes)
	Phytate/zinc molar ratio > 15
	High intake of inorganic calcium (> 1 g/day) potentiates the inhibitory effects of these diets, especially when animal protein intake is low

[a] The phytate content of foods is provided by Hallberg and Hulthen (2000). The zinc content of foods is available from the U.S. Department of Agriculture at http://www.nal.usda.gov/fnic/foodcomp.

Evidence of the efficacy of zinc lozenges in reducing the duration of common colds remains unclear.

Bioavailability

The bioavailability of zinc can be affected by many factors at many sites and is a function of the extent of digestion. The intestine is the major organ in which variations in bioavailability affect dietary zinc requirements. Dietary substances such as phytate can reduce zinc bioavailability (see "Dietary Interactions"). To date, a useful algorithm for establishing dietary zinc requirements based on the presence of other nutrients and food components has not been established, and much information is still needed to develop one that can predict zinc bioavailability. Algorithms for estimating dietary zinc bioavailability will need to include the dietary content of phytic acid, protein, zinc, and possibly calcium, iron, and copper. (Characteristics associated with diets varying in zinc bioavailability are summarized in Table 2.)

Dietary Interactions

There is evidence that zinc may interact with certain other nutrients and dietary substances (see Table 3).

TABLE 3 Potential Interactions with Other Dietary Substances

Substance	Potential Interaction	Notes
NUTRIENTS THAT AFFECT ZINC		
Iron	Iron may decrease zinc absorption.	In general, data indicate that high intakes of supplemental iron inhibit zinc absorption if both are taken without food, but do not inhibit zinc absorption if they are consumed with food. This relationship is of some concern in the management of iron supplementation during pregnancy and lactation.
Calcium and phosphorus	Calcium and phosphorus may decrease zinc absorption.	Dietary calcium may decrease zinc absorption, but there is not yet definitive evidence. Human studies have found that calcium phosphate supplements (1,360 mg/day of calcium) decreased zinc absorption, whereas calcium supplements in the form of a citrate–malate complex (1,000 mg/day of calcium) had no statistically significant effect on zinc absorption. Currently, data suggest that consuming a calcium-rich diet does not lower zinc absorption in people who consume adequate zinc. The effect of calcium on zinc absorption in people with low zinc intakes has not been extensively studied. Certain dietary sources of phosphorus, including phytate and phosphorus-rich proteins, such as milk casein, decrease zinc absorption.
Protein	Protein may affect zinc absorption.	The amount and type of dietary protein may affect zinc absorption. In general, zinc absorption is higher in diets rich in animal protein versus those rich in plant protein. The markedly greater bioavailability of zinc from human milk than from cow milk is an example of how protein digestibility, which is much lower in casein-rich cow milk than in human milk, influences zinc absorption.
Phytic acid and fiber	Phytic acid, or phytate, may reduce zinc absorption.	Phytic acid, which is found in many plant-based foods, including grains and legumes, binds to zinc and reduces its absorption in the gastrointestinal tract. Phytate binding of zinc has been demonstrated as a contributing factor for zinc deficiency related to the consumption of unleavened bread seen in certain population groups in the Middle East. Although high-fiber foods tend also to be phytate-rich, fiber alone may not have a major effect on zinc absorption.

TABLE 3 Continued

Substance	Potential Interaction	Notes
Picolinic acid	Picolinic acid may promote negative zinc balance.	Picolinic acid has a high metal binding affinity. People do not consume picolinic acid through food, but through dietary supplements, such as zinc picolinate or chromium picolinate. Zinc picolinate as a zinc source for humans has not received extensive investigation, but in an animal model, picolinic acid supplementation promoted negative zinc balance, presumably by promoting urinary zinc excretion.

ZINC AFFECTING OTHER NUTRIENTS

Copper	Increased zinc intake may lead to reduced copper absorption.	Reduced copper status has been associated with increased zinc intake. Doses of 60 mg/day (50 mg from supplements and 10 mg from food) for 10 weeks have shown this effect. This interaction also derives from the therapeutic effect of zinc in reducing copper absorption in patients with Wilson's disease.
Folate	Low zinc intake may decrease folate absorption.	Some studies have shown that low zinc intake may decrease folate absorption and folate status, whereas other studies have found that low zinc intake did not affect folate nutriture and that folate supplementation does not adversely affect zinc status. However, extensive studies on this potential relationship have not been carried out in women, and because both of the nutrients are important for fetal and postnatal development, further research is warranted.
Iron	Zinc may reduce iron absorption.	High intakes of supplemental zinc may reduce iron absorption. One study found a 56 percent decline in iron absorption when a supplemental dose of zinc and iron (administered in water) contained five times as much zinc as iron. However, when the same dose was given in a hamburger meal, no effect on iron absorption was noted.

INADEQUATE INTAKE AND DEFICIENCY

Overt human zinc deficiency is rare. Because zinc is involved in so many core areas of metabolism, the signs and symptoms of mild deficiency are diverse and inconsistent. Impaired growth velocity is the primary clinical feature and can be corrected with zinc supplementation. Other functions that respond to zinc supplementation include pregnancy outcome and immune function. Other basic and nonspecific signs and symptoms include the following:

- Growth retardation
- Alopecia
- Diarrhea
- Delayed sexual maturation and impotence
- Eye and skin lesions
- Impaired appetite

It is noteworthy that zinc homeostasis within the body is such that zinc deficiency can occur with only modest degrees of dietary zinc restriction, while circulating zinc concentrations are indistinguishable from normal.

Special Considerations

Individuals susceptible to zinc deficiency: People with malabsorption syndromes, including sprue, Crohn's disease, and short bowel syndrome are at risk of zinc deficiency due to malabsorption of zinc and increased urinary zinc losses. Acrodermatitis enteropathica, an autosomal recessive trait, is a zinc malabsorption problem of an undetermined genetic basis. The mutation causes severe skin lesions and cognitive dysfunction.

EXCESS INTAKE

There is no evidence of adverse effects from the excess intake of naturally occurring zinc in food. The adverse effects associated with chronic intake of supplemental zinc include suppression of the immune system, a decrease in high density lipoprotein (HDL) cholesterol, and reduced copper status. Other adverse effects include the following:

- *Acute effects:* Acute adverse effects of excess zinc include acute epigastric pain, nausea, vomiting, loss of appetite, abdominal cramps, diarrhea, and headaches. Doses of 225–450 mg of zinc have been estimated to cause vomiting. Gastrointestinal distress has been reported at doses of 50–150 mg/day of zinc

- *Impaired immune function:* Intake of 300 mg/day of supplemental zinc for 6 weeks has been shown to cause impaired immune function

SPECIAL CONSIDERATIONS

Individuals susceptible to adverse effects: People with Menke's disease may be distinctly susceptible to the adverse effects of excess zinc intake. Because Menke's disease is a defect in the ATPase involved in copper efflux from enterocytes, supplying extra zinc will likely further limit copper absorption.

KEY POINTS FOR ZINC

✓ Zinc functions as a component of various enzymes in the maintenance of the structural integrity of proteins and in the regulation of gene expression. Factors such as stress, acute trauma, and infection can cause plasma zinc levels to drop.

✓ In humans, plasma zinc concentrations will remain relatively stable when zinc intake is restricted or increased, unless these changes in intake are severe and prolonged.

✓ The adult requirements for zinc are based on metabolic studies of zinc absorption, defined as the minimum amount of dietary zinc necessary to offset total daily losses of zinc. The adverse effect of excess zinc on copper metabolism (i.e., reduced copper status) was chosen as the critical effect on which to base a UL for total daily intake of zinc from food, water, and supplements.

✓ The bioavailability of zinc in vegetarian diets is reduced if phytate content in the diet is high, which may result in low zinc status.

✓ Zinc interacts with many other nutrients and dietary substances. To date, a useful algorithm for establishing dietary zinc requirements based on the presence of other nutrients and food components has not been established, and much information is still needed to develop one that can predict zinc bioavailability.

✓ Zinc-rich foods include red meat, some seafood, whole grains, and some fortified breakfast cereals. Whole grains tend to be richer in zinc than unfortified refined grains. This is because zinc, mainly found in the germ and bran portions of grains, is lost during the milling process.

✓ Overt human zinc deficiency is rare.

✓ Because zinc is involved in so many core areas of metabolism, the signs and symptoms of mild deficiency are diverse and inconsistent. Impaired growth velocity is the primary clinical feature and can be corrected with zinc supplementation.

✓ The signs and symptoms of zinc deficiency include impaired growth, alopecia, diarrhea, delayed sexual maturation and impotence, eye and skin lesions, loss of appetite, altered immune function, and adverse pregnancy outcomes.

✓ It is noteworthy that zinc homeostasis within the body is such that zinc deficiency can occur with only modest degrees of dietary zinc restriction, while circulating zinc concentrations are indistinguishable from normal.

✓ People with malabsorption syndromes, including sprue, Crohn's disease, and short bowel syndrome are at risk of zinc deficiency due to malabsorption of zinc and increased urinary zinc losses.

✓ There is no evidence of adverse effects from the excess intake of naturally occurring zinc in food. The adverse effects associated with chronic intake of excess supplemental zinc include acute gastrointestinal effects and headaches, impaired immune function, changes in lipoprotein and cholesterol levels.

TABLE 1 Dietary Reference Intakes for Boron, Nickel, and Vanadium by Life Stage Group[a]

	DRI values (mg/day)		
	Boron	Nickel	Vanadium[c]
	UL[b]	UL	UL
Life stage group[d]			
0 through 6 mo	ND[e]	ND	ND
7 through 12 mo	ND	ND	ND
1 through 3 y	3	0.2	ND
4 through 8 y	6	0.3	ND
9 through 13 y	11	0.6	ND
14 through 18 y	17	1.0	ND
19 through 30 y	20	1.0	1.8
31 through 50 y	20	1.0	1.8
51 through 70 y	20	1.0	1.8
> 70 y	20	1.0	1.8
Pregnancy			
≤ 18 y	17	1.0	ND
19 through 50 y	20	1.0	ND
Lactation			
≤ 18 y	17	1.0	ND
19 through 50 y	20	1.0	ND

[a] Data were insufficient to set a UL for arsenic and for silicon. Although a UL was not determined for arsenic, there is no justification for adding it to food or supplements. In addition, although silicon has not been shown to cause adverse effects in humans, there is no justification for adding it to supplements.

[b] **UL** = Tolerable Upper Intake Level. Unless otherwise specified, the UL represents total intake from food, water, and supplements.

[c] Although vanadium in food has not been shown to cause adverse effects in humans, there is no justification for adding it to food, and vanadium supplements should be used with caution. The UL is based on adverse effects in laboratory animals and these data could be used to set a UL for adults, but not for children or adolescents.

[d] All groups except for Pregnancy and Lactation represent males and females.

[e] **ND** = Not determinable. This value is not determinable due to the lack of data of adverse effects in this age group and concern regarding the lack of ability to handle excess amounts. Source of intake should only be from food to prevent high levels of intake.

ARSENIC, BORON, NICKEL, SILICON, AND VANADIUM

There is evidence that the minerals arsenic, boron, nickel, silicon, and vanadium play a beneficial role in some physiological processes of certain animal species. For boron, silicon, and vanadium, measurable responses by human subjects to dietary intake variations have also been demonstrated. However, the available data were not as extensive and the responses were not as consistently observed as with vitamins and other minerals. Therefore, data were insufficient to determine Estimated Average Requirements (EARs), and thus Recommended Dietary Allowances (RDAs), for these minerals.

Estimates of dietary intakes of arsenic, boron, nickel, silicon, and vanadium by the North American adult population were available and could have been used to establish Adequate Intakes (AIs). However, establishing an AI also requires a clearly defined, reproducible indicator in humans who are sensitive to a range of intakes. Indicators that meet this criterion for establishing an AI were not available for any of these minerals, and therefore no AIs were set.

ULs were set for boron, nickel, and vanadium based on animal data. DRI values are listed by life stage group in Table 1. There were insufficient data to set Tolerable Upper Intake Levels (ULs) for arsenic and silicon.

Observations of deficiency effects (e.g., on growth and development) in multiple animal species and data from limited human studies suggest beneficial roles for arsenic, boron, nickel, silicon, and vanadium in human health. However, the data indicate a need for continued study of these elements to determine their metabolic role, identify sensitive indicators, and more fully characterize their specific functions in human health.

ARSENIC, BORON, NICKEL, SILICON, AND VANADIUM AND THE BODY

Function

Arsenic: There have been no studies performed to determine the nutritional importance of arsenic for humans. Animal studies suggest a role for arsenic in the metabolism of methionine, in growth and reproduction, and in gene expression.

Boron: A collective body of evidence has yet to establish a clear biological function for boron in humans. Although some evidence does suggest a role in the metabolism of vitamin D and estrogen, further research is necessary.

Nickel: The possible nutritional importance or biochemical function of nickel in humans has not been established. Nickel may serve as a cofactor or structural component of specific metalloenzymes of various functions, including hydrolysis and redox reactions and gene expression. Nickel may also serve as a cofactor facilitating iron absorption or metabolism.

Silicon: A functional role for silicon in humans has not yet been identified, although animal studies show that silicon may be involved in the formation of bone.

Vanadium: A functional role for vanadium in humans has not been identified. There are some reports that vanadium may increase the action of insulin, but the potential mechanism of action is uncertain. Vanadium also stimulates cell proliferation and differentiation and inhibits various ATPases, phosphatases, and phosphoryl-transfer enzymes.

Absorption, Metabolism, Storage, and Excretion

Arsenic: Approximately 90 percent of inorganic arsenic from water is absorbed by the body; the amount absorbed of dietary arsenic is approximately 60–70 percent. Once absorbed, inorganic arsenic is transported to the liver, where it is reduced to arsenite and then methylated. Most ingested arsenic is rapidly excreted in the urine.

Boron: With normal intakes, about 90 percent of dietary boron is absorbed. The mechanism of absorption has not been confirmed, but a passive (nonmediated) diffusion process is likely. The excretory form of boron has not been studied.

Nickel: The absorption of dietary nickel is less than 10 percent and is affected by certain foods, including milk, coffee, tea, orange juice, and ascorbic acid. Nickel is transported through the blood bound primarily to albumin. Most organs and tissues do not accumulate nickel, but in humans the thyroid and adrenal glands have relatively high concentrations. Because of the poor absorption of nickel, most ingested nickel is excreted in the feces. Absorbed nickel is excreted in the urine, with minor amounts secreted in the sweat and bile.

Silicon: Findings indicating that as much as 50 percent of ingested silicon is excreted in the urine suggest that some dietary forms of silicon are well absorbed. Silicon in the blood exists almost entirely as silicic acid and is not bound to proteins. Most body silicon is found in the various connective tissues including the aorta, trachea, bone, tendons, and skin. Excretion is primarily through the urine.

Vanadium: Less than 5 percent of ingested vanadium is absorbed. Absorbed vanadate is converted to the vanadyl cation, which can complex with ferritin and transferrin in plasma and body fluids. Very little absorbed vanadium remains in the body; whatever does remain is found primarily in the liver, kidneys, and bone. Because of the low absorption of ingested vanadium, most excretion occurs through the feces.

DETERMINING DRIS

Determining Requirements

Data were insufficient to estimate EARs, RDAs, or AIs for arsenic, boron, nickel, silicon, and vanadium.

The UL

The Tolerable Upper Intake Level (UL) is the highest level of daily nutrient intake that is likely to pose no risk of adverse health effects for almost all individuals. Although members of the general healthy population should be advised not to routinely exceed the UL, intake above the UL may be appropriate for investigation within well-controlled clinical trials. The UL is not meant to apply to individuals receiving any of these elements under medical supervision.

Arsenic: Data were insufficient to set a UL for arsenic. Although a UL was not determined for arsenic, there is no justification for adding it to food or supplements.

Although no UL was set for arsenic, there may be a risk of adverse effects with the consumption of organic arsenic in food or with the intake of inorganic arsenic in water supplies at the current maximum contamination level of 50 μg/L, set in the United States.

Boron: The UL for boron is based on reproductive and developmental effects in animals as the critical endpoint and represents intake from food, water, and supplements.

According to data from the Third National Health and Nutrition Examination Survey (NHANES III, 1988–1994) at the 95th percentile, intake of boron from the diet and supplements was approximately 2.8 mg/day. Adding to that a maximum intake from water of 2 mg/day provides a total intake of less then 5 mg/day of boron at this percentile. At the 95th percentile intake, no segment of the U.S. population had a *total* (dietary, water, and supplemental) intake greater than 5 mg/day, according to NHANES III and the Continuing Survey of Food Intakes by Individuals (CSFII, 1994–1996) data. Those who take body-building supplements could consume an additional 1.5–20 mg/day. Therefore, this supplemental intake may exceed the UL of 20 mg/day.

Nickel: The UL for nickel is based on general systemic toxicity (in the form of decreased body-weight gain reported in rat studies) as the critical endpoint. Because there were no data on the adverse effects of nickel consumption from a normal diet, the UL for nickel applies to excess nickel intake as soluble nickel salts.

Individuals with preexisting nickel hypersensitivity (from previous dermal exposure) and kidney dysfunction are distinctly susceptible to the adverse effects of excess nickel intake and may not be protected by the UL set for the general population.

Based on the Food and Drug Administration's (FDA's) Total Diet Study (1991–1997), 0.5 mg/day was the highest intake at the 99th percentile of nickel (from food) reported for any life stage and gender group; this was also the reported intake for pregnant females. Nickel intake from supplements provided only 9.6–15 µg/day at the 99th percentile for all age and gender groups, according to NHANES III. The risk of adverse effects resulting from excess intake of nickel from food and supplements appears to be very low at the highest intakes noted above. Increased risks are likely to occur from environmental exposures or from the consumption of contaminated water.

Silicon: Data were insufficient to set a UL for silicon. Although silicon has not been shown to cause adverse effects in humans, there is no justification for adding it to supplements.

Vanadium: The UL for vanadium is based on renal toxicity in animals as the critical adverse effect. Since the forms of vanadium found in food and supplements are the same, the UL applies to total vanadium intake from food, water, and supplements. Due to insufficient data, no UL was set for pregnant and lactating women, children, and infants. Caution should be exercised regarding the consumption of vanadium supplements by these individuals.

Because of the widespread use of high-dose (60 mg/day) supplemental vanadium by athletes and other subgroups (e.g., borderline diabetics) that are considered part of the apparently healthy general population, further research on vanadium toxicity is needed.

Vanadium in the forms of vanadyl sulfate (100 mg/day) and sodium metavanadate (125 mg/day) has been used as a supplement for diabetic patients. Although insulin requirements were decreased in patients with Type I diabetes, the doses of vanadium used in the supplements were about 100 times the usual intakes and greatly exceeded the UL for vanadium.

Although percentile data were not available for dietary vanadium intakes from U.S. surveys, the highest mean intake of vanadium for the U.S. population was 18 μg/day. The average intake of supplemental vanadium at the 99th percentile by adults was 20 μg/day, which is significantly lower than the adult UL. The risk of adverse effects resulting from excess intake of vanadium from food is very unlikely. Because of the high doses of vanadium present in some supplements, increased risks are likely to result from excess intake.

DIETARY SOURCES

Foods

Arsenic: Dairy products contribute as much as 31 percent of dietary arsenic; meat, poultry, fish, grains, and cereal products collectively contribute approximately 56 percent. Based on a national survey conducted in six Canadian cities from 1985 to 1988, the foods that contained the highest concentrations of arsenic were fish, meat and poultry, bakery goods and cereals, and fats and oils. Most of the arsenic found in fish is in the organic form. Major contributors of inorganic arsenic are raw rice, flour, grape juice, and cooked spinach.

Boron: Fruit-based beverages and products, tubers, and legumes have been found to have the highest concentrations of boron. Other studies have reported that the top ten foods with the highest concentration of boron were avocado, peanut butter, peanuts, prune and grape juices, chocolate powder, wine, pecans, and granola-raisin and raisin-bran cereals. When both content and total food consumption (amount and frequency) were considered, the five major contributors were found to be coffee, milk, apples, dried beans, and potatoes, which collectively accounted for 27 percent of the dietary boron consumption. Coffee and milk are generally low in boron, but they tend to be high dietary contributors because of the volume at which they are consumed.

Nickel: Nuts and legumes have the highest concentrations of nickel, followed by sweeteners, including chocolate powder and chocolate candy. Major contributors to nickel intake are mixed dishes and soups (19–30 percent), grains and grain products (12–30 percent), vegetables (10–24 percent), legumes (3–

16 percent), and desserts (4–18 percent). Major contributors of nickel to the Canadian diet include meat and poultry (37 percent), bakery goods and cereals (19 percent), soups (15 percent), and vegetables (11 percent). Cooking acidic foods in stainless-steel cookware can increase the nickel content of these foods.

Silicon: Plant-based foods contain higher concentrations of silicon than do animal-based foods. Beer, coffee, and water appear to be the major contributors of silicon to the diet, followed by grains and vegetables. Silicate additives that have been increasingly used as antifoaming and anticaking agents in foods can raise the silicon content of foods, but the bioavailability of these additives is low.

Vanadium: Foods rich in vanadium include mushrooms, shellfish, black pepper, parsley, dill seed, and certain prepared foods. Processed foods contain more vanadium than unprocessed foods. Beer and wine may also contribute appreciable amounts to the diet. The Total Diet Study showed grains and grain products contributed 13–30 percent of the vanadium in adult diets; beverages, which contributed 26–57 percent, were an important source for adults and elderly men. Canned apple juice and cereals have been shown to be major contributors to vanadium intake in infants and toddlers.

Dietary Supplements

Arsenic: This information was not provided at the time the DRI values for this nutrient were set.

Boron: In NHANES III, the adult median intake of boron from supplements was approximately 0.14 mg/day.

Nickel: In NHANES III, the adult median intake of nickel from supplements was approximately 5 µg/day.

Silicon: In NHANES III, the adult median intake of silicon from supplements was approximately 2 mg/day.

Vanadium: In NHANES III, the adult median intake of vanadium from supplements was approximately 9 µg/day.

Bioavailablility

This information was not provided at the time the DRI values for this nutrient were set.

INADEQUATE INTAKE AND DEFICIENCY

This information was not provided at the time the DRI values for these nutrients were set.

EXCESS INTAKE

Arsenic: Arsenic occurs in both inorganic and organic forms, with the inorganic forms that contain trivalent arsenite (III) or pentavalent arsenate (V) having the greatest toxicological significance. No data were found on the possible adverse effects, including cancer, of organic arsenic compounds from food. Because organic forms of arsenic are less toxic than inorganic forms, any increased health risks from the intake of organic arsenic from food is unlikely.

In contrast, inorganic arsenic is an established human poison, and acute adverse effects such as anemia and hepatotoxicity can occur in doses of 1 mg/kg/day or greater. The ingestion of acute doses greater than 10 mg/kg/day leads to encephalopathy and gastrointestinal symptoms. Chronic intake of 10 µg /kg/day or greater of inorganic arsenic produces arsenicism, a condition characterized by keratosis and the alteration of skin pigmentation. Intermediate and chronic exposures of arsenic up to levels of 11 mg/L of water are associated with symmetrical peripheral neuropathy.

The ingestion of inorganic arsenic is also associated with the risk of skin, bladder, and lung cancers. Most studies indicating a positive association with cancer involved intakes of inorganic arsenic from drinking water, as reported in areas of Taiwan, Japan, Argentina, and Chile. Studies of U.S. populations exposed to arsenic in drinking water have not identified cancer increases. Occupational exposure to inorganic forms of arsenic, in environments such as smelters and chemical plants, occurs primarily by inhalation (where the predominate form is arsenic trioxide dust).

Boron: No data were available on adverse health effects from ingestion of large amounts of boron from food and water. However, animal data suggest that reproductive and developmental effects may occur.

Nickel: There is no evidence in humans of adverse effects associated with exposure to nickel through a normal diet. The acute effects of ingesting large doses of soluble nickel salts include nausea, abdominal pain, diarrhea, vomiting, and shortness of breath. In animal studies, the signs and symptoms of general systemic toxicity include lethargy, ataxia, irregular breathing, hypothermia, and salivation, as well as decreased body-weight gain and impaired reproduction.

Silicon: There is no evidence that naturally occurring silicon in food and water produces adverse health effects. Limited reports indicate that magnesium trisilicate (6.5 mg of elemental silicon per tablet) used as an antacid in large amounts for long periods (i.e., several years) may be associated with the development of silicon-containing kidney stones.

Vanadium: There is no evidence of adverse effects associated with vanadium intake from food, which is the major source of exposure for the general population; no special subpopulations are distinctly susceptible. In animal studies, renal toxicity has occurred. Most vanadium toxicity reports involve industrial exposure to high levels of airborne vanadium. Vanadyl sulfate supplements are used by some weight-training athletes to increase performance; in addition, vanadium supplements have been studied for the treatment of diabetes. For these reasons, further research on vanadium toxicity is necessary.

KEY POINTS FOR ARSENIC, BORON, NICKEL, SILICON, AND VANADIUM

✓   Data were insufficient to set EARs, RDAs, or AIs for arsenic, boron, nickel, silicon, and vanadium.

✓   There were insufficient data to set ULs for arsenic and silicon. However, ULs based on animal data were set for boron, nickel, and vanadium.

✓   Although a UL was not determined for arsenic, there is no justification for adding it to food or supplements.

✓   Although silicon has not been shown to cause adverse effects in humans, there is no justification for adding it to supplements.

✓   Observations of deficiency effects (e.g., on growth and development) in multiple animal species and data from limited human studies suggest that there are beneficial roles for arsenic, boron, nickel, silicon, and vanadium in human health. However, the data indicate a need for continued study of these elements to determine their metabolic role, identify sensitive indicators, and more fully characterize their specific functions in human health.

Part IV
Appendixes

A

ACKNOWLEDGMENTS

The project consultants (see roster below and biographical sketches in Part IV, Appendix B) and IOM staff thank the individuals who shared their opinions about Dietary Reference Intakes and what should be included in a summary volume and in other ways contributed during the qualitative research phase that formed the basis for the development of this summary, including Jody Engel, Jeanne Goldberg, Ashli Greenwald, Liz Hill, Cheryl Koch, Maureen Leser, Martha Lynch, Madeline Sigman-Grant, Gloria Stables, and Peggy Turner. Thanks especially to Michelle Tuttle who managed, developed, and reported on this phase and to writers Jean Weininger and Gail Zyla who contributed to early drafts.

The support and participation of Danielle Brulé, Mary Bush, Margaret Cheney, Krista Esslinger, Linda Greene-Finestone, and Sylvie St-Pierre from Health Canada is gratefully acknowledged, as are the contributions of many Institute of Medicine and National Academies Press colleagues, named in the Preface.

Many volunteers spent countless hours and months developing the DRI paradigm, conducting the comprehensive nutrient reviews, and exploring how to appropriately use the new values. They were supported by a dedicated staff. This summary is a small reflection of their efforts. The members of the committees, subcommittee, and panels are listed below. We acknowledge many others who also contributed to this process, including Catherine Woteki who chaired the Food and Nutrition Board during the early DRI paradigm development; Cutberto Garza, who chaired the Food and Nutrition Board throughout the DRI process; and Allison Yates, who directed the Food and Nutrition Board and the Dietary Reference Intakes project essentially from beginning to completion.

Standing Committee on the Scientific Evaluation of Dietary Reference Intakes: Lindsay H. Allen, Stephanie A. Atkinson, Susan I. Barr, Benjamin Caballero, Robert J. Cousins, Johanna T. Dwyer, John W. Erdman, Jr. (chair), John D. Fernstrom, Cutberto Garza (also chair, Food and Nutrition Board), Scott M. Grundy, Charles H. Hennekens, Janet C. King, Sanford A. Miller, William M. Rand, Joseph V. Rodricks, Robert M. Russell (vice chair), Vernon Young (chair; deceased).

Subcommittee on Interpretation and Uses of Dietary Reference Intakes: Tanya D. Agurs-Collins, Lenore Arab, Susan I. Barr (chair), Susan T. Borra, Alicia Carriquiry, Ann M. Coulston, Barbara L. Devaney, Johanna T. Dwyer, Jean-Pierre Habicht, Janet R. Hunt, Janet C. King, Harriet Kuhnlein, Suzanne P. Murphy (chair), Valerie Tarasuk.

Subcommittee on Upper Reference Levels of Nutrients: Steven A. Abrams, G. Harvey Anderson, George C. Becking, Herbert Blumenthal (consultant), Elaine M. Faustman, Suzanne Hendrich, Renate D. Kimbrough, Walter Mertz (deceased), Rita B. Messing, Sanford A. Miller, Ian C. Munro (chair), Suzanne P. Murphy, Harris Pastides, Joseph V. Rodricks (chair), Irwin H. Rosenberg, Stephen L. Taylor, John A. Thomas, Robert H. Wasserman, Gary M. Williams.

Panel on Calcium and Related Nutrients: Steven A. Abrams, Burton M. Altura, Stephanie A. Atkinson (chair), Bess Dawson-Hughes, Robert P. Heaney, Michael F. Holick, Suzanne P. Murphy, Robert K. Rude, Bonny L. Specker, Connie M. Weaver, Gary M. Whitford.

Panel on Folate, Other B Vitamins, and Choline: Lindsay H. Allen, Lynn B. Bailey, Merton Bernfield (deceased), Phillipe De Wals, Ralph Green, Donald B. McCormick, Roy M. Pitkin (chair), Irwin H. Rosenberg, Robert M. Russell, Barry Shane, Steven H. Zeisel.

Panel on Dietary Antioxidants and Related Compounds: Gary R. Beecher, Raymond F. Burk, Alvin C. Chan, John W. Erdman, Jr., Robert A. Jacob, Ishwarlal Jialal, Laurence N. Kolonel, Norman I. Krinsky (chair), James R. Marshall, Susan Taylor Mayne, Ross L. Prentice, Kathleen Schwarz, Daniel Steinberg, Maret G. Traber.

Panel on Micronutrients: John L. Beard, Lewis Braverman (consultant), Robert J. Cousins, Francoise Delange (consultant), John T. Dunn, Guylaine Ferland, K. Michael Hambidge, Janet C. King, Sean Lynch, James G. Penland, A. Catharine Ross, Robert M. Russell (chair), Barbara J. Stoecker, John W. Suttie, Judith R. Turnlund, Keith P. West, Stanley H. Zlotkin.

Panel on Dietary Reference Intakes for Macronutrients: George A. Brooks, Nancy F. Butte, Benjamin Caballero, Jean-Pierre Flatt, Susan K. Fried, Peter J. Garlick, Scott M. Grundy, Sheila M. Innis, David J.A. Jenkins, Rachel K. Johnson, Ronald M. Krauss, Penny M. Kris-Etherton, Alice H. Lichtenstein, Joanne R. Lupton (chair), Sanford A. Miller (chair), Frank Q. Nuttall, Paul B. Pencharz,

F. Xavier Pi-Sunyer, William M. Rand, Peter J. Reeds (deceased), Eric B. Rimm, Susan B. Roberts.

Panel on the Definition of Dietary Fiber: George C. Fahey, Jr., Joanne R. Lupton (chair), David J.A. Jenkins, Judith A. Marlett, Leon Prosky (consultant), Joann L. Slavin, Alison Stephen (consultant), Jon A. Story, Christine Williams.

Panel on Dietary Reference Intakes for Electrolytes and Water: Lawrence J. Appel (chair), David H. Baker, Oded Bar-Or (deceased), Marshall Lindheimer, Kenneth Minaker, R. Curtis Morris, Jr., Lawrence M. Resnick (deceased), Michael N. Sawka, Stella L. Volpe, Myron H. Weinberger, Paul K. Whelton.

Dietary Reference Intakes Project Staff: Sandra Amamoo-Kakra, Kimberly A. Brewer, Carrie L. Holloway, Geraldine Kennedo, Donna M. Livingston, Sheila A. Moats, Karah Nazor, Mary Poos, Michele Ramsey, Crystal Rasnake, Elisabeth A. Reese, Sandra A. Schlicker, Gail Spears, Kimberly Stitzel, Carol W. Suitor, Paula R. Trumbo, Alice L. Vorosmarti, Allison A. Yates (also Food and Nutrition Board director).

CONSULTANTS TO THE SUMMARY REPORT OF THE DIETARY REFERENCE INTAKES

JOHANNA T. DWYER, Office of Dietary Supplements, NIH

RACHEL K. JOHNSON, College of Agriculture and Life Sciences, University of Vermont

RENA MENDELSON, School of Nutrition, Ryerson University

ESTHER F. MYERS, Scientific Affairs and Research, American Dietetic Association

SHARON M. NICKOLS-RICHARDSON, Department of Human Nutrition, Foods and Exercise, Virginia Polytechnic Institute and State University

LINDA SNETSELAAR, Department of Epidemiology, University of Iowa

HUGUETTE TURGEON-O'BRIEN, Departement des Sciences des Aliments et de Nutrition, Universite Laval Quebec

SUSAN WHITING, College of Pharmacy and Nutrition, University of Saskatchewan

WRITER

JENNIFER PITZI HELLWIG

DEVELOPMENTAL EDITOR/COPYEDITOR

MARY KALAMARAS

STAFF

LINDA D. MEYERS, Director, Food and Nutrition Board, Institute of Medicine

JENNIFER J. OTTEN, Study Director, Institute of Medicine

B
BIOGRAPHICAL SKETCHES

CONSULTANTS

Johanna T. Dwyer, D.Sc, R.D., is senior nutrition scientist in the National Institutes of Health Office of Dietary Supplements, a part time assignment she has held since October 2003, and professor of medicine (nutrition) and community health at Tufts University's Friedman School of Nutrition and School of Medicine. She directs the Frances Stern Nutrition Center at Tufts-New England Medical Center and is an adjunct professor at the Harvard School of Public Health. In 2001–2002, Dr. Dwyer served as assistant administrator for human nutrition in the Agricultural Research Service, U.S. Department of Agriculture. Dr. Dwyer's work is centered on dietary supplements, especially bioactive substances such as the flavonoids, life-cycle related concerns such as the prevention of diet-related disease in children and adolescents, and maximizing quality of life and health in the elderly. Dr. Dwyer is editor of *Nutrition Today*. She is past president of the American Society for Nutritional Sciences, past secretary of the American Society for Clinical Nutrition, and past president and fellow of the Society for Nutrition Education. She has served on numerous committees at the National Institutes of Health and the U.S. Department of Agriculture, and continues her interest in nutrition policy in her present position. She is a member of the Institute of Medicine (IOM), past councilor of the IOM and active as a member of IOM boards and committees, particularly those of the Food and Nutrition Board. A recipient of numerous honors and awards for her work in nutrition, Dr. Dwyer received the Conrad V. Elvejhem Award for Public Service of the American Society for Nutrition Sciences in 2005, and the Medallion Award of the American Dietetic Association in 2002. Dr. Dwyer earned a B.S. with distinction from Cornell University, an M.S. from the University of Wisconsin, and M.Sc. and D.Sc. degrees from the Harvard School of Public Health.

Rachel K. Johnson, Ph.D., M.P.H., R.D., is a professor of nutrition and dean of the College of Agriculture and Life Sciences and a distinguished University Scholar at the University of Vermont. Dr. Johnson's research expertise is in national nutrition policy, pediatric nutrition and obesity, dietary intake methodology, and energy metabolism. She has published numerous scholarly papers and book chapters on those and other topics. She has served on the Board of Editors for the *Journal of the American Dietetic Association, Nutrition Today,* and the *Nutrition Bulletin* and is the senior nutrition advisor for *EatingWell* magazine. Professional activities include serving as chair of the Commission on Dietetic Registration and the Board of Directors for the American Dietetic Association. She also served on the Year 2000 Dietary Guidelines Advisory Committee, the Additives and Ingredients Subcommittee of the U.S. Food and Drug Administration's (FDA) Food Advisory Committee, and Panel on Dietary Reference Intakes for Macronutrients of the Institute of Medicine. Dr. Johnson received her doctorate and bachelor's degrees in nutrition from the Pennsylvania State University, and a master of public health degree from the University of Hawaii. She completed a dietetic internship at the Indiana University Medical Center.

Rena Mendelson, M.S., D.Sc., R.D., is a professor of nutrition at Ryerson University where she recently completed a six-year term as associate vice president, academic, and dean of graduate studies. For more than 30 years, Dr. Mendelson has taught university students at Simmons College in Boston, the University of Toronto, and Ryerson University. She was the principal investigator for the Ontario Food Survey and chairs the board of the Canadian Council of Food and Nutrition. Her publications include scientific journals as well as popular books and newsletters. She recently completed a revised edition of *Food to Grow On* designed to promote healthy eating and physical activity for families of all ages. Dr. Mendelson completed her undergraduate studies at the University of Western Ontario and received her master's degree in nutrition at Cornell University before completing her doctorate in nutrition at the Harvard University School of Public Health.

Esther F. Myers, Ph.D., R.D., FADA, is an internationally known author, lecturer, educator, and researcher. She is well known to the members of the American Dietetic Association (ADA) in her present role in Research and Scientific Affairs. Dr. Myers has authored several papers describing evidence analysis processes and the ADA process and co-authored a chapter on systematic reviews of evidence for *Research: Successful Approaches*, edited by Elaine Monsen. Dr. Myers has presented on evidence analysis and an evidence-based approach to practice throughout the United States, and in Canada, Spain, and Malaysia and was a keynote speaker at the International Union of Nutritional Sciences (IUNS) meeting in South Africa. She is the staff liaison to the Standardized Language/Nutrition Care Process Committee of the American Dietetic Association and presented a poster session the Nutrition Care Process and nutrition diagnostic terminology at the IUNS meeting in South Africa. After retiring from the Air Force and serving as Chief Consultant to the USAF Surgeon General she joined the American Dietetic Association as Director of Research and Scientific Affairs in October 2000. Prior to joining ADA, she served as a site visitor for the Commission on Accreditation for Dietetics Education (CADE), a peer reviewer for *the Journal of the American Dietetic Association,* and a member of the Health Services Research Task Force overseeing dietetic outcomes research. She currently focuses efforts on research activities needed for the dietetics profession, nutrition care process/standardized language development, the ADA strategic leadership initiative in obesity, and the American Dietetic Association Foundation (ADAF) initiative, Healthy Weight for Kids.

Sharon M. (Shelly) Nickols-Richardson, Ph.D., R.D., is an associate professor in the Department of Human Nutrition, Foods and Exercise at Virginia Polytechnic Institute and State University. She is also an affiliate of the Center for Gerontology and has served as director of the didactic program in dietetics at the university. She has worked as a clinical dietitian and was chief of the clinical section of the dietetic service at the Harry S. Truman Memorial Veterans Affairs Medical Center in Columbia, Missouri. Dr. Nickols-Richardson serves as the Director of the Bone Metabolism, Osteoporosis, and Nutrition Evaluation Laboratory at Virginia Tech. Her research interests are related to the impact of weight loss, weight loss diets, and restrained eating on bone mineral density and bone metabolism, and the interaction of nutrient intake and resistance training on bone mineral density and bone quality. She is a member of a number of professional societies including the American Dietetic Association, American Association of Family and Consumer Sciences, American Society for Bone and Mineral Research, and American Society for Nutrition. She has served as an associate editor for the *Journal of Family and Consumer Sciences* and as a reviewer for several other professional journals. She has been recognized as a young dietitian of the year by the Georgia Dietetic Association and a future leader by the International Life Sciences Institute, North America, among other awards. Dr. Nickols-Richardson received a bachelor of science degree in nutritional sciences from Oklahoma State University and master's and doctoral degrees in foods and nutrition from the University of Georgia. She completed her dietetic internship at Presbyterian Hospital of Dallas.

Linda G. Snetselaar, Ph.D., R.D., is professor and endowed chair, preventive nutrition education, and director of the Nutrition Center in the Department of Epidemiology in the College of Public Health at the University of Iowa. She is also a faculty member in the Department of Internal Medicine, Division of Endocrinology. Dr. Snetselaar has served as a principal or co-principal investigator for several sentinel diet-related intervention studies including the Diabetes Control and Complications Trial, the Modification of Diet in Renal Disease study, Dietary Intake in Lipid Research, and the Women's Health Initiative. She has directed numerous counseling workshops for nutrition interventions. Her research interests include cardiovascular disease and diet, renal disease and diet, diabetes and diet, and cancer and diet. She holds an M.S. in nutrition and a Ph.D. in health sciences education, both from the University of Iowa.

Huguette Turgeon O'Brien, Ph.D., R.D., is professor of human nutrition and director of the master's and doctoral studies program in the Department of Food Science and Nutrition at Laval University, Québec, Canada. Her experience includes working as a community nutritionist for the Montreal Diet Dispensary and the Douglas Hospital in Montréal and as a research assistant for the Human Nutrition Research Centre in Laval University. She was co-responsible for the evaluation of the Canada Prenatal Nutrition Program (CPNP) for the province of Québec. She played a key role in the development of the Health Canada document *Nutrition for a Healthy Pregnancy—National Guidelines for the Child-bearing Years* (1999). She also participated in review of Canada's Food Guide to Healthy Eating and Health Canada's Policies concerning the addition of vitamins and minerals to foods. She serves on a number of advisory councils including the Scientific Advisory Board of the OLO Foundation for vulnerable pregnant women and the Advising Board for the Health Survey conducted among the Inuit of Northern-Québec. Dr. Turgeon O'Brien's primary research interest is in the area of prenatal nutrition and iron status of subgroups of the population. She is presently involved in research in Morocco, Benin, Burkina Faso, and Mali mainly on the effects of bioavailable dietary iron on iron status and parasitic infections. Her publications include articles in scientific journals as well as popular books. She completed her undergraduate degree at Laval University and a community nutrition internship at the Montreal Diet Dispensary before obtaining her M.Sc. in nutrition at the University of Montréal and her Ph.D. in nutrition at Laval University.

Susan Whiting, Ph.D., is professor of nutrition at the College of Pharmacy and Nutrition, University of Saskatchewan. She previously taught nutrition at Mount Saint Vincent University in Halifax prior to moving to the University of Saskatchewan where she has taught in the Nutrition and Dietetics program for 17 years. Dr. Whiting's areas of expertise involve the safety and effectiveness of calcium supplements, the role of nutrition in prevention and treatment of osteoporosis, vitamin D status, how nutrition affects bone development in children and young adults, dietary assessment methodology, and food policy with emphasis on socioeconomic factors. She is a consultant to the Scientific Advisory Board of the Osteoporosis Society and a member of the editorial board of the *British Journal of Nutrition*. She is a member of the Canadian Society of Nutritional Sciences and the American Society for Nutrition, serving as president of CSNS from 2002 to 2004. Dr. Whiting holds membership in several other professional organizations as well, including Dietitians of Canada and the American Society for Bone and Mineral Research. She served as a reviewer of the *Dietary Reference Intakes for Calcium, Phosphorus, Magnesium, Vitamin D, and Fluoride* report and as a member of the Committee on the Use of Dietary Reference Intakes in Nutrition Labeling.

WRITERS AND EDITORS

Jennifer Pitzi Hellwig, M.S., R.D., E.L.S., is a freelance writer, editor, and consultant specializing in health, medicine, food, and nutrition. Her work has appeared in several national consumer and professional publications. She is a former faculty member at the Tufts University Friedman School of Nutrition Science and Policy, where she taught a writing course for graduate students in nutrition and medicine. Ms. Hellwig holds a master's degree in nutrition communication from Tufts University and a bachelor's degree in dietetics from the University of Vermont.

Jennifer J. Otten, M.S., R.D., is a study director at the Institute of Medicine (IOM). Prior to serving as study director for this project, she worked for over seven years at the Institute of Medicine as communications director, communications officer, and communications specialist. Before joining the IOM, Ms. Otten was an assistant account executive in the food and nutrition division of Porter Novelli. A recipient of the IOM's Distinguished Service Individual Award and Distinguished Service Group Award, Ms. Otten is a member of the American Dietetic Association, Dietitians in Business and Communications, and the Society for Behavioral Medicine. Ms. Otten has a B.S. in nutritional sciences from Texas A&M University, a master's degree from Tufts University in nutrition communication, and completed her dietetic internship at Massachusetts General Hospital.

Linda D. Meyers, Ph.D., is director of the Food and Nutrition Board of the Institute of Medicine. She has also served as the deputy director and a senior program officer for the Board. Prior to joining the IOM in 2001, she worked for 15 years in the Office of Disease Prevention and Health Promotion in the Department of Health and Human Services as senior nutrition advisor, deputy director, and acting director. Dr. Meyers has received a number of awards for her contributions to public health, including the Secretary's Distinguished Service Award for *Healthy People 2010* and the Surgeon General's Medallion. Dr.

Meyers has a B.A. in health and physical education from Goshen College in Indiana, an M.S. in food and nutrition from Colorado State University, and a Ph.D. in nutritional sciences from Cornell University.

DEVELOPMENTAL EDITOR/COPYEDITOR

Mary Kalamaras is a freelance editor and writer living in the Boston area. She provides editorial services for clients who publish in the fields of science, medicine, and technology, including the *New England Journal of Medicine*. Prior to beginning her freelance career, she served as developmental editor at the National Academies Press, where her focus was on creating print- and Web-based publications that communicated the findings and recommendations of National Academies reports to the broader public. While at the Academies, she received a distinguished service award for creating and distributing more than 400,000 copies of a studies-based booklet and poster on childhood development aimed at child-care professionals. She also edited *Fed Up! Winning the War Against Childhood Obesity*, written by Susan Okie, M.D., a Harvard-trained family physician and contributing editor to the *New England Journal of Medicine*. Prior to her work for the Academies, Ms. Kalamaras served as senior editor at Discovery Channel Publishing, where she developed and managed book projects covering topics in science, technology, history, and travel. Her work there included *The Infinite Journey: Eyewitness Accounts of NASA and the Age of Space*, produced in cooperation with the National Aeronautics and Space Agency. Ms. Kalamaras began her publishing career in New York City, as an editor at Stewart, Tabori & Chang, an award-winning publisher of nonfiction illustrated books. She holds a B.A. in journalism and mass media from Douglass College, Rutgers University.

C
METHODS

The general methods for examining and interpreting the evidence on requirements for nutrients are presented in this appendix, with special attention given to approaches used to provide Dietary Reference Intakes (DRIs) where data are lacking for specific subgroups of the population (typically for infants, children, pregnant and lactating women, and older adults). Included as well are discussions of methodological problems in assessing requirements and estimating intakes from dietary survey data.

METHODOLOGICAL CONSIDERATIONS

Types of Data Used

The scientific data for developing the Dietary Reference Intakes (DRIs) have essentially come from observational and experimental studies in humans. Observational studies include single-case and case-series reports and cross-sectional, cohort, and case-control studies. Experimental studies include randomized and nonrandomized prevention trials and controlled dose–response, balance, turnover, and depletion–repletion physiological studies. Results from animal experiments are generally not applicable to the establishment of DRIs, but selected animal studies are considered in the absence of human data.

ANIMAL MODELS

Basic research using experimental animals affords considerable advantage in terms of control of nutrient exposures, environmental factors, and even genetics. In contrast, the relevance to free-living humans may be unclear. In addition, dose levels and routes of administration that are practical in animal experiments may differ greatly from those relevant to humans. Nevertheless, animal feeding experiments were sometimes included in the evidence reviewed to determine the ability to specify DRIs.

HUMAN FEEDING STUDIES

Controlled feeding studies, usually in a confined setting such as a metabolic unit, can yield valuable information on the relationship between nutrient consumption and health-related biomarkers. Much of the understanding of human nutrient requirements to prevent deficiencies is based on studies of this type. Studies in which the subjects are confined allow for close control of both intake and activities. Complete collections of nutrient losses through urine and feces are possible, as are recurring sampling of biological materials such as blood. Nutrient balance studies measure nutrient status in relation to intake. Depletion–repletion studies, by contrast, measure nutrient status while subjects are maintained on diets containing marginally low or deficient levels of a nutrient; then the deficit is corrected with measured amounts of that nutrient. Unfortunately, these two types of studies have several limitations. Typically they are limited in time to a few days or weeks, and so longer-term outcomes cannot be measured with the same level of accuracy. In addition, subjects may be confined, and findings are therefore not always generalizable to free-living individuals. Finally, the time and expense involved in such studies usually limit the number of subjects and the number of doses or intake levels that can be tested.

In spite of these limitations, feeding studies play an important role in understanding nutrient needs and metabolism. Such data were considered in the DRI process and were given particular attention in the absence of reliable data to directly relate nutrient intake to disease risk.

OBSERVATIONAL STUDIES

In comparison to human feeding studies, observational epidemiological studies are frequently of direct relevance to free-living humans, but they lack the controlled setting. Hence they are useful in establishing evidence of an association between the consumption of a nutrient and disease risk but are limited in their ability to ascribe a causal relationship. A judgment of causality may be supported by a consistency of association among studies in diverse populations, and it may be strengthened by the use of laboratory-based tools to measure exposures and confounding factors, such as personal interviews, rather than other means of data collection. In recent years, rapid advances in laboratory technology have made possible the increased use of biomarkers of exposure, susceptibility, and disease outcome in molecular epidemiological research. For example, one area of great potential in advancing current knowledge of the effects of diet on health is the study of genetic markers of disease susceptibility (especially polymorphisms in genes encoding metabolizing enzymes) in relation to dietary exposures. This development is expected to provide more accurate assessments of the risk associated with different levels of intake of both nutrients and nonnutritive food constituents.

While analytic epidemiological studies (studies that relate exposure to disease outcomes in individuals) have provided convincing evidence of an associative relationship between selected nondietary exposures and disease risk, there are a number of other factors that limit study reliability in research relating nutrient intakes to disease risk.

First, the variation in nutrient intake may be rather limited in populations selected for study. This feature alone may yield modest relative risk trends across intake categories in the population, even if the nutrient is an important factor in explaining large disease rate variations among populations.

A second factor, one that gives rise to particular concerns about confounding, is the human diet's complex mixture of foods and nutrients that includes many substances that may be highly correlated. Third, many cohort and case-control studies have relied on self-reports of diet, typically food records, 24-hour recalls, or diet history questionnaires. Repeated application of such instruments to the same individuals shows considerable variation in nutrient consumption estimates from one time period to another with correlations often in the 0.3 to 0.7 range. In addition, there may be systematic bias in nutrient consumption estimates from self-reports as the reporting of food intakes and portion sizes may depend on individual characteristics such as body mass, ethnicity, and age. For example, total energy consumption may tend to be substantially underreported (30 to 50 percent) among obese persons, with little or no underreporting among lean persons. Such systematic bias, in conjunction with random measurement error and limited intake range, has the potential to greatly impact analytic epidemiological studies based on self-reported dietary habits. Note that cohort studies using objective (biomarker) measures of nutrient intake may have an important advantage in the avoidance of systematic bias, though important sources of bias (e.g., confounding) may remain.

RANDOMIZED CLINICAL TRIALS

By randomly allocating subjects to the (nutrient) exposure of interest, clinical trials eliminate the confounding that may be introduced in observational studies by self-selection. The unique strength of randomized trials is that if the sample is large enough, the study groups will be similar with respect not only to those confounding variables known to the investigators, but also to any unknown factors that might be related to risk of the disease. Thus, randomized trials achieve a degree of control of confounding that is simply not possible with any observational design strategy, and thus they allow for the testing of small effects that are beyond the ability of observational studies to detect reliably.

Although randomized controlled trials represent the accepted standard for studies of nutrient consumption in relation to human health, they too possess important limitations. Specifically, persons agreeing to be part of a randomized trial may be a select subset of the population of interest, thus limiting the generalization of trial results. For practical reasons, only a small number of nutrients or nutrient combinations at a single intake level are generally studied in a randomized trial (although a few intervention trials to compare specific dietary patterns have been initiated in recent years). In addition, the follow-up period will typically be short relative to the preceding time period of nutrient consumption that may be relevant to the health outcomes under study, particularly if chronic disease endpoints are sought. Also, dietary intervention or supplementation trials tend to be costly and logistically difficult, and the maintenance of intervention adherence can be a particular challenge.

Because of the many complexities in conducting studies among free-living human populations and the attendant potential for bias and confounding, it is the totality of the evidence from both observational and intervention studies, appropriately weighted, that must form the basis for conclusions about causal relationships between particular exposures and disease outcomes.

WEIGHING THE EVIDENCE

As a principle, only studies published in peer-reviewed journals were used in the original DRI series and, thus, used as the basis for this book. However, studies published in other scientific journals or readily available reports were considered if they appeared to provide important information not documented elsewhere. To the extent possible, original scientific studies have been used to derive the DRIs. On the basis of a thorough review of the scientific literature, clinical, functional, and biochemical indicators of nutritional adequacy and excess were evaluated for each nutrient.

The quality of the study was considered in weighing the evidence. The characteristics examined included the study design and the representativeness of the study population; the validity, reliability, and precision of the methods used for measuring intake and indicators of adequacy or excess; the control of biases and confounding factors; and the power of the study to demonstrate a given difference or correlation. Publications solely expressing opinions were not used in setting DRIs. The assessment acknowledged the inherent reliability of each type of study design as described above, and it applied standard criteria from Hill concerning the strength, dose–response, and temporal pattern of estimated nutrient–disease or adverse effect associations, the consistency of associations among studies of various types, and the specificity and biological plausibility of the suggested relationships. For example, biological plausibility would not be sufficient in the presence of a weak association and lack of evidence that exposure preceded the effect.

Data were examined to determine whether similar estimates of the requirement resulted from the use of different indicators and different types of studies. In the DRI model described in Part I, for a single nutrient, the criterion for setting the Estimated Average Requirement (EAR) may differ from one life stage group to another because the critical function or the risk of disease may be different. When no or very poor data are available for a given life stage group, extrapolation is made from the EAR or Adequate Intake (AI) set for another group (see section later on extrapolation); explicit and logical assumptions on relative requirements were made. Because EARs can be used for multiple purposes, unlike AIs, they are established whenever sufficient supporting data were available.

DATA LIMITATIONS

Although the reference values in the original DRI report series were based on data, the data were often scanty or drawn from studies that had limitations in addressing the various questions that confronted the DRI panels. Therefore, many of the questions raised about the requirements for and recommended intakes of these nutrients cannot be answered fully. Apart from studies of overt deficiency diseases, there is a dearth of studies that address specific effects of inadequate intakes on specific indicators of health status, and thus a research agenda was proposed in each of the original DRI series reports. For many of the nutrients in the DRI reports, estimated requirements are based on factorial, balance, and biochemical indicator data because there is little information relating health status indicators to functional sufficiency or insufficiency. Thus, after careful review and analysis of the evidence, including examination of the extent of congruent findings, scientific judgment was used to determine the basis for establishing the values.

Method for Determining the Adequate Intake for Infants

The AI for young infants is generally taken to be the average intake by full-term infants who are born to healthy, well-nourished mothers and who are exclusively fed human milk. The extent to which intake of a nutrient from human milk may exceed the actual requirements of infants is not known, and ethics of experimentation preclude testing the levels known to be potentially inadequate. Using the infant exclusively fed human milk as a model is in keeping with the basis for earlier recommendations for intake. It also supports the recommendation that exclusive intake of human milk is the preferred method of feeding for normal full-term infants for the first 4 to 6 months of life. This recommendation has been made by the Canadian Paediatric Society, the American Academy of Pediatrics, the Institute of Medicine, and many other expert groups, even though most U.S. babies no longer receive human milk by age 6 months.

In general, this book does not cover possible variations in physiological need during the first month after birth or the variations in intake of nutrients from human milk that result from differences in milk volume and nutrient concentration during early lactation.

In keeping with the decision made by the Standing Committee on the Scientific Evaluation of Dietary Reference Intakes, there were not specific recommended intakes to meet the needs of formula-fed infants. The use of formula introduces a large number of complex issues, one of which is the bioavailability of different forms of the nutrient in different formula types.

AGES 0 THROUGH 6 MONTHS

To derive the AI for infants ages 0 through 6 months, the mean intake of a nutrient was calculated based on (1) the average concentration of the nutrient from 2 to 6 months of lactation using consensus values from several reported studies, if possible, and (2) an average volume of milk intake of 0.78 L/day. This volume was reported from studies that used test weighing of full-term infants. In this procedure, the infant is weighed before and after each feeding. Because there is variation in both the composition of milk and the volume consumed, the computed value represents the mean. It is expected that infants will consume increased volumes of human milk during growth spurts.

AGES 7 THROUGH 12 MONTHS

During the period of infant growth and gradual weaning to a mixed diet of human milk and solid foods from ages 7 through 12 months, there is no evidence for markedly different nutrient needs. The AI can be derived for this age group by calculating the sum of (1) the content of the nutrient provided by 0. 6 L/day of human milk, which is the average volume of milk reported from studies of infants receiving human milk in this age category and (2) that provided by the usual intakes of complementary weaning foods consumed by infants in this age category. Such an approach is in keeping with the current recommendations of the Canadian Paediatric Society, the American Academy of Pediatrics, and the Institute of Medicine for continued feeding of infants with human milk through 9 to 12 months of age with appropriate introduction of solid foods. The World Health Organization recommends the introduction of solid foods after 6 months of age.

For some of the nutrients in other DRI reports, two other approaches were considered as well: (1) extrapolation downward from the EAR for young adults by adjusting for metabolic or total body size and growth and adding a factor for variability and (2) extrapolation upward from the AI for infants ages 0 through 6 months by using the same type of adjustment. Both of these methods are described below. The results of the methods are evaluated in the process of setting the AI.

Method for Extrapolating Data from Younger to Older Infants

When information is not available on the nutrient intake of older infants, intake data can be extrapolated from young to older infants. Using the metabolic weight ratio method to extrapolate data from younger to older infants involves metabolic scaling but does not include an adjustment for growth because it is based on a value for a growing infant. To extrapolate from the AI for infants ages 0 through 6 months to an AI for infants ages 7 through 12 months, the following formula is used:

$$AI_{7-12 \text{ mo}} = AI_{0-6 \text{ mo}} \times F,$$

where $F = (Weight_{7-12 \text{ mo}}/Weight_{0-6 \text{ mo}})^{0.75}$.

Method for Extrapolating Data from Adults to Children

SETTING THE AI FOR CHILDREN

When data are lacking to set an EAR or AI for children and adolescents, the values can often be extrapolated from adult values. The EAR or AI can be extrapolated down by scaling requirements to the 0.75 power of body mass, which adjusts for metabolic differences demonstrated to be related to body weight. Other approaches include extrapolating down based on the reference body weights, which has been done in developing ULs for some nutrients, and extrapolating on the basis of energy intake.

Methods for Determining Increased Needs for Pregnancy

It is known that the placenta actively transports certain nutrients from the mother to the fetus against a concentration gradient. However, for many nutrients, experimental data that could be used to set an EAR and RDA or an AI for pregnancy are lacking. In these cases, the potential increased need for these nutrients during pregnancy is based on theoretical considerations, including obligatory fetal transfer, if data are available, and on increased maternal needs related to increases in energy or protein metabolism, as applicable. Thus, in some cases, the EAR can be determined by the additional weight gained during pregnancy.

Methods for Determining Increased Needs for Lactation

For most nutrients, it is assumed that the total nutrient requirements for lactating women equal the requirements for nonpregnant, nonlactating women of similar age plus an increment to cover the amount needed for milk production.

ESTIMATES OF NUTRIENT INTAKES

Reliable and valid methods of food composition analysis are crucial in determining the intake of a nutrient needed to meet a requirement.

Methodological Considerations

The quality of nutrient intake data varies widely across studies. The most valid intake data are those collected from the metabolic study protocols in which all food is provided by the researchers, amounts consumed are measured accurately, and the nutrient composition of the food is determined by reliable and valid laboratory analyses. Such protocols are usually possible with only a few subjects. Thus, in many studies, intake data are self-reported (e.g., through 24-hour recalls of food intake, diet records, or food frequency questionnaires).

Potential sources of error in self-reported intake data include over- or underreporting of portion sizes and frequency of intake, omission of foods, and inaccuracies related to the use of food composition tables. In addition, because a high percentage of the food consumed in the United States and Canada is not prepared from scratch in the home, errors can occur due to a lack of information on how a food was manufactured, prepared, and served. Therefore, the values reported by nationwide surveys or studies that rely on self-report are often inaccurate and possibly biased, with a greater tendency to underestimate actual intake.

Adjusting for Day-to-Day Variation

Because of day-to-day variation in dietary intakes, the distribution of 1-day (or 2-day) intakes for a group is wider than the distribution of usual intakes even though the mean of the intakes may be the same. To reduce this problem, statistical adjustments have been developed that require at least 2 days of dietary data from a representative subsample of the population of interest. However, no accepted method is available to adjust for the underreporting of intake, which may average as much as 20 percent for energy.

DIETARY INTAKES IN THE UNITED STATES AND CANADA

Sources of Dietary Intake Data

At the time the original DRI reports were published, the major sources of current dietary intake data for the U.S. population were the National Health and Nutrition Examination Survey (NHANES), which was conducted by the U.S. Department of Health and Human Services, and the Continuing Survey of Food Intakes by Individuals (CSFII), which was conducted by the U.S. Department of Agriculture (USDA). Both surveys used the food composition database developed by USDA to calculate nutrient intakes. National survey data for Canada for these nutrients was collected in 10 provinces.

Sources of Supplement Intake Data

Data on supplement use was obtained via the 1986 National Health Interview Survey, involving 11,558 adults and 1,877 children. Participants were asked about their use of supplements during the previous two weeks, and supplement composition was obtained from product labels whenever possible.

Food Sources

For some nutrients, two types of information are provided about food sources: identification of the foods that are the major contributors of the nutrients to diets in the United States and Canada and identification of the foods that contain the highest amounts of the nutrient. The determination of foods that are major contributors depends on both nutrient content of a food and total consumption of the food (amount and frequency). Therefore, a food that has a relatively low concentration of the nutrient might still be a large contributor to total intake if that food is consumed in relatively large amounts.

METHODS TO DETERMINE UPPER LEVELS

The Tolerable Upper Intake Level (UL) refers to the highest level of daily nutrient intake that is likely to pose no risk of adverse health effects for almost all people in a population. As intake increases above the UL, the potential risk of adverse effects increases.

Risk Assessment Model

The model used to derive the ULs consists of a set of scientific factors that are considered explicitly. The factors are organized into a framework called risk

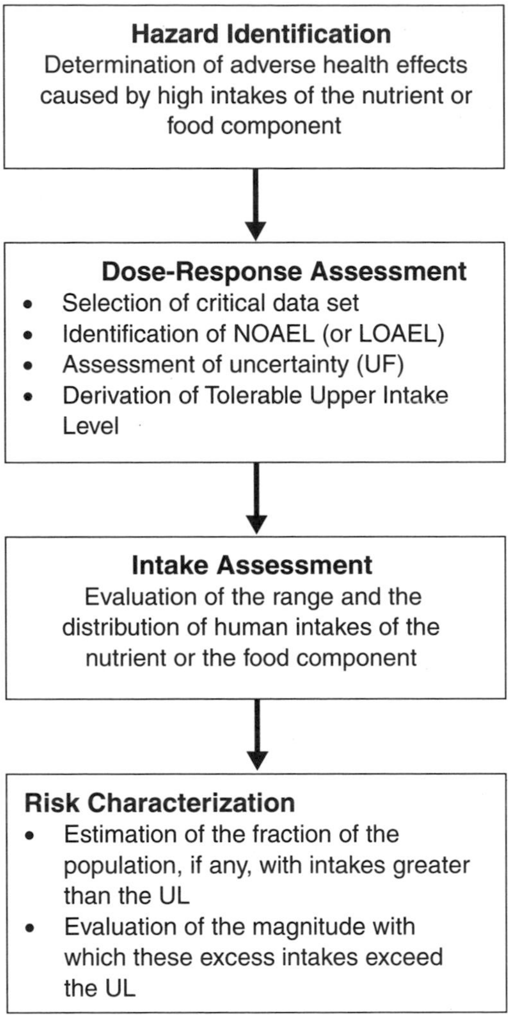

FIGURE C-1 Risk assessment model for nutrient toxicity.

assessment. In determining ULs, risk assessment is used to systematically evaluate the likelihood of adverse effects due to excess exposure to a nutrient.

The steps used in risk assessment are summarized in Figure C-1 and explained in more detail in the text that follows.

STEP 1: HAZARD IDENTIFICATION

In this step, a thorough review of the scientific literature is conducted to identify adverse health effects caused by consuming excess amounts of the nutrient in question. Data from human, animal, and in vitro research is examined, and scientific judgment is used to determine which observed effects are adverse. In addition, adverse nutrient–nutrient interactions are considered in defining an adverse effect. When available, data regarding the rate of nutrient absorption, distribution, metabolism, and excretion may also be used to help identify potential hazards. Any available knowledge of the molecular and cellular mechanisms by which a nutrient causes an adverse effect may also be identified. The scientific quality and quantity of the database evaluated as well. Finally, distinct subgroups that are highly sensitive to the adverse effects of high nutrient intake are identified.

STEP 2: DOSE–RESPONSE ASSESSMENT

At this stage, the most critical data pertaining to the UL are selected. These data are chosen based on their relevance to human route of expected intake, and expected magnitude and duration of intake.

Once the critical data have been chosen, a threshold "dose," or intake, is determined. For nutrients, a key assumption underlying risk assessment is that no risk of adverse effects is expected unless the threshold dose, or intake, is exceeded.

When possible, a no-observed-adverse-effect level (NOAEL) is identified. This is the highest intake (or experimental oral dose) of a nutrient at which no adverse effects have been observed in the people studied. If there are not enough data to select a NOAEL, then a lowest-observed-adverse-effect level (LOAEL) may be used. The LOAEL is the lowest intake (or experimental dose) at which an adverse effect has been identified.

Uncertainty Factors

Because the UL is intended to be an estimate of the level of intake that will protect the health of virtually all healthy members of a population, a critical part of risk assessment is accounting for uncertainty that is inherent in the process. In addition, the fact that excessive levels of a nutrient can cause more than one adverse effect must be considered. The NOAELs and LOAELs for these unique effects will typically differ.

To help account for such variations, an uncertainty factor (UF) is selected. The UF is intended to incorporate all potential sources of uncertainties. In general, the UFs are lower when the available data are high quality and when the adverse effects of the nutrient are extremely mild and reversible. When determining a UF, the following potential sources of uncertainty are generally considered:

- Individual variations in sensitivity to a nutrient
- Extrapolation from data from experimental animal studies to humans, when animal data constitute the primary evidence available
- Absence of NOAEL (to account for uncertainty of deriving a UL from the LOAEL)
- Use of data showing effects of subchronic nutrient exposures (NOAEL) to predict the potential effects of chronic exposure

The UL is derived by dividing the NOAEL (or LOAEL) by a single UF that incorporates all the relevant uncertainties. Scientific judgment is used to derive the appropriate NOAELs, LOAELs, and UFs. The considerations and uncertainties that are accounted for in the setting of ULs are detailed in the original DRI reports.

STEP 3: INTAKE ASSESSMENT

Information on the nutrient intake of the population is assessed. In cases where the UL pertains only to supplemental intake of the nutrient (as opposed to intake from food), the assessment is directed at supplement intakes only.

STEP 4: RISK CHARACTERIZATION

Several factors are considered to determine whether nutrient intakes create a risk of adverse effects to a population:

- The fraction of the group consistently consuming the nutrient at levels in excess of the UL
- The seriousness of the adverse effects associated with the nutrient
- The extent to which the effect is reversible when intakes are reduced to levels less than the UL
- The fraction of the population with consistent intakes above the NOAEL or even the LOAEL

D
GLOSSARY AND ACRONYMS

AAP	American Academy of Pediatrics
ACC	Acetyl-CoA carboxylase
Accommodation	An adaptative response that allows survival, but at the expense of some more or less serious consequences on health or physiological function
ACE	Angiotensin converting enzyme
Action	Demonstrated effects in various biological systems that may or may not have physiological significance
Acute exposure	An exposure to a toxin or excess amount of a nutrient that is short term, perhaps as short as one day or one dose. In this report it generally refers to total exposure (diet plus supplements) on a single day.
Adaptation	Maintenance of essentially unchanged functional capacity despite some alterations in steady-state conditions
ADD	Attention deficit disorder
Adequacy of nutrient intake	Intake of a nutrient that meets the individual's requirement for that nutrient
ADP	Adenosine diphosphate
Adverse effect	Any significant alteration in the structure or function of the human organism, or any impairment of a physiologically important function, that could lead to an adverse health effect
AI	Adequate Intake; a category of Dietary Reference Intakes
AITD	Autoimmune thyroid disease
AMDR	Acceptable Macronutrient Distribution Range
ANP	Atrial natriuretic peptide
Antioxidant	See Dietary Antioxidant
ARB	Angiotensin II receptor blocker
Association	Potential interaction derived from epidemiological studies of the relationship between a specific nutrient and chronic disease
ASTDR	Agency for Toxic Substances and Disease Registry
ATBC	Alpha-Tocopherol, Beta-Carotene (Cancer Prevention Study)

ATP	Adenosine triphosphate
AUC	Area under the curve
BEE	Basal energy expenditure
Bias	Used in a statistical sense, referring to a tendency of an estimate to deviate from a true value (as by reason of nonrandom sampling). To be unbiased, a statistic would have an expected value equal to a population parameter being estimated.
Bioavailability	Accessibility of a nutrient to participate in unspecified metabolic or physiological processes
BMI	Body mass index
BMR	Basal metabolic rate
CARET	Carotene and Retinol Efficacy Trial
Carotenodermia	Yellow discoloration of the skin with elevated plasma carotene concentrations
CDC	Centers for Disease Control and Prevention; an agency of the U.S. Department of Health and Human Services
CF	Cystic fibrosis
CHAOS	Cambridge Heart Antioxidant Study
CHD	Coronary heart disease
Chronic exposure	Exposure to a chemical compound such as a nutrient for a long period of time, perhaps as long as every day for the lifetime of an individual
CI	Confidence interval
CID	Cold-induced diuresis
CLAS	Cholesterol Lowering Atherosclerosis Study
Cluster analysis	A general approach to multivariate problems, the aim of which is to determine whether individuals fall into groups or clusters
CoA	Coenzyme A
Cr	Elemental symbol for chromium
CRBP	Cellular retinol binding protein
CSFII	Continuing Survey of Food Intakes by Individuals; a survey conducted periodically by the Agricultural Research Service, U.S. Department of Agriculture
Cut-point	The exact point when something stops or changes. The EAR is used as a cut-point in the EAR cut-point method of assessing the prevalence of inadequacy for a group.
CV	Coefficient of variation—standard deviation divided by the square root of n, where n is the sample size
CVD	Cardiovascular disease; includes heart disease and stroke

DASH Diet	Dietary Approaches to Stop Hypertension Diet; a diet rich in fruits, vegetables, and low-fat diary products and reduced in saturated fat, total fat, and cholesterol
DASH-Sodium Trial	A clinical trial that tested the effects on blood pressure of three different sodium levels in two distinct diets
DASH Trial	A clinical trial that tested the effects of different dietary patterns on blood pressure
DDS	Delayed dermal sensitivity
Deficiency	An abnormal physiological condition resulting from inadequate intake of a nutrient or multiple nutrients.
Dehydration	The process of decreasing total body water; lower than normal total body water (euhydration) (see Hypohydration)
DEXA	Dual energy X-ray absorptiometry
DFE	Dietary folate equivalent
DHA	Docosahexaenoic acid
Dietary antioxidant	A dietary antioxidant is a substance in foods that significantly decreases the adverse effects of reactive species, such as reactive oxygen and nitrogen species, on normal physiological function in humans.
Dietary status	The condition of an individual or group as a result of food and nutrient intake. Dietary status also refers to the sum of dietary intake measurements for an individual or a group.
Disappearance data	Data that refer to food and nutrients that disappear from the marketplace. The term refers to food and nutrient availability for a population that is calculated from national or regional statistics by the inventory-style method. Usually taken into account are the sum of food remaining from the previous year, food imports, and agricultural production; from this sum is subtracted the sum of food remaining at the end of the year, food exports, food waste, and food used for non-food purposes. Disappearance data do not always take account of food that does not enter commerce, such as home food production, wild food harvests, etc.
Distribution of observed intakes	The observed dietary or nutrient intake distribution representing the variability of *observed* intakes in the population of interest. For example, the distribution of observed intakes may be obtained from dietary survey data such as 24-hour recalls.
Distribution of requirements	The distribution reflecting the individual-to-individual variability in requirements. Variability exists because not all individuals in a (sub) population have the same requirements for a nutrient (even if individuals are grouped into homogeneous classes, such as Hispanic men aged 19 to 50 years).

Distribution of usual intakes	The distribution of long-run average dietary or nutrient intakes of individuals in the population. The distribution should reflect only the individual-to-individual variability in intakes. Statistical procedures may be used to adjust the distribution of observed intakes by partially removing the day-to-day variability in individual intakes, so the adjusted distribution more closely reflects a usual intake distribution.
DLW	Doubly labeled water
DNA	Deoxyribonucleic acid
Dose–response assessment	Second step in a risk assessment in which the relationship between nutrient intake and an adverse effect (in terms of incidence or severity of the effect) is determined
DRI	Dietary Reference Intakes
DTH	Delayed-type hypersensitivity
EAR	Estimated Average Requirement; a category of Dietary Reference Intakes
EAR cut-point method	A method of assessing the nutrient adequacy of groups. It consists of assessing the proportion of individuals in the group whose usual nutrient intakes are below the EAR.
ECF	Extracellular fluid
ECG	Electrocardiogram
EEG	Electroencephalogram
EEPA	Energy expenditure of physical activity
EER	Estimated energy requirement
EGR	Erythrocyte glutathione reductase
EGRAC	Erythrocyte glutathione reductase activity coefficient
EPA	U.S. Environmental Protection Agency
EPOC	Excess post-exercise oxygen consumption
Error in measurement	Mistake made in the observation or recording of data
Erythrocyte	A red blood cell
Euhydration	Normal hydration
FAO	Food and Agriculture Organization of the United Nations
FASEB	Federation of American Societies for Experimental Biology
FDA	Food and Drug Administration; an agency of the U.S. Department of Health and Human Services
Fe	Elemental symbol for iron
FFA	Free fatty acids
FFM	Fat-free mass
FM	Fat mass
FNB	Food and Nutrition Board; a division of the Institute of Medicine of the National Academies

Food balance sheet	See Disappearance data
Fore milk	Human milk collected at the beginning of an infant feeding
Former RDA and RNI	Recommended daily dietary intake level of a nutrient sufficient to meet the nutrient requirement of nearly all healthy persons in a particular life stage and gender group. These standards were last issued in the United States in 1989 (RDA, Recommended Dietary Allowance) and in Canada in 1990 (RNI, Recommended Nutrient Intake).
FQ	Food quotient
Function	Role played by a nutrient in growth, development, and maturation
GFR	Glomerular filtration rate
Gravid	Pregnant
H_2O_2	Hydrogen peroxide
Hazard identification	First step in a risk assessment, which is concerned with the collection, organization, and evaluation of all information pertaining to the toxic properties of a nutrient
HDL	High density lipoprotein
Health Canada	The federal department in Canada responsible for maintaining and improving the health of Canadian people.
Hind milk	Human milk collected at the end of an infant feeding
HIV	Human immunodeficiency virus
HOPE	Heart Outcomes Prevention Evaluation
Household	Individuals sharing in the purchase, preparation, and consumption of foods. Usually this will represent individuals living as a family in one home, including adults and children. A household may be the unit of observation rather than the independent individuals within it.
HPLC	High-performance liquid chromatography
HPV	Human papilloma virus
HRT	Hormone replacement therapy
Hyperhydration	Higher than normal total body water (euhydration)
Hyperkalemia	Serum potassium concentration > 5.0 mEq/L or mmol/L
Hypernatremia	Serum sodium concentration > 145 mEq/L or mmol/L
Hypertension	Systolic blood pressure ≥ 140 or diastolic blood pressure ≥ 90 mm Hg
Hypohydration	Lower than normal total body water (euhydration) (see Dehydration)
Hypokalemia	Serum potassium concentration < 3.5 mEq/L or mmol/L
Hyponatremia	Serum sodium concentration < 135 mEq/L or mmol/L

IAEA	International Atomic Energy Agency
IARC	International Agency for Research on Cancer
ICC	Indian childhood cirrhosis
ICCIDD	International Council for the Control of Iodine Deficiency Disorders
ICF	Intracellular fluid
ICT	Idiopathic copper toxicosis
IM	Intramuscular
Inadequacy of nutrient intake	Intake of a nutrient that fails to meet the individual's requirement for that nutrient
Interindividual variability	Variability from person to person
Intraindividual variability	Variability within one person. The term is generally used to refer to day-to-day variation in reported intakes, also called the within-person variation or standard deviation within (SD_{within}).
IOM	Institute of Medicine
IPCS	International Programme on Chemical Safety
IR	Insulin receptor
IRE	Iron response element
IRP	Iron response proteins
IU	International unit
Joint distribution	Simultaneous distribution of both requirements (y-axis) and usual intakes (x-axis) for a single nutrient by individuals within a population or group
Kashin-Beck disease	Human cartilage disease found in some of the low-selenium intake areas in Asia
Keshan disease	Human cardiomyopathy that occurs only in selenium-deficient children
Lacto-ovo-vegetarian	A person who consumes milk (lacto), eggs (ovo), and plant foods and products, but no meat or fish
LBM	Lean body mass
LCAT	Lecithin-cholesterol acyltransferase
LDL	Low-density lipoprotein
Likelihood	Probability
LMWCr	Low molecular weight chromium-binding substance
LOAEL	Lowest-observed-adverse-effect level; the lowest intake (or experimental dose) of a nutrient at which an adverse effect has been identified
LPL	Lipoprotein lipase
LSRO	Life Sciences Research Office
Lycopenodermia	Deep orange discoloration of the skin resulting from high intakes of lycopene-rich food

MAP	Mean arterial pressure; diastolic pressure times 2 plus systolic pressure over 3; the average pressure during a cardiac cycle
MCH	Mean corpuscular hemoglobin—the amount of hemoglobin in erythrocytes (red blood cells)
MCL	Maximum contaminant level; a level set by the U.S. Environmental Protection Agency for environmental contaminants
MCV	Mean corpuscular volume—the volume of the average erythrocyte
Mean intake	Average intake of a particular nutrient or food for a group or population of individuals. Also average intake of a nutrient or food over two or more days for an individual.
Mean requirement	Average requirement of a particular nutrient for a group or population of individuals.
MET	Metabolic equivalent—a rate of energy expenditure sustained by a rate of oxygen consumption of 3.5 mL/kg of body weight/min
MHC	Major histocompatibility complex
MI	Myocardial infarction
Mn	Elemental symbol for manganese
MPOD	Macular pigment optical density
MUFA	Monounsaturated fatty acid
MVP	Mitral valve prolapse
NAD	Nicotinamide adenine dinucleotide
NADH	Nicotinamide adenine dinucleotide hydride; a coenzyme
NADPH	Nicotinamide adenine dinucleotide phosphate
NAS	National Academy of Sciences
NE	Niacin equivalent
NEC	Necrotizing enterocolitis
NFCS	Nationwide Food Consumption Survey; a food consumption survey conducted through 1965 by the U.S. Department of Agriculture
NHANES	National Health and Nutrition Examination Survey; a survey conducted periodically by the National Center for Health Statistics, Centers for Disease Control and Prevention
NHIS	National Health Interview Survey
NO	Nitric oxide
NOAEL	No-observed-adverse-effect level; the highest intake (or experimental dose) of a nutrient at which no adverse effect has been observed

Normal distribution	In the statistical sense, refers to a specific type of distribution of the values for a parameter within a group or population. The distribution is symmetrical and the mean ± 2 standard deviations will encompass the parameter for 95 percent of the individuals in the group.
NRC	National Research Council
NTD	Neural tube defect
Nutrient requirement	The lowest continuing intake level of a nutrient that will maintain a defined level of nutriture in a healthy individual; also called individual requirement
Nutritional status	Condition of an individual or group resulting from nutrient intake and utilization of a nutrient at the tissue level
ORAC	Oxygen radical absorbance capacity
OTA	Office of Technology Assessment
Oxidative stress	Imbalance between the production of various reactive species and the ability of the organism's natural protective mechanisms to cope with these reactive compounds and prevent adverse effects
OxLDL	Oxidized low density lipoprotein
PAI	Physical activity index
PAL	Physical activity level
PAPS	3′-Phosphoadenosine-5′-phosphosulfate
Phylloquinone	Plant form of vitamin K and a major form of this vitamin in the human diet
PHS	Physicians' Health Study
PL	Pyridoxal
PLP	Pyridoxal phosphate
PM	Pyridoxamine
PMP	Pyridoxamine phosphate
PN	Pyridoxine
PNP	Pyridoxine phosphate
Population	A large group; in this report, a large group of people
Prevalence	The percentage of a defined population that is affected by a specific condition at the same time
Prevalence of inadequate intakes	The percentage of a population that has intakes below requirements
Probability approach	A method of assessing the nutrient adequacy of groups. It uses the distribution of usual intakes and the distribution of requirements to estimate the prevalence of inadequate intakes in a group. Also known as the NRC approach.

Probability of inadequacy	Outcome of a calculation that compares an individual's usual intake to the distribution of requirements for persons of the same life stage and gender to determine the probability that the individual's intake does not meet his or her requirement.
Provitamin A carotenoids	α-Carotene, β-carotene, and β-cryptoxanthin
Psychogenic polydipsia	The excessive consumption of fluid, especially water, among chronic psychiatric patients, particularly those with schizophrenia
PUFA	Polyunsaturated fatty acid
RAR	Retinoic acid receptor
RBC	Red blood cell
RDA	Recommended Dietary Allowance; a category of Dietary Reference Intakes
RE	Retinol equivalent
REE	Resting Energy Expenditure
Requirement	The lowest continuing intake level of a nutrient that will maintain a defined level of nutriture in a healthy individual
Rhabdomyolysis	Injury to skeletal muscle tissue that results in the destruction of skeletal muscle cells and allows for the escape of cellular contents into the extracellular fluid, leading to renal failure and compartment syndromes
Risk	The probability or likelihood that some unwanted effect will occur; in this report, refers to an unwanted effect from too small or too large an intake of a nutrient
Risk assessment	The organized framework for evaluating scientific information that has as its objective a characterization of the nature and likelihood of harm resulting from excess human exposure to an environmental agent (in this case, a nutrient); it includes the development of both qualitative and quantitative expressions of risk
Risk characterization	The final step in a risk assessment, which summarizes the conclusions from steps 1 through 3 of the assessment (hazard identification, dose response, and estimate of exposure) and evaluates the risk; this step also includes a characterization of the degree of scientific confidence that can be placed in the Tolerable Upper Intake Level
Risk curve	Used to demonstrate inadequacy or excess of a particular nutrient. As defined in the usual statistical sense, a risk curve is in contrast to the concept of probability curve.

Risk management	Process by which risk assessment results are integrated with other information to make decisions about the need for, method of, and extent of risk reduction; in addition, it considers such issues as the public health significance of the risk, the technical feasibility of achieving various degrees of risk control, and the economic and social costs of this control
Risk of excess	In relation to the DRIs, the likelihood that an individual will exceed the UL for a particular nutrient
Risk of exposure	In the toxicological sense, the likelihood that individuals will experience contact with a toxin (or consume levels of a nutrient above the UL)
Risk of inadequacy	The likelihood that an individual will have usual intake of a particular nutrient that is less than the individual's requirement
RMR	Resting metabolic rate
RNA	Ribonucleic acid
RNI	Recommended Nutrient Intake
RNS	Reactive nitrogen species
ROS	Reactive oxygen species
RQ	Respiratory quotient
RXR	Retinoid X receptor
Salt sensitivity	The extent of blood pressure change in response to a reduction in salt intake; the term "salt-sensitive blood pressure" applies to those individuals or subgroups who experience the greatest reduction in blood pressure from a given reduction in salt intake
SD	Standard deviation
SDA	Specific dynamic action
SE	Standard error
Selenite and selenate	Inorganic selenium, the forms found in many dietary supplements
Selenomethionine and selenocysteine	Major dietary forms of selenium
Selenosis	Selenium toxicity characterized by hair loss and nail sloughing
SEM	Standard error of the mean
Sensitivity analysis	Technique of varying the implicit assumptions or presumed conditions of an analysis approach to see how much this affects the overall outcome
SHRSP	Stroke-prone spontaneously hypertensive (inbred strain of rats)
Skewed distribution	A distribution that is not symmetrical around its mean. For example, a skewed distribution can have a long tail to the right (right-skewed distribution) or to the left (left-skewed distribution).

SMR	Sleeping metabolic rate
SOD	Superoxide dismutase
sTfR	Soluble transferrin receptor
Symmetrical distribution	A distribution that has the same number of values (observations) above and below the mean and has equal proportions of these values around the mean
TBW	Total body water
TDS	Total Diet Study; a study conducted by the Food and Drug Administration
α-TE	α-Tocopherol equivalent
TEE	Total energy expenditure
TEF	Thermic effect of food
Threshold	The point in a dose–response curve that is accepted as the point beyond which a risk of adverse effects occurs
TIBC	Total iron binding capacity
TMA	Trimethylamine
α-Tocopherol	The only form of vitamin E that is maintained in human plasma and thus it is the only form utilized to estimate the vitamin E requirement
Total water	Includes drinking water, water in beverages, and water that is part of food
Toxicity	An adverse condition relating to or caused by a toxin
TPN	Total parenteral nutrition
TPP	Thiamin pyrophosphate
TRH	Thyrotropin-releasing hormone
True prevalence	The actual prevalence of a condition assuming no error in measurement of either requirements or intakes that would result in false negative or false positive classifications
TSH	Thyroid stimulating hormone, also known as thyrotropin
α-TTP	α-Tocopherol transfer protein
UF	Uncertainty factor; the number by which the NOAEL (or LOAEL) is divided to obtain the Tolerable Upper Intake Level; the size of the UF varies depending on the confidence in the data and the nature of the adverse effect
UL	Tolerable Upper Intake Level; a category of Dietary Reference Intakes
Unit of observation	The level of aggregation at which data are collected. For example, the unit of observation for dietary assessment may be the individual, the household, or the population
Univariate distribution	The distribution of a single variable
USDA	U.S. Department of Agriculture
USP	U.S. Pharmacopeia

Usual intake

The long-run average intake of food, nutrients, or a specific nutrient for an individual

Variance of usual intakes or requirements

In the statistical sense, reflects the spread of the distribution of usual intakes or requirements on both sides of the mean intake or requirement. When the variance of a distribution is low, the likelihood of seeing values that are far away from the mean is low; in contrast, when the variance is large, the likelihood of seeing values that are far away from the mean is high. For usual intakes and requirements, variance reflects the person-to-person variability in the group.

Vitamin E

The 2R-stereoisomeric forms of α-tocopherol (RRR-, RSR-, RRS-, and RSS-α-tocopherol)

VLDL

Very low density lipoprotein

WHO

World Health Organization

E

DRI VALUES FOR INDISPENSABLE AMINO ACIDS BY LIFE STAGE AND GENDER GROUP

AI for Infants Ages 0 through 6 Months

0–6 mo
214 mg/d or 36 mg/kg/d of histidine
529 mg/d or 88 mg/kg/d of isoleucine
938 mg/d or 156 mg/kg/d of leucine
640 mg/d or 107 mg/kg/d of lysine
353 mg/d or 59 mg/kg/d of methionine + cysteine
807 mg/d or 135 mg/kg/d of phenylalanine + tyrosine
436 mg/d or 73 mg/kg/d of threonine
167 mg/d or 28 mg/kg/d of tryptophan
519 mg/d or 87 mg/kg/d of valine

Infants Ages 7 through 12 Months

EAR for 7–12 mo
22 mg/kg/d of histidine
30 mg/kg/d of isoleucine
65 mg/kg/d of leucine
62 mg/kg/d of lysine
30 mg/kg/d of methionine + cysteine
58 mg/kg/d of phenylalanine + tyrosine
34 mg/kg/d of threonine
9 mg/kg/d of tryptophan
39 mg/kg/d of valine

RDA for 7–12 mo

32 mg/kg/d of histidine
43 mg/kg/d of isoleucine
93 mg/kg/d of leucine
89 mg/kg/d of lysine
43 mg/kg/d of methionine + cysteine
84 mg/kg/d of phenylalanine + tyrosine
49 mg/kg/d of threonine
13 mg/kg/d of tryptophan
58 mg/kg/d of valine

Children Ages 1 through 3 Years

EAR for 1–3 y

16 mg/kg/d of histidine
22 mg/kg/d of isoleucine
48 mg/kg/d of leucine
45 mg/kg/d of lysine
22 mg/kg/d of methionine + cysteine
41 mg/kg/d of phenylalanine + tyrosine
24 mg/kg/d of threonine
6 mg/kg/d of tryptophan
28 mg/kg/d of valine

RDA for 1–3 y

21 mg/kg/d of histidine
28 mg/kg/d of isoleucine
63 mg/kg/d of leucine
58 mg/kg/d of lysine
28 mg/kg/d of methionine + cysteine
54 mg/kg/d of phenylalanine + tyrosine
32 mg/kg/d of threonine
8 mg/kg/d of tryptophan
37 mg/kg/d of valine

Children Ages 4 through 8 Years

EAR for 4–8 y

13 mg/kg/d of histidine
18 mg/kg/d of isoleucine
40 mg/kg/d of leucine
37 mg/kg/d of lysine
18 mg/kg/d of methionine + cysteine
33 mg/kg/d of phenylalanine + tyrosine
19 mg/kg/d of threonine
5 mg/kg/d of tryptophan
23 mg/kg/d of valine

RDA for 4–8 y   16 mg/kg/d of histidine
                                       22 mg/kg/d of isoleucine
                                       49 mg/kg/d of leucine
                                       46 mg/kg/d of lysine
                                       22 mg/kg/d of methionine + cysteine
                                       41 mg/kg/d of phenylalanine + tyrosine
                                       24 mg/kg/d of threonine
                                       6 mg/kg/d of tryptophan
                                       28 mg/kg/d of valine

Boys Ages 9 through 13 Years

BOYS

EAR for 9–13 y   13 mg/kg/d of histidine
                                       18 mg/kg/d of isoleucine
                                       40 mg/kg/d of leucine
                                       37 mg/kg/d of lysine
                                       18 mg/kg/d of methionine + cysteine
                                       33 mg/kg/d of phenylalanine + tyrosine
                                       19 mg/kg/d of threonine
                                       5 mg/kg/d of tryptophan
                                       23 mg/kg/d of valine

BOYS

RDA for 9–13 y   17 mg/kg/d of histidine
                                       22 mg/kg/d of isoleucine
                                       49 mg/kg/d of leucine
                                       46 mg/kg/d of lysine
                                       22 mg/kg/d of methionine + cysteine
                                       41 mg/kg/d of phenylalanine + tyrosine
                                       24 mg/kg/d of threonine
                                       6 mg/kg/d of tryptophan
                                       28 mg/kg/d of valine

Girls Ages 9 through 13 Years

GIRLS

EAR for 9–13 y   12 mg/kg/d of histidine
                                       17 mg/kg/d of isoleucine

38 mg/kg/d of leucine
35 mg/kg/d of lysine
17 mg/kg/d of methionine + cysteine
31 mg/kg/d of phenylalanine + tyrosine
18 mg/kg/d of threonine
5 mg/kg/d of tryptophan
22 mg/kg/d of valine

GIRLS

RDA for 9-13 y

15 mg/kg/d of histidine
21 mg/kg/d of isoleucine
47 mg/kg/d of leucine
43 mg/kg/d of lysine
21 mg/kg/d of methionine + cysteine
38 mg/kg/d of phenylalanine + tyrosine
22 mg/kg/d of threonine
6 mg/kg/d of tryptophan
27 mg/kg/d of valine

Boys Ages 14 through 18 Years

BOYS

EAR for 14–18 y

12 mg/kg/d of histidine
17 mg/kg/d of isoleucine
38 mg/kg/d of leucine
35 mg/kg/d of lysine
17 mg/kg/d of methionine + cysteine
31 mg/kg/d of phenylalanine + tyrosine
18 mg/kg/d of threonine
5 mg/kg/d of tryptophan
22 mg/kg/d of valine

BOYS

RDA for 14–18 y

15 mg/kg/d of histidine
21 mg/kg/d of isoleucine
47 mg/kg/d of leucine
43 mg/kg/d of lysine
21 mg/kg/d of methionine + cysteine

38 mg/kg/d of phenylalanine + tyrosine
22 mg/kg/d of threonine
6 mg/kg/d of tryptophan
27 mg/kg/d of valine

Girls Ages 14 through 18 Years

GIRLS

EAR for 14–18 y

12 mg/kg/d of histidine
16 mg/kg/d of isoleucine
35 mg/kg/d of leucine
32 mg/kg/d of lysine
16 mg/kg/d of methionine + cysteine
28 mg/kg/d of phenylalanine + tyrosine
17 mg/kg/d of threonine
4 mg/kg/d of tryptophan
20 mg/kg/d of valine

GIRLS

RDA for 14–18 y

14 mg/kg/d of histidine
19 mg/kg/d of isoleucine
44 mg/kg/d of leucine
40 mg/kg/d of lysine
19 mg/kg/d of methionine + cysteine
35 mg/kg/d of phenylalanine + tyrosine
21 mg/kg/d of threonine
5 mg/kg/d of tryptophan
24 mg/kg/d of valine

Adults Ages 19 Years and Older

EAR FOR ADULTS

19 y and older

11 mg/kg/d of histidine
15 mg/kg/d of isoleucine
34 mg/kg/d of leucine
31 mg/kg/d of lysine
15 mg/kg/d of methionine + cysteine
27 mg/kg/d of phenylalanine + tyrosine
16 mg/kg/d of threonine

4 mg/kg/d of tryptophan
19 mg/kg/d of valine

RDA FOR ADULTS

19 y and older

14 mg/kg/d of histidine
19 mg/kg/d of isoleucine
42 mg/kg/d of leucine
38 mg/kg/d of lysine
19 mg/kg/d of methionine + cysteine
33 mg/kg/d of phenylalanine + tyrosine
20 mg/kg/d of threonine
5 mg/kg/d of tryptophan
24 mg/kg/d of valine

Pregnancy

EAR FOR PREGNANCY

For all ages

15 mg/kg/d of histidine
20 mg/kg/d of isoleucine
45 mg/kg/d of leucine
41 mg/kg/d of lysine
20 mg/kg/d of methionine + cysteine
36 mg/kg/d of phenylalanine + tyrosine
21 mg/kg/d of threonine
5 mg/kg/d of tryptophan
25 mg/kg/d of valine

RDA FOR PREGNANCY

For all ages

18 mg/kg/d of histidine
25 mg/kg/d of isoleucine
56 mg/kg/d of leucine
51 mg/kg/d of lysine
25 mg/kg/d of methionine + cysteine
44 mg/kg/d of phenylalanine + tyrosine
26 mg/kg/d of threonine
7 mg/kg/d of tryptophan
31 mg/kg/d of valine

Lactation

EAR for Lactation

For all ages

15 mg/kg/d of histidine
24 mg/kg/d of isoleucine
50 mg/kg/d of leucine
42 mg/kg/d of lysine
21 mg/kg/d of methionine + cysteine
41 mg/kg/d of phenylalanine + tyrosine
24 mg/kg/d of threonine
7 mg/kg/d of tryptophan
28 mg/kg/d of valine

RDA for Lactation

For all ages

19 mg/kg/d of histidine
30 mg/kg/d of isoleucine
62 mg/kg/d of leucine
52 mg/kg/d of lysine
26 mg/kg/d of methionine + cysteine
51 mg/kg/d of phenylalanine + tyrosine
30 mg/kg/d of threonine
9 mg/kg/d of tryptophan
35 mg/kg/d of valine

TABLE F-1 Conversions

Water
1 L = 33.8 fluid oz; 1 L = 1.06 qt; 1 cup = 8 fluid oz

Vitamin A and Carotenoids
- µg RAE = 1 µg all-*trans*-retinol
- µg RAE = 2 µg supplemental all-*trans*-β-carotene
- µg RAE = 12 µg dietary all-*trans*-β-carotene
- µg RAE = 24 µg other dietary provitamin A carotenoids
- µg RAE = µg RE in foods containing only preformed Vitamin A (retinol)
- µg RAE = µg RE in foods containing only plant sources (provitamin A carotenoids) of vitamin A (e.g., carrots) ÷ 2
- One IU of retinol = 0.3 µg of retinol, or 0.3 µg RAE
- One IU of supplemental β-carotene = 0.5 IU of retinol or 0.15 µg RAE (0.3 × 0.5)
- One IU of dietary β-carotene = 0.165 IU retinol or 0.05 µg RAE (0.3 × 0.165)
- One IU of other dietary provitamin A carotenoids = 0.025 µg RAE

Vitamin D
1 µg cholecalciferol = 40 IU vitamin D

Vitamin E
- mg of α-tocopherol in a meal = mg of α-tocopherol equivalents in a meal × 0.8
- mg of α-tocopherol in food, fortified food, or multivitamin

$$= \text{IU of the } RRR\text{-}\alpha\text{-tocopherol compound} \times 0.67$$

or

$$= \text{IU of the } all\ rac\text{-}\alpha\text{-tocopherol compound} \times 0.45$$

Folate

1 µg of DFEs	= 1.0 µg of food folate
	= 0.6 µg of folate added to foods (as a fortificant or folate supplement with food)
	= 0.5 µg of folate taken as a supplement (without food).
1 µg of food folate	= 1.0 µg of DFEs
1 µg of folate added as a fortificant or as a supplement consumed with meals	= 1.7 µg of DFEs
1 µg of folate supplement taken without food	= 2.0 µg of DFEs.

Niacin
As niacin equivalents (NEs). 1 mg of niacin = 60 mg of tryptophan

F
CONVERSIONS

WATER

Conversion factors: 1 L = 33.8 fluid oz; 1 L = 1.06 qt; 1 cup = 8 fluid oz.

VITAMIN A AND CAROTENOIDS

A major change in the extent to which provitamin A carotenoids can be used to form vitamin A is the replacement of retinol equivalents (µg RE) with retinol activity equivalents (µg RAE) for the provitamin A carotenoids. The RAEs for dietary α-carotene, β-carotene, and β-cryptoxanthin are 12, 24, and 24 µg, respectively, compared to corresponding REs of 6, 12, and 12 µg reported by the National Research Council in 1989.

DETERMINING THE VITAMIN A CONTENT OF FOODS WITH SOME NUTRIENT DATABASES

Newer nutrient databases provide vitamin A activity in RAE. Even if a database does not, it is still possible to estimate total vitamin A activity in µg RAE from existing tables using µg RE. For foods, such as liver, containing only vitamin A activity from preformed vitamin A (retinol), no adjustment is necessary. Vitamin A values for foods containing only plant sources (provitamin A carotenoids) of vitamin A (e.g., carrots) can be adjusted by dividing the µg RE by two. For foods that are mixtures containing both plant and animal sources of vitamin A (e.g., a casserole containing meat and vegetables), the adjustment process is more complex. If the recipe for a mixture is known, the new vitamin A value may be calculated after adjusting the vitamin A content of each ingredient, as necessary. Alternatively, if the nutrient database contains values as µg RE for both total vitamin A and carotenoids, then it is possible to calculate a new value both for carotenoids and for total vitamin A. To determine a revised total vitamin A value, the retinol value is calculated as the difference between the original total vitamin A value and the original carotenoid value. The revised total vitamin A content is then calculated as the sum of the retinol value and the adjusted carotenoid value, which is the original carotenoid value in µg RE divided by two. As discussed in the following section, this same procedure may be used to adjust intake data that have been analyzed using other databases.

Supplemental β-carotene has a higher bioconversion to vitamin A than does dietary β-carotene. With low doses, the conversion is as high as 2:1. Little is known about the bioconversion of the forms of β-carotene that are added to foods, so fortification forms of β-carotene should be assumed to have the same bioconversion as food forms, which is 12:1. Food and supplement labels usually state vitamin A levels in International Units (IU). One IU of retinol is equivalent to 0.3 μg of retinol, or 0.3 μg RAE. One IU of β-carotene in supplements is equivalent to 0.5 IU of retinol or 0.15 μg RAE (0.3 × 0.5). One IU of dietary β-carotene is equivalent to 0.165 IU retinol or 0.05 μg RAE (0.3 × 0.165). One IU of other dietary provitamin A carotenoids is equivalent 0.025 μg RAE.

INTERPRETING PUBLISHED DATA ON VITAMIN A INTAKES OF VARIOUS POPULATION GROUPS

Existing data on vitamin A intakes of individuals and groups will need to be reinterpreted because of the changes in the retinol molar equivalency ratios for carotenoids to μg RAE. Two scenarios are possible: (1) the existing data provide values for both total vitamin A and carotenoid intake, and (2) the existing data provide values only for total vitamin A intake.

EXISTING DATA PROVIDE VALUES FOR BOTH TOTAL VITAMIN A AND CAROTENOIDS

The data manipulations required depend on the type of information that is sought (for example, mean intakes versus the proportion of a group with inadequate intakes). A way to approximate the mean intake of a group follows:

1a.   Find the group mean intake for total vitamin A intake (e.g., for women aged 30 to 39 years in the Continuing Survey of Food Intakes by Individuals [CSFII, 1994–1996], mean intake was 895 μg RE). Subtract the group mean intake of carotenoids (e.g., for women aged 30 to 39 years in the CSFII, mean carotene intake was 500 μg RE). Thus, preformed vitamin A intake would be estimated as 395 μg (895 − 500).

1b.   Divide the group mean intake of carotenoids by 2 (in this example, 500 ÷ 2 = 250 μg RAE). This represents the corrected value for provitamin A intake.

1c.   Add the corrected provitamin A intake determined in Step 1b to the preformed vitamin A intake determined in Step 1a. In this example, the mean vitamin A intake of women aged 30 to 39 years in the CSFII would be 645 μg RAE (250 + 395).

Existing Data Provide Values for Only Total Vitamin A Intake

In this situation, there will be more uncertainty associated with estimates of both group mean intakes and the proportion of a group with inadequate intakes. This is because of the lack of information on the proportion of the total vitamin A intake that was derived from carotenoids. In this situation, a possible approach to approximating group mean intakes follows:

2a.   Use other published data from a similar subject life stage and gender group that provide intakes of both total vitamin A and carotenoids to perform the calculations in Steps 1a through 1c above. For example, if the group of interest was 30- to 39-year-old women, data for this group from the CSFII could be used.

2b.   Calculate the adjusted vitamin A intake for this group as a percentage of the unadjusted mean intake. For the example of 30- to 39-year-old women, the adjusted mean intake was 645 µg, and the unadjusted mean was 895 µg. Thus the adjusted vitamin A intake would be 0.72 (645 ÷ 895), or 72 percent.

2c.   Apply the adjustment factor to the mean intake of the group of interest. For example, if the group's mean intake had been reported as 1,100 µg, the adjusted intake would be 792 µg (1,100 × 0.72).

Implications Arising from the Development of Retinol Activity Equivalents (RAE)

The vitamin A activity of provitamin A carotenoids found in darkly colored fruits and green leafy vegetables is half that previously assumed. Consequently, individuals who rely on plant foods for the majority of their vitamin A needs should ensure that they consume foods that are rich in carotenoids (specifically, deep yellow and green vegetables and fruits) on a regular basis.

Another implication of the reduced contribution from the provitamin A carotenoids is that vitamin A intakes of most population groups are lower than was previously believed. For example, in the CSFII survey, the reported mean proportion of vitamin A derived from carotenoids was 47 percent. Using the new conversion factors would thus reduce the population mean vitamin A intake by about 23 to 24 percent, or from 982 µg RE to 751 µg RAE.

VITAMIN D

As cholecalciferol. 1 µg cholecalciferol = 40 IU vitamin D.

VITAMIN E

The EARs, RDAs, and AIs for vitamin E are based on α-tocopherol only and do not include amounts obtained from the other seven naturally occurring forms of vitamin E (β-, γ-, δ-tocopherol and the four tocotrienols). Although absorbed, these forms do not contribute to meeting the vitamin E requirement because they are not converted to α-tocopherol. Only the 2R-stereoisomeric forms of α-tocopherol are preferentially secreted by the liver into the plasma for transport to tissues. Since the 2S-stereoisomeric forms of α-tocopherol are not maintained in human plasma or tissues, vitamin E is defined in this publication as limited to the 2R-stereoisomeric forms of α-tocopherol to establish recommended intakes. However, all eight stereoisomers of supplemental α-tocopherol are used as the basis for establishing the Tolerable Upper Intake Level (UL) for vitamin E.

Newer nutrient databases provide values for α-tocopherol. Older ones do not distinguish among all the different forms of vitamin E in food. These databases often present the data as α-tocopherol equivalents (α-TE) and thus include the contribution of all eight naturally occurring forms of vitamin E, after adjustment for bioavailability using previously determined equivalencies (e.g., α-tocopherol has been usually assumed to have only 10 percent of the availability of α-tocopherol) based on fetal resorption assays. It is recommended that the use of α-TE be abandoned due to the lack of evidence of bioavailability via transport in plasma or tissues. Because these other forms of vitamin E occur in foods (e.g., γ-tocopherol is present in widely consumed oils such as soybean and corn oils), the intake of α-TE is greater than the intake of α-tocopherol alone.

All α-tocopherol in foods is *RRR*-α-tocopherol, but the *all rac*-α-tocopherol in fortified foods and supplements is an equal mix of the 2R- and 2S-stereoisomers. The EARs, RDAs, and AIs given in the Vitamin E chapter apply only to the intake of the *RRR*-α-tocopherol from food and the 2R-stereoisomeric forms of α-tocopherol (*RRR*-, *RSR*-, *RRS*-, and *RSS*-α-tocopherol) that occur in fortified foods and supplements. The UL applies to all eight stereoisomeric forms of α-tocopherol that occur in fortified foods and supplements.

Conversion Factor for Vitamin E in Food and Supplements

To estimate the α-tocopherol intake from food surveys in the United States in which food intake data are presented as α-TE, the α-TE should be multiplied by 0.8.

$$\text{mg of } \alpha\text{-tocopherol in a meal} =$$
$$\text{mg of } \alpha\text{-tocopherol equivalents in a meal} \times 0.8.$$

In addition, the amount of chemically synthesized *all rac*-α-tocopherol compounds added to foods and multivitamin supplements in milligrams should be estimated at 50 percent to calculate the intake of the 2*R*-stereoisomers of α-tocopherol when assessing intakes to meet requirements.

If vitamin E in foods, fortified foods, and multivitamin supplements is reported in international units (IUs), the activity in milligrams of α-tocopherol may be calculated by multiplying the number of IUs by 0.67 if the form of vitamin E is *RRR*-α-tocopherol (natural vitamin E) (historically and incorrectly labeled *d*-α-tocopherol), and by 0.45 if the form is *all rac*-α-tocopherol (synthetic vitamin E) (historically and incorrectly labeled *dl*-α-tocopherol compounds).

$$\text{mg of α-tocopherol in food, fortified food, or multivitamin}$$
$$= \text{IU of the } RRR\text{-α-tocopherol compound} \times 0.67$$
$$\text{or}$$
$$= \text{IU of the } all\ rac\text{-α-tocopherol compound} \times 0.45$$

For example, a person with intake from food of 15 mg/day of α-TE would have consumed approximately 12 mg/day of α-tocopherol ($15 \times 0.8 = 12$). If this person took a daily multivitamin supplement with 30 IU of *RRR*-α-tocopheryl acetate, an additional 20 mg/day of α-tocopherol would have been consumed ($30 \times 0.67 = 20$). Thus, this person would have an effective total intake of 32 mg/day of α-tocopherol (12 + 20). If the daily multivitamin supplement contained 30 IU of *all rac*-α-tocopherol, it would be equivalent to 13.5 mg/day of α-tocopherol ($30 \times 0.45 = 13.5$), and the person's total intake of α-tocopherol would be 25.5 mg/day (12 + 13.5).

FOLATE

Dietary Folate Equivalents and Folate Sources

Currently, nutrition labels do not distinguish between sources of folate (food folate and folic acid) or express the folate content of food in dietary folate equivalents (DFEs), which take into account the different bioavailabilities of folate sources. DFEs and types of folate are related as follows:

1 μg of DFEs	=	1.0 μg of food folate
	=	0.6 μg of folate added to foods (as a fortificant or folate supplement with food)
	=	0.5 μg of folate taken as a supplement (without food)

1 µg of food folate   = 1.0 µg of DFEs
1 µg of folate added as
a fortificant or as a
supplement consumed
with meals   = 1.7 µg of DFEs

1 µg of folate supplement
taken without food   = 2.0 µg of DFEs

Diet Assessment of Individuals. When intakes of folate in the diet of an individual are assessed, it is possible to approximate the DFE intake by estimating the amount added in fortification and the amount present naturally as food folate by using the relationship 1 µg of folate added as a fortificant = 1.7 µg of DFEs (the reciprocal of 1 µg of DFEs = 0.6 µg folate added to food).

The following four-step method is proposed to approximate DFEs when estimating the dietary intake of an individual:

1. Group foods into (a) fortified cereal grain foods and specially fortified foods and (b) all others.

2. If other current data are not available for cereal grains, assume the following levels of fortification (read the label of the product to determine whether folate has been added in amounts greater than the required fortification level; this primarily refers to cereals):

- one slice of bread provides 20 µg of added folate;
- one serving (about 1 cup) of cooked pasta provides 60 µg of added folate; and
- one serving (about 1 cup) of cooked cereal or rice provides 60 µg of added folate.

Moderately fortified ready-to-eat cereals provide approximately 25 percent of the daily value per serving according to the product label, which is currently equivalent to 100 µg of added folate (25 percent of 400 µg). Highly fortified ready-to-eat cereals provide 100 percent of the daily value per serving, or 400 µg of added folate. Serving sizes of ready-to-eat cereals vary widely.

3. Combine the folate contributed by all the fortified cereal grains and multiply the result by 1.7 to obtain DFEs from folate added to foods.

4. Add DFEs from cereal grains to the folate content (in µg) from all other foods obtained from existing nutrient databases to obtain the total folate content in DFEs. For example, if the fortified cereal grains consumed were

- 8 slices of bread at 20 μg of added folate per slice (160 μg of total folate),
- 1 serving of moderately fortified ready-to-eat cereal (100 μg of folate), and
- 1 one-cup serving of pasta (60 μg of folate).

the total content would be 320 μg of added folate. The other foods in the diet—fruits, vegetables, meats, legumes, and milk products—provide 250 μg of food folate as determined by food composition data.

Therefore, total folate intake in DFEs = $(1.7 \times 320) + 250 = 794$ μg of DFEs.

Diet Assessment of Populations. If dietary folate intake has been reported for groups without adjusting for DFEs and if members of the group have consumed foods fortified with folate, the amount of available folate will be higher than reported for those group members. Adjustments can be made only at the individual level, not at the group level.

NIACIN

As niacin equivalents (NEs). 1 mg of niacin = 60 mg of tryptophan.

G

Iron Intakes and Estimated Percentiles of the Distribution of Iron Requirements from the Continuing Survey of Food Intakes by Individuals (CSFII), 1994–1996

TABLE G-1 Iron Content of Foods Consumed by Infants 7 to 12 Months of Age, CSFII, 1994–1996

Foods	Iron Content (mg/100 kcal)	Absorption (%)	Amount of Iron[a]	Estimate of Iron Absorbed (mg)	Weighted Mean Absorption (%)[b]
Human breast milk[c]	0.04	50	0.18	0.09	0.65
Meat and poultry	1.2	20	0.36	0.07	0.52
Fruits	0.4	5	0.27	0.13	0.10
Vegetables	1.2	5	0.56	0.03	0.20
Cereals[d]	8.75	6	12.1	0.73	5.24
Noodles	0.6	5	0.38	0.02	0.14
Total			13.85	1.07	6.85

[a] Based on a total daily energy intake of 845 kcal.
[b] Calculation based on the proportion of iron in each of the six food groups.
[c] Assumes an intake of 670 mL/day.
[d] Refers to iron-fortified infant cereals containing 35 mg iron/100 g of dry cereal.

TABLE G-2 Contribution of Iron from the 14 Food Groups for Children Aged 1 to 3 and 4 to 8 Years, CSFII, 1994–1996

Food Group	Iron Content (mg/100 kcal)[a]	Amount of Iron (mg) 1–3 y[b]	Amount of Iron (mg) 4–8 y[c]
Meat	1.19	1.57	2.17
Fruits	0.36	0.23	0.25
Vegetables	1.22	1.14	1.87
Cereals	2.65	8.64	11.98
Vegetables plus meat	0.7	0.17	0.18
Grain plus meat	0.78	1.12	1.53
Cheese	0.15	0.04	0.05
Eggs	0.9	0.22	0.19
Ice cream, yogurt, etc.	0.13	0.06	0.01
Fats, candy	0.05	0.03	0.05
Milk	0.08	0.18	0.15
Formula	1.8	0.18	0.00
Juices	0.44	0.34	0.22
Other beverages	0.11	0.07	0.12
Total		14.27	18.77

[a] Source: Whitney EN, Rolfes SR. 1996. *Understanding Nutrition*, 7th ed. St. Paul: West Publishing; Pennington JAT. 1998. *Bowes and Church's Food Values of Portions Commonly Used*, 17th ed. Philadelphia: Lippincott

[b] The CSFII database provides total food energy (average of 2 days) and the proportion of energy from each of 14 food groups. The iron content of each food was determined from appropriate references (expressed as iron content per 100 kcal), thus the iron content of each food was calculated. The results are based on a total daily energy intake of 1,345 kcal (*n* = 1,868) as reported in CSFII.

[c] Calculated as shown above. Based on a total daily energy intake of 1,665 kcal (*n* = 1,711) as reported in CSFII. According to the Third National Health and Nutrition Examination Survey, the median intake of iron by infants is 15.5 mg/day; the iron mainly comes from fortified formulas and cereals, with smaller amounts from vegetables, pureed meats, and poultry. It is estimated that the absorption of iron from fortified cereals is in the range of 6 percent, from breast milk 50 percent, and from meat 20 percent.

TABLE G-3 Estimated Percentiles of the Distribution of Iron Requirements (mg/d) in Young Children and Adolescent and Adult Males, CSFII, 1994–1996

Estimated Percentile of Requirements	Young Children, Both Sexes[a]			Male Adolescents and Adults		
	0.5–1 y[b]	1–3 y[c]	4–8 y[c]	9–13 y[c]	14–18 y[c]	Adult[c]
2.5	3.01	1.01	1.33	3.91	5.06	3.98
5	3.63	1.24	1.64	4.23	5.42	4.29
10	4.35	1.54	2.05	4.59	5.85	4.64
20	5.23	1.96	2.63	5.03	6.43	5.09
30	5.87	2.32	3.13	5.36	6.89	5.44
40	6.39	2.66	3.62	5.64	7.29	5.74
50[d]	6.90	3.01	4.11	5.89	7.69	6.03
60	7.41	3.39	4.65	6.15	8.08	6.32
70	7.93	3.82	5.27	6.43	8.51	6.65
80	8.57	4.39	6.08	6.76	9.03	7.04
90	9.44	5.26	7.31	7.21	9.74	7.69
95	10.15	6.06	8.45	7.58	10.32	8.06
97.5[e]	10.78	6.81	9.52	7.91	10.83	8.49

[a] Based on pooled estimates of requirement components; presented Estimated Average Requirement (EAR) and Recommended Dietary Allowance (RDA) based on the higher estimates obtained for males.

[b] Based on 10 percent bioavailability.

[c] Based on 18 percent bioavailability.

[d] Fiftieth percentile = EAR.

[e] Ninety-seven and one-half percentile = RDA.

TABLE G-4 Estimated Percentiles of the Distribution of Iron Requirements (mg/d) for Female Adolescents and Adults, CSFII, 1994–1996

Estimated Percentile of Requirement	9–13 y	14–18 y	Oral Contraceptive User,[a] Adolescent
2.5	3.24	4.63	4.11
5	3.60	5.06	4.49
10	4.04	5.61	4.97
20	4.59	6.31	5.57
30	4.98	6.87	6.05
40	5.33	7.39	6.48
50[c]	5.66	7.91	6.89
60	6.00	8.43	7.34
70	6.36	9.15	7.84
80	6.78	10.03	8.47
90	7.38	11.54	9.47
95	7.88	13.08	10.42
97.5[d]	8.34	14.80	11.44

[a] Based on 60 percent reduction in menstrual blood loss.

[b] Mixed population assumes 17 percent oral contraceptive users, 83 percent nonusers, all menstruating.

[c] Fiftieth percentile = Estimated Average Requirement.

[d] Ninety-seven and one-half percentile = Recommended Dietary Allowance.

Mixed Adolescent Population[b]	Menstruating Adult	Oral Contraceptive User,[a] Adult	Mixed Adult Population[b]	Post Menopause
4.49	4.42	3.63	4.18	2.73
4.92	4.88	4.00	4.63	3.04
5.45	5.45	4.45	5.19	3.43
6.14	6.22	5.06	5.94	3.93
6.69	6.87	5.52	6.55	4.30
7.21	7.46	5.94	7.13	4.64
7.71	8.07	6.35	7.73	4.97
8.25	8.76	6.79	8.39	5.30
8.92	9.63	7.27	9.21	5.68
9.77	10.82	7.91	10.36	6.14
11.21	13.05	8.91	12.49	6.80
12.74	15.49	9.90	14.85	7.36
14.39	18.23	10.94	17.51	7.88

TABLE G-5 Probabilities of Inadequate Iron Intakes[a] and Associated Ranges of Usual Intake for Infants and Children 1 through 8 Years, CSFII, 1994–1996

Probability of Inadequacy	Associated Range of Usual Intakes (mg/d)		
	Infants 8–12 mo	Children 1–3 y	Children 4–8 y
1.0[b]	< 3.01	< 1.0	< 1.33
0.96	3.02–3.63	1.1–1.24	1.34–1.64
0.93	3.64–4.35	1.25–1.54	1.65–2.05
0.85	4.36–5.23	1.55–1.96	2.07–2.63
0.75	5.24–5.87	1.97–2.32	2.64–3.13
0.65	5.88–6.39	2.33–2.66	3.14–3.62
0.55	6.40–6.90	2.67–3.01	3.63–4.11
0.45	6.91–7.41	3.02–3.39	4.12–4.64
0.35	7.42–7.93	3.40–3.82	4.65–5.27
0.25	7.94–8.57	3.83–4.38	5.28–6.08
0.15	8.58–9.44	4.39–5.25	6.09–7.31
0.08	9.45–10.17	5.26–6.06	7.32–8.45
0.04	10.18–10.78	6.07–6.81	8.46–9.52
0[b]	> 10.78	> 6.81	> 9.52

[a] Probability of inadequate intake = probability that requirement is greater than the usual intake. Derived from Table G-3.

[b] For population assessment purposes, a probability of 1 has been assigned to all usual intakes falling below the two and one-half percentile of requirement and a probability of 0 has been assigned to all usual intakes falling above the ninety-seven and one-half percentile of requirement. This enables the assessment of population risk where precise estimates are impractical and effectively without impact.

TABLE G-6 FOLLOWS

TABLE G-6 Probabilities of Inadequate Iron Intakes[a] (mg/d) and Associated Ranges of Usual Intake in Adolescent Males and in Girls Using or Not Using Oral Contraceptives (OC), CSFII, 1994–1996

Probability of Inadequacy	9–13 y	
	Male	Female
1.0[d]	< 3.91	< 3.24
0.96	3.91–4.23	3.24–3.60
0.93	4.24–4.59	3.61–4.04
0.85	4.60–5.03	4.05–4.59
0.75	5.04–5.36	4.60–4.98
0.65	5.37–5.64	4.99–5.33
0.55	5.65–5.89	5.34–5.66
0.45	5.90–6.15	5.67–6.00
0.35	6.16–6.43	6.01–6.36
0.25	6.44–6.76	6.37–6.78
0.15	6.77–7.21	6.79–7.38
0.08	7.22–7.58	7.39–7.88
0.04	7.59–7.91	7.89–8.34
0[d]	> 7.91	> 8.34

[a] Probability of inadequate intake = probability that requirement is greater than the usual intake. May be used in simple computer programs to evaluate adjusted distributions of usual intakes. See Institute of Medicine. 2000. *Dietary Reference Intakes: Applications in Dietary Assessment*. Washington, DC: National Academy Press, for method of adjusting observed intake distributions. Not to be applied in the assessment of individuals. Derived from Tables G-3 and G-4.

[b] Assumes 60 percent reduction in menstrual iron loss.

[c] Mixed population represents 17 percent oral contraceptive users and 83 percent nonoral contraceptive users.

[d] For population assessment purposes, a probability of 1 has been assigned to all usual intakes falling below the two and one-half percentile of requirement and a probability of 0 has been assigned to all usual intakes falling above the ninety-seven and one-half percentile of requirement. This enables the assessment of population risk where precise estimates are impractical and effectively without impact.

14–18 y			
Male	Female		
	Non-OC Users	OC Users[b]	Mixed Population[c]
< 5.06	< 4.63	< 4.11	< 4.49
5.06–5.42	4.64–5.06	4.11–4.49	4.49–4.92
5.43–5.85	5.07–5.61	4.50–4.97	4.93–5.45
5.86–6.43	5.62–6.31	4.98–5.57	5.46–6.14
6.44–6.89	6.32–6.87	5.58–6.05	6.15–6.69
6.90–7.29	6.88–7.39	6.06–6.48	6.70–7.21
7.30–7.69	7.40–7.91	6.49–6.89	7.22–7.71
7.70–8.08	7.92–8.48	6.90–7.34	7.72–8.25
8.09–8.51	8.49–9.15	7.35–7.84	8.26–8.92
8.52–9.03	9.16–10.03	7.85–8.47	8.93–9.77
9.04–9.74	10.04–11.54	8.48–9.47	9.78–11.21
9.75–10.32	11.55–13.08	9.48–10.42	11.22–12.74
10.33–10.83	13.09–14.80	10.43–11.44	12.75–14.39
> 10.83	> 14.80	> 11.44	> 14.39

TABLE G-7 Probabilities of Inadequate Iron Intakes[a] (mg/d) and Associated Ranges of Usual Intake in Adult Men and Women Using and Not Using Oral Contraceptives (OC) , CSFII, 1994–1996

| Probability of Inadequacy | Adult Men | Menstruating Women | | | Postmenopausal Women |
		Non-OC Users	OC Users[b]	Mixed Population[c]	
1.0[d]	< 3.98	< 4.42	< 3.63	< 4.18	< 2.73
0.96	3.98–4.29	4.42–4.88	3.63–4.00	4.18–4.63	2.73–3.04
0.93	4.30–4.64	4.89–5.45	4.01–4.45	4.64–5.19	3.05–3.43
0.85	4.65–5.09	5.46–6.22	4.46–5.06	5.20–5.94	3.44–3.93
0.75	5.10–5.44	6.23–6.87	5.07–5.52	5.95–6.55	3.94–4.30
0.65	5.45–5.74	6.88–7.46	5.53–5.94	6.56–7.13	4.31–4.64
0.55	5.75–6.03	7.47–8.07	5.95–6.35	7.14–7.73	4.65–4.97
0.45	6.04–6.32	8.08–8.76	6.36–6.79	7.74–8.39	4.98–5.30
0.35	6.33–6.65	8.77–9.63	6.80–7.27	8.40–9.21	5.31–5.68
0.25	6.66–7.04	9.64–10.82	7.28–7.91	9.22–10.36	5.69–6.14
0.15	7.05–7.69	10.83–13.05	7.92–8.91	10.37–12.49	6.15–6.80
0.08	7.70–8.06	13.06–15.49	8.92–9.90	12.50–14.85	6.81–7.36
0.04	8.07–8.49	15.50–18.23	9.91–10.94	14.86–17.51	7.37–7.88
0[d]	> 8.49	> 18.23	> 10.94	> 17.51	> 7.88

[a] Probability of inadequate intake = probability that requirement is greater than the usual intake. May be used in simple computer programs to evaluate adjusted distributions of usual intakes. See Institute of Medicine. 2000. *Dietary Reference Intakes: Applications in Dietary Assessment*. Washington, DC: National Academy Press, for method of adjusting observed intake distributions. Not to be applied in the assessment of individuals. Derived from Tables G-3 and G-4.

[b] Assumes 60 percent reduction in menstrual iron loss.

[c] Mixed population represents 17 percent oral contraceptive users and 83 percent nonoral contraceptive users.

[d] For population assessment purposes, a probability of 1 has been assigned to all usual intakes falling below the two and one-half percentile of requirement and a probability of 0 has been assigned to all usual intakes falling above the ninety-seven and one-half percentile of requirement. This enables the assessment of population risk where precise estimates are impractical and effectively without impact.

H

STANDARD DEVIATION OF REQUIREMENTS FOR NUTRIENTS WITH AN EAR

Standard Deviation (SD) of requirements is calculated from the Coefficient of Variation (CV) and the Estimated Average Requirement (EAR) as:

$$SD = CV \times EAR$$

Nutrient with an EAR	CV (percent)	Basis if not 10 percent[a]
MACRONUTRIENTS		
Dietary Carbohydrate	15	Variation in brain glucose utilization
Protein	12	Skewed distribution; calculated as half distance from 16th to 84th percentile of protein requirement distribution[b]
VITAMINS		
Vitamin A	20	Half-life for liver vitamin A in adults
Vitamin B_6	10	
Vitamin B_{12}	10	
Vitamin C	10	
Vitamin E	10	
Folate	10	

Nutrient with an EAR	CV (percent)	Basis if not 10 percent[a]
Niacin	15	Limited studies suggest greater variation than 10 percent, partly from wide variation in conversion efficiency of tryptophan to niacin
Riboflavin	10	
Thiamin	10	
MINERALS		
Copper	15	Limited data to set EAR
Iodine	20	Calculation that subtracts out variation due to experimental design
Iron		Skewed distribution; calculated by modeling components of requirement distribution, estimating the requirement for absorbed iron at the 97.5 percentile, and with use of an upper limit of 18 percent iron absorption, and rounding
Magnesium	10	
Molybdenum	15	Limited data to set EAR (few Mo levels in depletion/repletion study and small number of subjects)
Phosphorus	10	
Selenium	10	
Zinc	10	

[a] The assumption of 10 percent is based on extensive data on the variation in basal metabolic rate and on a similar CV of 12 percent for protein requirements in adults.

[b] Rand and colleagues demonstrated that the natural logarithm of requirements in mg nitrogen/kg/day has a normal distribution with a mean of 4.65 and a standard deviation of 0.12. From this and because the skewness is not extreme, an approximate standard deviation can be calculated.

I
ESTIMATES OF WITHIN-SUBJECT VARIATION IN INTAKE

TABLE I-1 Estimates of Within-Subject Variation in Intake, Expressed as Standard Deviation (SD)[a] and Coefficient of Variation (CV) for Vitamins and Minerals in Adults Aged 19 and Over

Nutrient[b]	Adults Ages 19–50 y				Adults, Ages 51 y and Over			
	Females (n = 2,480)[c]		Males (n = 2,538)		Females (n = 2,162)		Males (n = 2,280)	
	SD	CV (%)	SD	CV (%)	SD	CV (%)	SD	CV (%)
Vitamin A (µg)	1,300	152	1,160	115	1,255	129	1,619	133
Carotene (RE)	799	175	875	177	796	147	919	153
Vitamin E (mg)	5	76	7	176	6	65	9	60
Vitamin C (mg)	73	87	93	92	61	69	72	71
Thiamin (mg)	0.6	47	0.9	46	0.5	41	0.7	40
Riboflavin (mg)	0.6	50	1.0	44	0.6	42	0.8	40
Niacin (mg)	9	47	12	44	7	42	9	39
Vitamin B_6 (mg)	0.8	53	1.0	48	0.6	44	0.8	42
Folate (µg)[d]	131	62	180	61	12	52	150	53
Vitamin B_{12} (µg)	12	294	13	212	10	237	14	226
Calcium (mg)	325	51	492	54	256	44	339	44
Phosphorus (mg)	395	39	573	38	313	33	408	32
Magnesium (mg)	86	38	122	38	74	33	94	32
Iron (mg)	7	53	9	51	5	44	7	44
Zinc (mg)	6	61	9	63	5	58	8	66
Copper (mg)	0.6	53	0.7	48	0.5	53	0.7	56
Sodium (mg)	1,839	44	1,819	43	1,016	41	1,323	38
Potassium (mg)	851	38	1,147	36	723	31	922	31

NOTE: When the CV is larger than 60 to 70 percent the distribution of daily intakes is nonnormal and the methods presented here are unreliable.

[a] Square root of the residual variance after accounting for subject, and sequence of observation (gender and age controlled by classifications).

[b] Nutrient intakes are for food only, data do not include intake from supplements.

[c] Sample size was inadequate to provide separate estimates for pregnant or lactating women.

[d] Folate reported in µg rather than as the new dietary folate equivalents (DFE).

SOURCE: Data from Continuing Survey of Food Intakes by Individuals 1994–1996.

TABLE I-2 Estimates of Within-Subject Variation in Intake, Expressed as Standard Deviation (*SD*)[a] and Coefficient of Variation (*CV*) for Vitamins and Minerals in Adolescents and Children

| Nutrient[b] | Adolescents, Ages 9–18 y | | | | Children, Ages 4–8 y | | | |
| | Females (n = 1,002) | | Males (n = 998) | | Females (n = 817) | | Males (n = 883) | |
	SD	CV (%)	SD	CV (%)	SD	CV (%)	SD	CV (%)
Vitamin A (µg)	852	109	898	91	808	103	723	86
Carotene (RE)	549	180	681	197	452	167	454	166
Vitamin E (mg)	4	67	5	62	3	54	3	57
Vitamin C (mg)	81	90	93	89	61	69	74	76
Thiamin (mg)	0.6	43	0.8	42	0.5	35	0.5	37
Riboflavin (mg)	0.7	42	1.0	41	0.6	35	0.7	35
Niacin (mg)	8	46	11	43	6	36	7	38
Vitamin B_6 (µg)	0.7	49	1.0	49	0.6	42	0.7	43
Folate (µg)[c]	128	58	176	60	99	48	117	50
Vitamin B_{12} (µg)	5.5	142	5.0	93	9.6	254	4.7	118
Calcium (mg)	374	48	505	48	313	40	353	41
Phosphorus (mg)	410	38	542	37	321	32	352	32
Magnesium (mg)	86	41	109	39	61	31	71	33
Iron (mg)	6	47	9	50	5	45	6	43
Zinc (mg)	5	50	8	58	3	41	4	42
Copper (mg)	0.5	52	0.6	48	0.4	47	0.4	41
Sodium (mg)	1,313	45	1,630	42	930	38	957	35
Potassium (mg)	866	41	1,130	41	631	32	750	35

NOTE: When the *CV* is larger than 60 to 70 percent the distribution of daily intakes is nonnormal and the methods presented here are unreliable.

[a] Square root of the residual variance after accounting for subject, and sequence of observation (gender and age controlled by classifications).

[b] Nutrient intakes are for food only, data do not include intake from supplements.

[c] Folate reported in µg rather than as the new dietary folate equivalents (DFE).

SOURCE: Data from Continuing Survey of Food Intakes by Individuals 1994–1996.

TABLE I-3 Estimates of Within-Subject Variation in Intake, Expressed as Standard Deviation (SD)[a] and Coefficient of Variation (CV) for Macronutrients in Adults Aged 19 and Over

| Nutrient[b] | Adults, Ages 19–50 y | | | | Adults, Ages 51 y and Over | | | |
| | Females (n = 2,480)[c] | | Males (n = 2,583) | | Females (n = 2,162) | | Males (n = 2,280) | |
	SD	CV (%)	SD	CV (%)	SD	CV (%)	SD	CV (%)
Energy (kcal)	576	34	854	34	448	31	590	29
Fat (total, g)	29.9	48	42.7	44	24.0	45	31.8	42
Fat (saturated, g)	10.9	52	15.9	49	8.6	50	11.4	45
Fat (mono-unsaturated, g)	12.0	50	17.4	46	9.7	48	13.0	44
Fat (poly-unsaturated, g)	8.4	64	11.3	59	7.0	61	8.8	57
Carbohydrate (g)	75.2	35	109	35	59.9	32	79.5	32
Protein (g)	26.6	42	40.4	41	22.1	37	28.6	35
Fiber (g)	6.5	49	9.2	51	5.9	43	7.7	43
Cholesterol (mg)	168	77	227	66	144	70	201	66

NOTE: When the CV is larger than 60 to 70 percent the distribution of daily intakes is nonnormal and the methods presented here are unreliable.

[a] Square root of the residual variance after accounting for subject, and sequence of observation (gender and age controlled by classifications).

[b] Nutrient intakes are for food only, data do not include intake from supplements.

[c] Sample size was inadequate to provide separate estimates for pregnant or lactating women.

SOURCE: Data from Continuing Survey of Food Intakes by Individuals 1994–1996.

TABLE I-4 Estimates of Within-Subject Variation in Intake, Expressed as Standard Deviation (SD)^a and Coefficient of Variation (CV) for Macronutrients in Adolescents and Children

| Nutrient^b | Adolescents Ages 9–18 y | | | | Children Ages 4–8 y | | | |
| | Females (n = 1,002) | | Males (n = 998) | | Females (n = 817) | | Males (n = 833) | |
	SD	CV (%)	SD	CV (%)	SD	CV (%)	SD	CV (%)
Energy (kcal)	628	34	800	33	427	27	478	27
Fat (total, g)	29.8	45	38.2	42	21.3	37	23.9	37
Fat (saturated, g)	11.3	48	15.3	48	8.5	40	9.6	40
Fat (mono- unsaturated, g)	12.4	48	15.5	44	8.6	39	9.9	41
Fat (poly- unsaturated, g)	7.3	60	8.7	55	5.1	52	5.5	52
Carbohydrate (g)	88.1	35	113	35	61.7	29	70.8	30
Protein (g)	26.2	42	33.9	39	19.2	34	20.4	33
Fiber (g)	6.2	51	8.7	56	4.6	43	5.3	45
Cholesterol (mg)	145	72	199	71	129	70	137	66

NOTE: When the CV is larger than 60 to 70 percent the distribution of daily intakes is nonnormal and the methods presented here are unreliable.

^{a} Square root of the residual variance after accounting for subject, and sequence of observation (gender and age controlled by classifications).

^{b} Nutrient intakes are for food only, data do not include intake from supplements.

SOURCE: Data from Continuing Survey of Food Intakes by Individuals 1994–1996.

INDEX

W

Summary Tables, Dietary Reference Intakes

Dietary Reference Intakes (DRIs): Estimated Average Requirements
Food and Nutrition Board, Institute of Medicine, National Academies

Life Stage Group	CHO (g/d)	Protein (g/kg/d)	Vit A (µg/d)[a]	Vit C (mg/d)	Vit E (mg/d)[b]	Thiamin (mg/d)	Ribo-flavin (mg/d)	Niacin (mg/d)[c]	Vit B$_6$ (mg/d)
Infants									
7–12 mo		1.0							
Children									
1–3 y	100	0.87	210	13	5	0.4	0.4	5	0.4
4–8 y	100	0.76	275	22	6	0.5	0.5	6	0.5
Males									
9–13 y	100	0.76	445	39	9	0.7	0.8	9	0.8
14–18 y	100	0.73	630	63	12	1.0	1.1	12	1.1
19–30 y	100	0.66	625	75	12	1.0	1.1	12	1.1
31–50 y	100	0.66	625	75	12	1.0	1.1	12	1.1
51–70 y	100	0.66	625	75	12	1.0	1.1	12	1.4
> 70 y	100	0.66	625	75	12	1.0	1.1	12	1.4
Females									
9–13 y	100	0.76	420	39	9	0.7	0.8	9	0.8
14–18 y	100	0.71	485	56	12	0.9	0.9	11	1.0
19–30 y	100	0.66	500	60	12	0.9	0.9	11	1.1
31–50 y	100	0.66	500	60	12	0.9	0.9	11	1.1
51–70 y	100	0.66	500	60	12	0.9	0.9	11	1.3
> 70 y	100	0.66	500	60	12	0.9	0.9	11	1.3
Pregnancy									
14–18 y	135	0.88	530	66	12	1.2	1.2	14	1.6
19–30 y	135	0.88	550	70	12	1.2	1.2	14	1.6
31–50 y	135	0.88	550	70	12	1.2	1.2	14	1.6
Lactation									
14–18 y	160	1.05	885	96	16	1.2	1.3	13	1.7
19–30 y	160	1.05	900	100	16	1.2	1.3	13	1.7
31–50 y	160	1.05	900	100	16	1.2	1.3	13	1.7

NOTE: An Estimated Average Requirement (EAR) is the average daily nutrient intake level estimated to meet the requirements of half of the healthy individuals in a group. EARs have not been established for vitamin D, vitamin K, pantothenic acid, biotin, choline, calcium, chromium, fluoride, manganese, or other nutrients not yet evaluated via the DRI process.

[a] As retinol activity equivalents (RAEs). 1 RAE = 1 µg retinol, 12 µg β-carotene, 24 µg α-carotene, or 24 µg β-cryptoxanthin. The RAE for dietary provitamin A carotenoids is twofold greater than retinol equivalents (RE), whereas the RAE for preformed vitamin A is the same as RE.

[b] As α-tocopherol. α-Tocopherol includes *RRR*-α-tocopherol, the only form of α-tocopherol that occurs naturally in foods, and the *2R*-stereoisomeric forms of α-tocopherol (*RRR*-, *RSR*-, *RRS*-, and *RSS*-α-tocopherol) that occur in fortified foods and supplements. It does not include the *2S*-stereoisomeric forms of α-tocopherol (*SRR*-, *SSR*-, *SRS*-, and *SSS*-α-tocopherol), also found in fortified foods and supplements.

Folate (µg/d)[d]	Vit B$_{12}$ (µg/d)	Copper (µg/d)	Iodine (µg/d)	Iron (mg/d)	Magnesium (mg/d)	Molybdenum (µg/d)	Phosphorus (mg/d)	Selenium (µg/d)	Zinc (mg/d)
				6.9					2.5
120	0.7	260	65	3.0	65	13	380	17	2.5
160	1.0	340	65	4.1	110	17	405	23	4.0
250	1.5	540	73	5.9	200	26	1,055	35	7.0
330	2.0	685	95	7.7	340	33	1,055	45	8.5
320	2.0	700	95	6	330	34	580	45	9.4
320	2.0	700	95	6	350	34	580	45	9.4
320	2.0	700	95	6	350	34	580	45	9.4
320	2.0	700	95	6	350	34	580	45	9.4
250	1.5	540	73	5.7	200	26	1,055	35	7.0
330	2.0	685	95	7.9	300	33	1,055	45	7.3
320	2.0	700	95	8.1	255	34	580	45	6.8
320	2.0	700	95	8.1	265	34	580	45	6.8
320	2.0	700	95	5	265	34	580	45	6.8
320	2.0	700	95	5	265	34	580	45	6.8
520	2.2	785	160	23	335	40	1,055	49	10.5
520	2.2	800	160	22	290	40	580	49	9.5
520	2.2	800	160	22	300	40	580	49	9.5
450	2.4	985	209	7	300	35	1,055	59	10.9
450	2.4	1,000	209	6.5	255	36	580	59	10.4
450	2.4	1,000	209	6.5	265	36	580	59	10.4

[c] As niacin equivalents (NE). 1 mg of niacin = 60 mg of tryptophan.

[d] As dietary folate equivalents (DFE). 1 DFE = 1 µg food folate = 0.6 µg of folic acid from fortified food or as a supplement consumed with food = 0.5 µg of a supplement taken on an empty stomach.

SOURCES: *Dietary Reference Intakes for Calcium, Phosphorous, Magnesium, Vitamin D, and Fluoride* (1997); *Dietary Reference Intakes for Thiamin, Riboflavin, Niacin, Vitamin B$_6$, Folate, Vitamin B$_{12}$, Pantothenic Acid, Biotin, and Choline* (1998); *Dietary Reference Intakes for Vitamin C, Vitamin E, Selenium, and Carotenoids* (2000); *Dietary Reference Intakes for Vitamin A, Vitamin K, Arsenic, Boron, Chromium, Copper, Iodine, Iron, Manganese, Molybdenum, Nickel, Silicon, Vanadium, and Zinc* (2001), and *Dietary Reference Intakes for Energy, Carbohydrate, Fiber, Fat, Fatty Acids, Cholesterol, Protein, and Amino Acids* (2002/2005). These reports may be accessed via www.nap.edu.

Dietary Reference Intakes (DRIs): Recommended Dietary Allowances and Adequate Intakes, Vitamins

Food and Nutrition Board, Institute of Medicine, National Academies

Life Stage Group	Vitamin A (μg/d)[a]	Vitamin C (mg/d)	Vitamin D (μg/d)[b,c]	Vitamin E (mg/d)[d]	Vitamin K (μg/d)	Thiamin (mg/d)
Infants						
0–6 mo	400*	40*	5*	4*	2.0*	0.2*
7–12 mo	500*	50*	5*	5*	2.5*	0.3*
Children						
1–3 y	300	15	5*	6	30*	0.5
4–8 y	400	25	5*	7	55*	0.6
Males						
9–13 y	600	45	5*	11	60*	0.9
14–18 y	900	75	5*	15	75*	1.2
19–30 y	900	90	5*	15	120*	1.2
31–50 y	900	90	5*	15	120*	1.2
51–70 y	900	90	10*	15	120*	1.2
> 70 y	900	90	15*	15	120*	1.2
Females						
9–13 y	600	45	5*	11	60*	0.9
14–18 y	700	65	5*	15	75*	1.0
19–30 y	700	75	5*	15	90*	1.1
31–50 y	700	75	5*	15	90*	1.1
51–70 y	700	75	10*	15	90*	1.1
> 70 y	700	75	15*	15	90*	1.1
Pregnancy						
14–18 y	750	80	5*	15	75*	1.4
19–30 y	770	85	5*	15	90*	1.4
31–50 y	770	85	5*	15	90*	1.4
Lactation						
14–18 y	1,200	115	5*	19	75*	1.4
19–30 y	1,300	120	5*	19	90*	1.4
31–50 y	1,300	120	5*	19	90*	1.4

NOTE: This table (taken from the DRI reports, see www.nap.edu) presents Recommended Dietary Allowances (RDA) in **bold type** or Adequate Intakes (AI) in ordinary type followed by an asterisk (*). An RDA is the average daily dietary intake level sufficient to meet the nutrient requirements of nearly all (97-98 percent) healthy individuals in a group. It is calculated from an Estimated Average Requirement (EAR). If sufficient scientific evidence is not available to establish an EAR, and thus calculate an RDA, an AI is usually developed. For healthy breastfed infants, the AI is the mean intake. The AI for other life stage and gender groups is believed to cover the needs of all healthy individuals in the group, but lack of data or uncertainty in the data prevent being able to specify with confidence the percentage of individuals covered by this intake.

[a] As retinol activity equivalents (RAEs). 1 RAE = 1 μg retinol, 12 μg β-carotene, 24 μg α-carotene, or 24 μg β-cryptoxanthin. The RAE for dietary provitamin A carotenoids is twofold greater than retinol equivalents (RE), whereas the RAE for preformed vitamin A is the same as RE.

[b] As cholecalciferol. 1 μg cholecalciferol = 40 IU vitamin D.

[c] In the absence of adequate exposure to sunlight.

[d] As α-tocopherol. α-Tocopherol includes *RRR*-α-tocopherol, the only form of α-tocopherol that occurs naturally in foods, and the *2R*-stereoisomeric forms of α-tocopherol (*RRR*-, *RSR*-, *RRS*-, and *RSS*α-tocopherol) that occur in fortified foods and supplements. It does not include the *2S*-stereoisomeric forms of α-tocopherol (*SRR*-, *SSR*-, *SRS*-, and *SSS*α-tocopherol), also found in fortified foods and supplements.

[e] As niacin equivalents (NE). 1 mg of niacin = 60 mg of tryptophan; 0–6 months = preformed niacin (not NE).

Riboflavin (mg/d)	Niacin (mg/d)[e]	Vitamin B_6 (mg/d)	Folate (μg/d)[f]	Vitamin B_{12} (μg/d)	Pantothenic Acid (mg/d)	Biotin (μg/d)	Choline (mg/d)[g]
0.3*	2*	0.1*	65*	0.4*	1.7*	5*	125*
0.4*	4*	0.3*	80*	0.5*	1.8*	6*	150*
0.5	6	0.5	150	0.9	2*	8*	200*
0.6	8	0.6	200	1.2	3*	12*	250*
0.9	12	1.0	300	1.8	4*	20*	375*
1.3	16	1.3	400	2.4	5*	25*	550*
1.3	16	1.3	400	2.4	5*	30*	550*
1.3	16	1.3	400	2.4	5*	30*	550*
1.3	16	1.7	400	2.4[h]	5*	30*	550*
1.3	16	1.7	400	2.4[h]	5*	30*	550*
0.9	12	1.0	300	1.8	4*	20*	375*
1.0	14	1.2	400[i]	2.4	5*	25*	400*
1.1	14	1.3	400[i]	2.4	5*	30*	425*
1.1	14	1.3	400[i]	2.4	5*	30*	425*
1.1	14	1.5	400	2.4[h]	5*	30*	425*
1.1	14	1.5	400	2.4[h]	5*	30*	425*
1.4	18	1.9	600[j]	2.6	6*	30*	450*
1.4	18	1.9	600[j]	2.6	6*	30*	450*
1.4	18	1.9	600[j]	2.6	6*	30*	450*
1.6	17	2.0	500	2.8	7*	35*	550*
1.6	17	2.0	500	2.8	7*	35*	550*
1.6	17	2.0	500	2.8	7*	35*	550*

[f] As dietary folate equivalents (DFE). 1 DFE = 1 μg food folate = 0.6 μg of folic acid from fortified food or as a supplement consumed with food = 0.5 μg of a supplement taken on an empty stomach.

[g] Although AIs have been set for choline, there are few data to assess whether a dietary supply of choline is needed at all stages of the life cycle, and it may be that the choline requirement can be met by endogenous synthesis at some of these stages.

[h] Because 10 to 30 percent of older people may malabsorb food-bound B_{12}, it is advisable for those older than 50 years to meet their RDA mainly by consuming foods fortified with B_{12} or a supplement containing B_{12}.

[i] In view of evidence linking folate intake with neural tube defects in the fetus, it is recommended that all women capable of becoming pregnant consume 400 μg from supplements or fortified foods in addition to intake of food folate from a varied diet.

[j] It is assumed that women will continue consuming 400 μg from supplements or fortified food until their pregnancy is confirmed and they enter prenatal care, which ordinarily occurs after the end of the periconceptional period—the critical time for formation of the neural tube.

SOURCES: *Dietary Reference Intakes for Calcium, Phosphorous, Magnesium, Vitamin D, and Fluoride* (1997); *Dietary Reference Intakes for Thiamin, Riboflavin, Niacin, Vitamin B6, Folate, Vitamin B12, Pantothenic Acid, Biotin, and Choline* (1998); *Dietary Reference Intakes for Vitamin C, Vitamin E, Selenium, and Carotenoids* (2000); *Dietary Reference Intakes for Vitamin A, Vitamin K, Arsenic, Boron, Chromium, Copper, Iodine, Iron, Manganese, Molybdenum, Nickel, Silicon, Vanadium, and Zinc* (2001); *and Dietary Reference Intakes for Water, Potassium, Sodium, Chloride, and Sulfate* (2005). These reports may be accessed via http://www.nap.edu.

**Dietary Reference Intakes (DRIs): Recommended Dietary Allowances and
Adequate Intakes, Elements**
Food and Nutrition Board, Institute of Medicine, National Academies

Life Stage Group	Calcium (mg/d)	Chromium (μg/d)	Copper (μg/d)	Fluoride (mg/d)	Iodine (μg/d)	Iron (mg/d)	Magnesium (mg/d)
Infants							
0–6 mo	210*	0.2*	200*	0.01*	110*	0.27*	30*
7–12 mo	270*	5.5*	220*	0.5*	130*	11	75*
Children							
1–3 y	500*	11*	340	0.7*	90	7	80
4–8 y	800*	15*	440	1*	90	10	130
Males							
9–13 y	1,300*	25*	700	2*	120	8	240
14–18 y	1,300*	35*	890	3*	150	11	410
19–30 y	1,000*	35*	900	4*	150	8	400
31–50 y	1,000*	35*	900	4*	150	8	420
51–70 y	1,200*	30*	900	4*	150	8	420
> 70 y	1,200*	30*	900	4*	150	8	420
Females							
9–13 y	1,300*	21*	700	2*	120	8	240
14–18 y	1,300*	24*	890	3*	150	15	360
19–30 y	1,000*	25*	900	3*	150	18	310
31–50 y	1,000*	25*	900	3*	150	18	320
51–70 y	1,200*	20*	900	3*	150	8	320
> 70 y	1,200*	20*	900	3*	150	8	320
Pregnancy							
14–18 y	1,300*	29*	1,000	3*	220	27	400
19–30 y	1,000*	30*	1,000	3*	220	27	350
31–50 y	1,000*	30*	1,000	3*	220	27	360
Lactation							
14–18 y	1,300*	44*	1,300	3*	290	10	360
19–30 y	1,000*	45*	1,300	3*	290	9	310
31–50 y	1,000*	45*	1,300	3*	290	9	320

NOTE: This table (taken from the DRI reports, see www.nap.edu) presents Recommended Dietary Allowances (RDA) in **bold type** or Adequate Intakes (AI) in ordinary type followed by an asterisk (*). An RDA is the average daily dietary intake level sufficient to meet the nutrient requirements of nearly all (97-98 percent) healthy individuals in a group. It is calculated from an Estimated Average Requirement (EAR). If sufficient scientific evidence is not available to establish an EAR, and thus calculate an RDA, an AI is usually developed. For healthy breastfed infants, the AI is the mean intake. The AI for other life stage and gender groups is believed to cover the needs of all healthy individuals in the group, but lack of data or uncertainty in the data prevent being able to specify with confidence the percentage of individuals covered by this intake.

Manganese (mg/d)	Molybdenum (µg/d)	Phosphorus (mg/d)	Selenium (µg/d)	Zinc (mg/d)	Potassium (g/d)	Sodium (g/d)	Chloride (g/d)
0.003*	2*	100*	15*	2*	0.4*	0.12*	0.18*
0.6*	3*	275*	20*	3	0.7*	0.37*	0.57*
1.2*	17	460	20	3	3.0*	1.0*	1.5*
1.5*	22	500	30	5	3.8*	1.2*	1.9*
1.9*	34	1,250	40	8	4.5*	1.5*	2.3*
2.2*	43	1,250	55	11	4.7*	1.5*	2.3*
2.3*	45	700	55	11	4.7*	1.5*	2.3*
2.3*	45	700	55	11	4.7*	1.5*	2.3*
2.3*	45	700	55	11	4.7*	1.3*	2.0*
2.3*	45	700	55	11	4.7*	1.2*	1.8*
1.6*	34	1,250	40	8	4.5*	1.5*	2.3*
1.6*	43	1,250	55	9	4.7*	1.5*	2.3*
1.8*	45	700	55	8	4.7*	1.5*	2.3*
1.8*	45	700	55	8	4.7*	1.5*	2.3*
1.8*	45	700	55	8	4.7*	1.3*	2.0*
1.8*	45	700	55	8	4.7*	1.2*	1.8*
2.0*	50	1,250	60	12	4.7*	1.5*	2.3*
2.0*	50	700	60	11	4.7*	1.5*	2.3*
2.0*	50	700	60	11	4.7*	1.5*	2.3*
2.6*	50	1,250	70	13	5.1*	1.5*	2.3*
2.6*	50	700	70	12	5.1*	1.5*	2.3*
2.6*	50	700	70	12	5.1*	1.5*	2.3*

SOURCES: *Dietary Reference Intakes for Calcium, Phosphorous, Magnesium, Vitamin D, and Fluoride* (1997); *Dietary Reference Intakes for Thiamin, Riboflavin, Niacin, Vitamin B6, Folate, Vitamin B12, Pantothenic Acid, Biotin, and Choline* (1998); *Dietary Reference Intakes for Vitamin C, Vitamin E, Selenium, and Carotenoids* (2000); *Dietary Reference Intakes for Vitamin A, Vitamin K, Arsenic, Boron, Chromium, Copper, Iodine, Iron, Manganese, Molybdenum, Nickel, Silicon, Vanadium, and Zinc* (2001); and *Dietary Reference Intakes for Water, Potassium, Sodium, Chloride, and Sulfate* (2005). These reports may be accessed via http://www.nap.edu.

Dietary Reference Intakes (DRIs): Recommended Dietary Allowances and Adequate Intakes, Total Water and Macronutrients
Food and Nutrition Board, Institute of Medicine, National Academies

Life Stage Group	Total Water[a] (L/d)	Carbohydrate (g/d)	Total Fiber (g/d)	Fat (g/d)	Linoleic Acid (g/d)	α-Linolenic Acid (g/d)	Protein[b] (g/d)
Infants							
0–6 mo	0.7*	60*	ND	31*	4.4*	0.5*	9.1*
7–12 mo	0.8*	95*	ND	30*	4.6*	0.5*	**11.0**+
Children							
1–3 y	1.3*	**130**	19*	ND[c]	7*	0.7*	**13**
4–8 y	1.7*	**130**	25*	ND	10*	0.9*	**19**
Males							
9–13 y	2.4*	**130**	31*	ND	12*	1.2*	**34**
14–18 y	3.3*	**130**	38*	ND	16*	1.6*	**52**
19–30 y	3.7*	**130**	38*	ND	17*	1.6*	**56**
31–50 y	3.7*	**130**	38*	ND	17*	1.6*	**56**
51–70 y	3.7*	**130**	30*	ND	14*	1.6*	**56**
> 70 y	3.7*	**130**	30*	ND	14*	1.6*	**56**
Females							
9–13 y	2.1*	**130**	26*	ND	10*	1.0*	**34**
14–18 y	2.3*	**130**	26*	ND	11*	1.1*	**46**
19–30 y	2.7*	**130**	25*	ND	12*	1.1*	**46**
31–50 y	2.7*	**130**	25*	ND	12*	1.1*	**46**
51–70 y	2.7*	**130**	21*	ND	11*	1.1*	**46**
> 70 y	2.7*	**130**	21*	ND	11*	1.1*	**46**
Pregnancy							
14–18 y	3.0*	**175**	28*	ND	13*	1.4*	**71**
19–30 y	3.0*	**175**	28*	ND	13*	1.4*	**71**
31–50 y	3.0*	**175**	28*	ND	13*	1.4*	**71**
Lactation							
14–18 y	3.8*	**210**	29*	ND	13*	1.3*	**71**
19–30 y	3.8*	**210**	29*	ND	13*	1.3*	**71**
31–50 y	3.8*	**210**	29*	ND	13*	1.3*	**71**

NOTE: This table (taken from the DRI reports, see www.nap.edu) presents Recommended Dietary Allowances (RDA) in **bold type** or Adequate Intakes (AI) in ordinary type followed by an asterisk (*). An RDA is the average daily dietary intake level sufficient to meet the nutrient requirements of nearly all (97-98 percent) healthy individuals in a group. It is calculated from an Estimated Average Requirement (EAR). If sufficient scientific evidence is not available to establish an EAR, and thus calculate an RDA, an AI is usually developed. For healthy breastfed infants, the AI is the mean intake. The AI for other life stage and gender groups is believed to cover the needs of all healthy individuals in the group, but lack of data or uncertainty in the data prevent being able to specify with confidence the percentage of individuals covered by this intake.

[a] *Total* water includes all water contained in food, beverages, and drinking water.

[b] Based on g protein per kg of body weight for the reference body weight, e.g., for adults 0.8 g/kg body weight for the reference body weight.

[c] Not determined.

SOURCES: *Dietary Reference Intakes for Energy, Carbohydrate, Fiber, Fat, Fatty Acids, Cholesterol, Protein, and Amino Acids* (2002/2005); *Dietary Reference Intakes for Water, Potassium, Sodium, Chloride, and Sulfate* (2005). These reports may be accessed via http://www.nap.edu.

Dietary Reference Intakes (DRIs): Acceptable Macronutrient Distribution Ranges
Food and Nutrition Board, Institute of Medicine, National Academies

Macronutrient	Range (percent of energy)		
	Children, 1–3 y	Children, 4–18 y	Adults
Fat	30–40	25–35	20–35
n-6 Polyunsaturated fatty acids[a]			
(linoleic acid)	5–10	5–10	5–10
n-3 Polyunsaturated fatty acids[a]			
(α-linolenic acid)	0.6–1.2	0.6–1.2	0.6–1.2
Carbohydrate	45–65	45–65	45–65
Protein	5–20	10–30	10–35

[a] Approximately 10 percent of the total can come from longer-chain n-3 or n-6 fatty acids.

SOURCE: *Dietary Reference Intakes for Energy, Carbohydrate, Fiber, Fat, Fatty Acids, Cholesterol, Protein, and Amino Acids* (2002/2005).

Dietary Reference Intakes (DRIs): Additional Macronutrient Recommendations
Food and Nutrition Board, Institute of Medicine, National Academies

Macronutrient	Recommendation
Dietary cholesterol	As low as possible while consuming a nutritionally adequate diet
Trans fatty acids	As low as possible while consuming a nutritionally adequate diet
Saturated fatty acids	As low as possible while consuming a nutritionally adequate diet
Added sugars[a]	Limit to no more than 25% of total energy

[a] Not a recommended intake. A daily intake of added sugars that individuals should aim for to achieve a healthful diet was not set.

SOURCE: *Dietary Reference Intakes for Energy, Carbohydrate, Fiber, Fat, Fatty Acids, Cholesterol, Protein, and Amino Acids* (2002/2005).

Dietary Reference Intakes (DRIs): Tolerable Upper Intake Levels, Vitamins
Food and Nutrition Board, Institute of Medicine, National Academies

Life Stage Group	Vitamin A (µg/d)[a]	Vitamin C (mg/d)	Vitamin D (µg/d)	Vitamin E (mg/d)[b,c]	Vitamin K	Thiamin
Infants						
0–6 mo	600	ND[e]	25	ND	ND	ND
7–12 mo	600	ND	25	ND	ND	ND
Children						
1–3 y	600	400	50	200	ND	ND
4–8 y	900	650	50	300	ND	ND
Males, Females						
9–13 y	1,700	1,200	50	600	ND	ND
14–18 y	2,800	1,800	50	800	ND	ND
19–70 y	3,000	2,000	50	1,000	ND	ND
> 70 y	3,000	2,000	50	1,000	ND	ND
Pregnancy						
14–18 y	2,800	1,800	50	800	ND	ND
19–50 y	3,000	2,000	50	1,000	ND	ND
Lactation						
14–18 y	2,800	1,800	50	800	ND	ND
19–50 y	3,000	2,000	50	1,000	ND	ND

NOTE: A Tolerable Upper Intake Level (UL) is the highest level of daily nutrient intake that is likely to pose no risk of adverse health effects to almost all individuals in the general population. Unless otherwise specified, the UL represents total intake from food, water, and supplements. Due to lack of suitable data, ULs could not be established for vitamin K, thiamin, riboflavin, vitamin B$_{12}$, pantothenic acid, biotin, and carotenoids. In the absence of a UL, extra caution may be warranted in consuming levels above recommended intakes. Members of the general population should be advised not to routinely exceed the UL. The UL is not meant to apply to individuals who are treated with the nutrient under medical supervision or to individuals with predisposing conditions that modify their sensitivity to the nutrient.

[a] As preformed vitamin A only.

[b] As α-tocopherol; applies to any form of supplemental α-tocopherol.

[c] The ULs for vitamin E, niacin, and folate apply to synthetic forms obtained from supplements, fortified foods, or a combination of the two.

Ribo-flavin	Niacin (mg/d)[c]	Vitamin B_6 (mg/d)	Folate (μg/d)[c]	Vitamin B_{12}	Pantothenic Acid	Biotin	Choline (g/d)	Carote-noids[d]
ND	ND	ND	ND	ND	ND	ND	ND	ND
ND	ND	ND	ND	ND	ND	ND	ND	ND
ND	10	30	300	ND	ND	ND	1.0	ND
ND	15	40	400	ND	ND	ND	1.0	ND
ND	20	60	600	ND	ND	ND	2.0	ND
ND	30	80	800	ND	ND	ND	3.0	ND
ND	35	100	1,000	ND	ND	ND	3.5	ND
ND	35	100	1,000	ND	ND	ND	3.5	ND
ND	30	80	800	ND	ND	ND	3.0	ND
ND	35	100	1,000	ND	ND	ND	3.5	ND
ND	30	80	800	ND	ND	ND	3.0	ND
ND	35	100	1,000	ND	ND	ND	3.5	ND

[d] β-Carotene supplements are advised only to serve as a provitamin A source for individuals at risk of vitamin A deficiency.

[e] ND = Not determinable due to lack of data of adverse effects in this age group and concern with regard to lack of ability to handle excess amounts. Source of intake should be from food only to prevent high levels of intake.

SOURCES: *Dietary Reference Intakes for Calcium, Phosphorous, Magnesium, Vitamin D, and Fluoride* (1997); *Dietary Reference Intakes for Thiamin, Riboflavin, Niacin, Vitamin B6, Folate, Vitamin B12, Pantothenic Acid, Biotin, and Choline* (1998); *Dietary Reference Intakes for Vitamin C, Vitamin E, Selenium, and Carotenoids* (2000); and *Dietary Reference Intakes for Vitamin A, Vitamin K, Arsenic, Boron, Chromium, Copper, Iodine, Iron, Manganese, Molybdenum, Nickel, Silicon, Vanadium, and Zinc* (2001). These reports may be accessed via http://www.nap.edu.

Dietary Reference Intakes (DRIs): Tolerable Upper Intake Levels, Elements
Food and Nutrition Board, Institute of Medicine, National Academies

Life Stage Group	Arse- nic[a]	Boron (mg/d)	Calci- um (g/d)	Chro- mium	Copper (μg/d)	Fluo- ride (mg/d)	Iodine (μg/d)	Iron (mg/d)	Magne- sium (mg/d)[b]
Infants									
0–6 mo	ND[e]	ND	ND	ND	ND	0.7	ND	40	ND
7–12 mo	ND	ND	ND	ND	ND	0.9	ND	40	ND
Children									
1–3 y	ND	3	2.5	ND	1,000	1.3	200	40	65
4–8 y	ND	6	2.5	ND	3,000	2.2	300	40	110
Males, Females									
9–13 y	ND	11	2.5	ND	5,000	10	600	40	350
14–18 y	ND	17	2.5	ND	8,000	10	900	45	350
19–70 y	ND	20	2.5	ND	10,000	10	1,100	45	350
> 70 y	ND	20	2.5	ND	10,000	10	1,100	45	350
Pregnancy									
14–18 y	ND	17	2.5	ND	8,000	10	900	45	350
19–50 y	ND	20	2.5	ND	10,000	10	1,100	45	350
Lactation									
14–18 y	ND	17	2.5	ND	8,000	10	900	45	350
19–50 y	ND	20	2.5	ND	10,000	10	1,100	45	350

NOTE: A Tolerable Upper Intake Level (UL) is the highest level of daily nutrient intake that is likely to pose no risk of adverse health effects to almost all individuals in the general population. Unless otherwise specified, the UL represents total intake from food, water, and supplements. Due to lack of suitable data, ULs could not be established for vitamin K, thiamin, riboflavin, vitamin B₁₂, pantothenic acid, biotin, and carotenoids. In the absence of a UL, extra caution may be warranted in consuming levels above recommended intakes. Members of the general population should be advised not to routinely exceed the UL The UL is not meant to apply to individuals who are treated with the nutrient under medical supervision or to individuals with predisposing conditions that modify their sensitivity to the nutrient.

[a] Although the UL was not determined for arsenic, there is no justification for adding arsenic to food or supplements.

[b] The ULs for magnesium represent intake from a pharmacological agent only and do not include intake from food and water.

[c] Although silicon has not been shown to cause adverse effects in humans, there is no justification for adding silicon to supplements.

Manganese (mg/d)	Molybdenum (µg/d)	Nickel (mg/d)	Phosphorus (g/d)	Potassium	Selenium (µg/d)	Silicon[e]	Sulfate	Vanadium (mg/d)[d]	Zinc (mg/d)	Sodium (g/d)	Chloride (g/d)
ND	ND	ND	ND	ND	45	ND	ND	ND	4	ND	ND
ND	ND	ND	ND	ND	60	ND	ND	ND	5	ND	ND
2	300	0.2	3.0	ND	90	ND	ND	ND	7	1.5	2.3
3	600	0.3	3.0	ND	150	ND	ND	ND	12	1.9	2.9
6	1,100	0.6	4.0	ND	280	ND	ND	ND	23	2.2	3.4
9	1,700	1.0	4.0	ND	400	ND	ND	ND	34	2.3	3.6
11	2,000	1.0	4.0	ND	400	ND	ND	1.8	40	2.3	3.6
11	2,000	1.0	3.0	ND	400	ND	ND	1.8	40	2.3	3.6
9	1,700	1.0	3.5	ND	400	ND	ND	ND	34	2.3	3.6
11	2,000	1.0	3.5	ND	400	ND	ND	ND	40	2.3	3.6
9	1,700	1.0	4.0	ND	400	ND	ND	ND	34	2.3	3.6
11	2,000	1.0	4.0	ND	400	ND	ND	ND	40	2.3	3.6

[d] Although vanadium in food has not been shown to cause adverse effects in humans, there is no justification for adding vanadium to food and vanadium supplements should be used with caution. The UL is based on adverse effects in laboratory animals and these data could be used to set a UL for adults but not children and adolescents.

[e] ND = Not determinable due to lack of data of adverse effects in this age group and concern with regard to lack of ability to handle excess amounts. Source of intake should be from food only to prevent high levels of intake.

SOURCES: *Dietary Reference Intakes for Calcium, Phosphorous, Magnesium, Vitamin D, and Fluoride* (1997); *Dietary Reference Intakes for Thiamin, Riboflavin, Niacin, Vitamin B6, Folate, Vitamin B12, Pantothenic Acid, Biotin, and Choline* (1998); *Dietary Reference Intakes for Vitamin C, Vitamin E, Selenium, and Carotenoids* (2000); *Dietary Reference Intakes for Vitamin A, Vitamin K, Arsenic, Boron, Chromium, Copper, Iodine, Iron, Manganese, Molybdenum, Nickel, Silicon, Vanadium, and Zinc* (2001); and *Dietary Reference Intakes for Water, Potassium, Sodium, Chloride, and Sulfate* (2005). These reports may be accessed via http://www.nap.edu.

REFERENCES

Full references, which also appear in the parent report series, the *Dietary Reference Intakes*, are not printed in this book but are provided online at http://www.nap.edu/catalog/11537.html.